The Daily Telegraph

COMPLETE PREGNANCY & CHILDBIRTH ANSWERS

by

Joe Kabyemela MD MRCOG

and

Leanne Bricker MB BCh MRCOG

Robinson
LONDON

For James, Eric, Jane and Fischer: with love undying

Foreword

The book shop shelves are already packed with so many excellent books on pregnancy and childbirth it would take something exceptional to justify yet another. But this book is, I believe, exceptional and its original, simple format works so well, it is only surprising no one has thought of it before.

It is a truism about medical matters that one can never ask enough questions and equally those to whom they are addressed, even with the best will in the world, would never be able to do their jobs properly if they spent all their time answering these queries. There will thus always be something of an information deficit on the part of the prospective mother and her spouse. Dr Joe Kabyemela and Leanne Bricker had the brilliant idea of collecting together all the questions they had ever been asked – almost 1400 in all – to which they have prepared lucid and intelligent answers. It permits them to provide much more information, spiced with good sense, than any comparable volume. The originality and effectiveness of this format is well illustrated by the section on 'Labour Monitoring of Fetal Well-being' though could apply equally to any other section. It is difficult to imagine any pregnant woman would be in a position to pose all 51 questions to her doctor or midwife and yet each is important and it is useful to know the answer. Further, the conversational tone of the dialogue, as readers will readily appreciate, makes the manner in which the authors answer the questions extremely clear which, it must be said, is often not the case in real life.

Altogether this is a most impressive achievement and I commend it highly to all mothers-to-be and their spouses and indeed any family member who has interest in the outcome of the greatest of all natural miracles – pregnancy and childbirth.

Dr James Le Fanu

Contents

CONTENTS

CONTENTS

CONTENTS

List of illustrations

1. Nine months in a nutshell

Pregnancy and childbirth may be a daily event in society but it is not an everyday run-of-the-mill occurrence. Nor does it need any hyperbole to describe it.

The wonders of childbirth need to be experienced to be believed.

It is easy to fall in the trap of assuming that pregnancy is riddled with risks and to approach it with trepidation.

It is human nature to put emphasis on the out-of-ordinary and hence the preponderance, even in this book, of chapters dealing with problems that may be associated with pregnancy and childbirth. It is, of course, true that the odds are stacked *against* anything going wrong in pregnancy. Roughly four out of five pregnancies will be problem-free. This means most women will go through pregnancy and birth without any major hitch.

But, of course, there are people who already have health problems on which pregnancy might have a profound effect. Then there are people who develop unique pregnancy problems, and finally there are problems which occur during pregnancy, at delivery, or after, where they were completely unexpected. These need to be understood. Being informed removes undue anxiety and, even where the outlook is not so good, it enables the individual and her family to come to terms with what may be in store.

Then there is the fact that pregnancy, even when completely normal, will be different from anything any woman has experienced before, unless it is another pregnancy. It is therefore useful to explain the changes that she is experiencing and what to expect as the pregnancy advances.

There is also the fact that many women get the little information they do have from family, friends and acquaintances. All doctors and midwives will tell you of their recurrent frustrations upon hearing the ubiquitous "my neighbour . . .", "my sister . . ." or "my friend . . .".

One normal pregnancy could be spectacularly different from another normal pregnancy. *"Normal"*, applied to pregnancy, is a very elastic term. It is of enormous benefit, therefore, for an expectant mother to know what a normal pregnancy may encompass.

A woman in her second or subsequent pregnancy should not necessarily expect a repeat of the same experience. Things may be completely different. This is another myth which brings out the common "but surely there must be something wrong: I didn't have this in my last pregnancy". No, not necessarily, madam. Every pregnancy is different. While doctors should and will look at – and probably even perform – tests, to rule out any potential complication, more often than not, it is just a variant of the norm.

So, as you read this book, sit back and relax and allow yourself to become an expert on this subject, or at least the next best thing.

Specific subjects are dealt with in the subsequent chapters. Here we set out to give you an overview of what pregnancy and childbirth is all about.

Pre-pregnancy (pre-conception)

Most pregnancies are unplanned. When it happens, the reaction may be that of stunned joy, confusion, mixed feelings or panic.

Symptoms of pregnancy do not occur until at least a week or so after missing a period. A pregnancy test nowadays can confirm pregnancy, even before symptoms start. For those with regular periods, a test performed a day after the period was due will confirm the pregnancy. This, however, depends on the quality of the test kit. Some of the cheaper ones on the market may not be very sensitive and, at this stage of the pregnancy, the hormone level may not be high enough to be detected. Test kits used in hospitals are sensitive enough to detect a pregnancy at this very early stage.

For those couples who plan their pregnancy, there are some general things they may want to observe before trying to conceive. Overall, the woman needs to be in good general health, preferably not on medication and, of course, not taking any form of contraception.

It just will not do to plan pregnancy while on a diet, for instance. Nor will it be helpful for an athlete who is in a punishing exercise regime, in preparation for a major competition. It only means that conception is less likely to happen. For somebody who is dieting, there is also the possibility that her programme may entail some nutritional deficiencies, which could in turn pose a risk to the formed embryo.

There are a number of considerations when the prospective mother suffers from a chronic condition such as hypertension (raised blood pressure), epilepsy, cystic fibrosis, sickle cell disease or diabetes. All these conditions and many more have been covered extensively in this book.

Early pregnancy

Historically, it has been found to be convenient – and in practice, useful – to divide the period of pregnancy into three sections. These are called "trimesters". Since a pregnancy, on average, lasts for forty weeks, trimesters will be about thirteen weeks each. A reference to the first trimester (also called the "early" trimester), will therefore refer to the first thirteen weeks (three months). The second trimester is also called the "mid-trimester"; it starts at the end of the first trimester and will conclude at the end of twenty-six weeks. Thence commences the "last" trimester (somehow, it is not called "late") or the third trimester. Because of the quirks of nature, the third trimester could possibly be shorter or longer than thirteen weeks in real life. This is in those instances where the baby arrives well before the calculated due date or when the due date is overrun by several days. Both these situations are quite common.

Fertilization
In natural (spontaneous) conception, an act of sexual intercourse leads to fusion of the male gamete (the spermatozoa) and the female egg (ovum). Fertilization has effectively taken place.

After being released, an egg can survive for only a few hours, probably not more than twenty-four and in most cases less than this. What this means is that, in the entire cycle of about twenty-eight days (for most women), there is only a small window when conception can take place. Male gametes (spermatozoa) do survive considerably longer, even though most die within twenty-four hours. In theory, sexual intercourse tonight could lead to fertilization tomorrow in a case where spermatozoa are deposited in the woman's genital tract. If, by coincidence, ovulation takes place within the critical 24–36 hour period when some healthy spermatozoa may be still lurking about, conception will occur. This, however, is an over-simplification of a very complex process. There are a lot of other factors that come into play in order for fertilization to lead to an established pregnancy. Any of these, if not right, could thwart the conception.

It should not surprise anybody that people don't always end up conceiving as soon as they plan, just because they are having regular intercourse, minus contraception. It is estimated that regular intercourse for a healthy couple has a 25 per cent chance of leading to pregnancy each "month" or menstrual cycle.

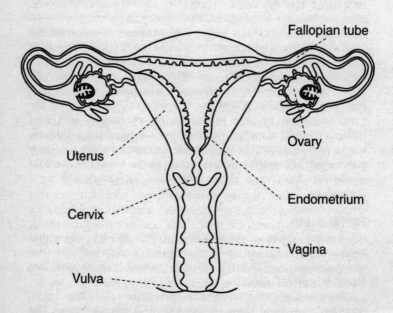

Fig 1 The female urino-genital tract

Surprisingly, the term "regular intercourse" seems to mean different things to different men and women. It should be regarded to mean having sexual intercourse on average three or four times a week, evenly spaced out. Clustered acts of intercourse, followed by several days of abstinence, cannot be regarded as regular, whatever the total number might say.

It has happened

Once the "winning" male sperm fuses with the female egg, a "zygote" is formed. It is effectively one cell formed from the two gametes. It has forty-six chromosomes, like each of the resultant billions of body cells that will result from its divisions. In effect, the nine-month journey to form a new human being has started.

Cell division starts in about thirty hours, when the first division of the zygote takes place to give two cells and, within four to five days, this will have reached a sixty-cell stage. All this time, the zygote is making its way through the tube towards the womb, and is now called a "morula".

Implantation will start taking place towards the end of the week and, within two weeks, this too is complete. Up until then, the woman is completely unaware she is pregnant. In fact, this is about the time she will be expecting her period. When it does not arrive, then her suspicions that something may be afoot start to surface.

Two things could delay the discovery of the pregnancy at this stage. A woman who has irregular periods may regard this as just another late one and file it away at the back of her mind. Her suspicions may not surface again for weeks, until she misses yet another period or tell-tale symptoms start.

Another thing that may mislead a newly pregnant (but still unaware) woman is light vaginal bleeding that may occur at the time of implantation. Since this is about the time she is expecting her period, the bleeding may be dismissed as just a light period. Again, she may remain oblivious of the momentous process taking place in her body until the next "period" fails to arrive or she starts getting nauseous for no apparent reason.

Things happen at a steady and fast pace and, by the end of the fourth week, the tiny fetus has its own circulation. Make no mistake, this fetus is still very small: it cannot be seen on the scan. In fact, strictly speaking, this is still an embryo and will remain as such for another four weeks or so before it is appropriately termed a fetus.

The fetus's neural tube will close by the end of six weeks. This is significant where there is a worry about spina bifida. The advice to take folic acid, to reduce the probability of spinda bifida, is quite a valid one. However, timing is crucial. If the folic acid is taken starting a week or two after missing a period (or later) it is really useless for this particular purpose. This is why, for those at risk (such as mothers who have previously had a spina bifida baby or pregnancy), the advice is to plan their pregnancy and to start the supplements before conception. Of course, you cannot guarantee when conception will take place, which may mean taking folic acid for several months. However, this should not be regarded as some kind of burden. Folic acid has so many other benefits.

Sex of the baby

The sex of the baby is determined at conception.

It all depends on the chromosomal make up of the male gamete (sperm) fertilizing the egg.

A woman will always contribute an egg with the same chromosomal constituent, which is 23X. The sperm will either be 23X or 23Y. Of the millions of sperms released at ejaculation, the distribution of the two types is roughly fifty-fifty. Of course, of the millions, only a few hundred reach the egg, and only one will get the privilege of fertilizing it. If it is 23X, the baby will be female; if it is 23Y, the baby will be male. It is that simple.

Sometimes, genetic defects occur which lead to sexual ambiguity. These are very complex and quite uncommon. We would not attempt to address these in this text. However, one interesting fact that deserves mention is that the early gonadal (sex organs) development for both male and female fetuses is indistinguishable. Before the eighth week, the gonads cannot be recognized as male or female.

Can a pregnancy test identify whether the fetus is male or female? The answer is no. A pregnancy test detects a hormone which is the same, whatever the sex of the fetus might be.

Can an ultrasound scan tell the sex of the baby? Yes, but this does not occur until well into the second trimester. If an expectant mother is having a scan in the first trimester, even at

12–13 weeks, she should not expect the baby's sex to be identifiable on the scan. Even when the image is very clear, the external genitalia of the fetus is so ambiguous at this stage, it is impossible to tell. This is a mere glimpse of what we have tackled in greater detail in the book.

All those changes

Changes to the mother's body tend to start quite early. They are all hormonally driven. Some of those hormones are actually produced by the fetus. This means, even though it is completely dependent on the mother, the fetus actively influences how the mother's body is going to function, to make the environment favourable for it.

Size and weight

The pace of change for the fetus is quite impressive. While it will weigh a mere 5 g at ten weeks, it will be about 300 g at twenty weeks – that's sixty times its weight, ten weeks earlier. The rate of increase then slows down steadily and it will increase in weight only about five times in the subsequent ten weeks (to 1500 g) and only about two and a half times after that (to about 3.5–4.0 kg at forty weeks).

The rate of weight increase for the fetus differs from person to person but the general pattern is the same. In fact, the speed of the change of weight in the later part of the second trimester and the whole of the third trimester is an important indicator of the health of the fetus.

As for the length of the body, many parents are shocked to learn how tiny the fetus is in the early part. An ultrasound scan at seven weeks will show the fetus very clearly if conditions are ideal. *Yet, its actual length is 1 cm from top to toe*! Even at twelve weeks, when limbs and even fingers can be made out as well as fetal activity appreciated on the scan, it is actually only about 5.5 cm (two inches) long.

Second trimester

The second trimester starts at fourteen weeks. Nothing earth-shattering happens at this point. Pregnancy is a smooth continuum and these divisions into trimesters are arbitrary, and only meant to facilitate care of the pregnancy. They are artificial milestones in many respects. However, for those with troublesome nausea and vomiting, this is about the time they should expect to put it all behind them. A word of caution. It is unusual (but not unknown) for nausea to persist beyond this stage, and for particularly unlucky mothers, it could carry on till the eve of labour. The reason for this remains unclear.

At the start of the second trimester, the mother is still unaware of fetal movements, even though the fetus is very active. This is to do with size. It is still too small. She will start feeling the movements from about sixteen weeks (at the earliest) if she has had a previous pregnancy. For first-timers, it doesn't happen before about eighteen weeks and in some cases not until twenty weeks.

Contentions of feeling movements at fourteen weeks are as misplaced as anxiety of lack of movements at eighteen weeks, where the scan shows normal findings.

Small and large babies

As the second trimester draws to a close at about twenty-six weeks, for normal babies in a normal pregnancy, genes and the environment start to exert their influence on the eventual size of the baby.

In the second trimester – let's say at twenty weeks – it is impossible to tell by the scan findings whether the baby will be small, average-sized or large. In fact, at this stage, fetuses of the same gestational age will be quite similar in size. Those destined to be big by their genetic inheritance will start pulling away from the pack in the third trimester. Trying to determine the gestational age accurately using an ultrasound scan in the third trimester is a futile exercise. The best you can hope for is a very rough guide.

What of the mother's tummy?

Examination of the abdomen in the first and second trimester is pretty accurate in determining the gestational age as long as the examiner knows what he or she is looking for. This also depends on things being normal with a singleton pregnancy. It is pretty useless in this respect for multiple pregnancy. Of course, examination of the abdomen is still valid for all the other purposes, even in multiple pregnancy.

For most of the first trimester, the womb is inside the pelvic cavity and abdominal examination will be negative. This is until near the end of the first trimester. In fact, the fundus (top) of the uterus just emerges at the bikini-line level at twelve weeks.

It is not uncommon to see a celebrity photographed showing an apparent *"three-months bump"*. There is nothing like a three-months bump, unless the lucky mother-to-be is carrying triplets.

Third trimester

The fetus continues to increase in size and the various organs are maturing functionally. The amount of water (amniotic fluid) is also increasing. It follows that the fundus of the uterus will continue rising and therefore the belly grows bigger. The womb's ability to increase in size and accommodate the weight of its contents is quite amazing. At conception, the uterus is about the size of a small fist, weighing about 50 g. By the end of the third trimester, it will extend from inside the pelvis to the diaphragm beneath the ribs, weighing about 1000 g – twenty times its original weight, and that is minus its contents!

In a few weeks after delivery, the uterus will shrink back to its original size, or very close to it.

Contractions

Braxton-Hicks contractions are common and could start as early as middle of the second trimester. A person examining the abdomen may feel these, but the mother is mostly unaware of them. She may start feeling them in the third trimester. They are usually irregular, unpredictable, short-lived and painless. The frequency may increase towards the end of pregnancy, to the extent of causing anxiety of impending labour. If one is unlucky, this stage may last three or four weeks, a grim prospect. Fortunately, this is unusual.

Term

This is where a lot of people tie themselves in a twist. What does a phrase like "a baby born two weeks premature" mean? In fact, it doesn't mean anything!

"Term" is a period stretching a good five weeks. Once a pregnancy reaches thirty-seven completed weeks, it is already term. A week or four weeks later, if the baby hasn't arrived yet, it will still be "term" and still normal. Any baby born in the period stretching from thirty-seven to forty-two weeks will therefore be born at "term". It also means, a parent who makes a reference to a child that was born "five days late", implying that he or she arrived five days after the calculated due date (EDD) is right, in a figure of speech. However, it is a technically misleading term, because it may create the impression that the baby arrived after "term", which is incorrect.

It is therefore appropriate to refer to the actual duration of pregnancy (thirty-four weeks, thirty-eight weeks, forty-one weeks, etc.) rather than to extrapolate figures from the expected date of delivery.

Term is characterized by differing degrees of discomfort, but discomfort there will be. There is also a tendency for the fetal movements to appear reduced. This is mostly because the baby has increased in size and the amount of amniotic fluid is continually decreasing, a phenomenon that starts at around thirty-six weeks. The effect is that of reduced room and restricted freedom for the baby. It is imperative, however, that any pregnant woman who feels that there is significant change in the rate of fetal activity should consult her GP to have the situation verified. If it happens today, it should be looked at today, not tomorrow or the day after.

About 80 per cent of babies will arrive at term but only a tiny proportion of these will arrive on the calculated expected date of delivery (EDD). Should this happen, it should be regarded as a pleasant bonus but should never be focused on as a realistic prospect. When an EDD is calculated, it should be made clear that the baby is expected to arrive around that date, maybe within about two weeks either way.

Braxton-Hicks contractions may start becoming more uncomfortable. The frequency may also increase. This has led many women to think they are going into labour, particularly those without previous experience. The visits to the loo increase as the womb maintains its siege on the bladder, which can hardly store a respectable amount of water before the urge to urinate arises.

Labour

Many women are told that they are not actually in labour when they are convinced they are. This is why stories of "I was in labour for five days" abound. Nobody is ever in labour for five days; it is not even physically possible! The misconception has a lot to do with the parents not getting the right amount of information antenatally of what might happen at the end of the pregnancy.

There is a phase loosely termed "the latent phase of labour". This can be mild, easily whiled away with a drink, a lengthy soak in the bath and a favourite activity. It can also be quite distressingly painful, requiring use of very strong painkillers in hospital. It can last less than an hour but may also go on for eighteen to twenty-four hours. This is all normal.

When a midwife or doctor performs a vaginal examination for the first time on a woman who is supposedly in labour, the aim is to establish the stage of labour. Sometimes the findings do not amount to the minimum requirement for diagnosing labour – regular contractions and the cervix dilated over 3 cm. If the findings are conveyed inappropriately, this may add to her distress – which is, of course, genuine. "You are not in labour," may, quite rightly, upset the woman, because she may take it to imply an accusation of feigning her distress. This person will most probably be in the latent phase and not in *established* labour. This needs to be explained, plus the fact that its duration cannot be predicted. This is unless she has been in labour before, in which case her previous experience is a fairly good guide.

Once labour is established, the progress is expected to be steady with regular contractions, the descent of the baby down the pelvis towards the outside world, and the continual dilatation of the cervix. In the majority of cases, this is exactly what happens. In a few, the process is so fast that the mother and the midwife looking after her barely have time to register what is happening. This is termed "precipitate labour". In other cases, the process is slow or may appear to stall altogether.

It is impossible to predict with absolute certainty who will have a successful vaginal delivery. It is, however, possible to predict where difficulties are likely to be encountered. Having said that, it is most unusual for a woman in her first pregnancy with a baby in a normal position (head first) to be advised not to aim for a vaginal delivery. It is amazing how, in some cases where things look improbable, labour is smooth and vaginal delivery successful. Conversely, everybody in the business has encountered cases where labour stalls for no apparent cause and defies all efforts to correct it. That is nature for you. Modern labour management is so efficient that the element of unpredictability is not regarded as a significant challenge.

Labour is divided into three stages. The first stage ends when the cervix is fully dilated and pushing can commence. The second stage is where the pushing is done. It ends with delivery of the baby and here commences the third and final stage. The third stage, that most mothers are scarcely aware of nor interested in, ends with the delivery of the placenta (afterbirth). The form of labour management adopted can influence the length of each of these stages.

Oh, baby, oh!

"*Isn't she wonderful?*" So sang Stevie Wonder. It may be a he (or both) but the sentiment is the same. The end of an odyssey that is unique in its intensity and emotions. It is also the beginning of motherhood proper. The experiences of the immediate postnatal period will differ from person to person but will always be challenging. Each milestone is a wonder to behold and any mother will tell you – it is all worth it.

The goals

In this book, we have tackled subjects that will encompass and address the questions of 95 per cent of all pregnant women, probably more.

In this book, we have steered clear of judging anybody. The book is meant to inform, because we believe this is the only genuine form of empowerment.

In a book of this nature, it is impossible to escape using terms that are not in everyday use in the English language. Opposite, we have set out to explain the many such unfamiliar terms and words that may be encountered in this book. If you, the reader, happen to know all or most of these, do not regard this to be an exercise in condescension. It is just part of the overall endeavour to get the message across.

Glossary

AFP: This stands for *alpha-fetal protein*, which is one of the key chemicals used to diagnose various conditions that may affect the fetus in the uterus. The two conditions which this could detect are Down's syndrome and spina bifida. It can help detect several other less common conditions. It is produced by the fetus.

Amniocentesis: The act of drawing water from around the baby. In most cases, this is for diagnostic purposes, but it may, in some cases, be used to relieve tension when there is an excessive amount of water (amniotic fluid).

Amnion: This is the name of the membranes which form the bag that contains water and the fetus. Also called *amniotic membranes*.

Amniotic fluid: The water around the baby. Also called *liquor*.

Antenatal: This literally means 'before birth'. The antenatal period is the pregnancy period, from conception to onset of labour. The other term for antenatal is *"prenatal"*, mostly used in the USA.

Anterior: To the front. The opposite is posterior, which is "to the back".

Areola: The dark area surrounding the nipple on the breast.

Bartholin's abscess: An abscess, which may form on either side of the vaginal entrance. It affects a gland which goes by the same name: the gland's natural function is to produce lubricating secretions during sexual intercourse.

Binovular twins: Non-identical twins, arising from separate eggs. The opposite is *monovular* twins, i.e. those arising from one egg and therefore identical.

Biophysical profile: This is a way of assessing the fetal well-being by looking at physical activity attributes. These are assessed by using ultrasound scanning. Things like muscle tone, limb movements, amniotic fluid volume and movement of the diaphragm as well as the pattern of the fetal heartbeat are collectively assessed to give a "biophysical profile score". The maximum score is 10. A score of 8–10 is good. A score of 6 is a cause for some concern and normally will prompt a plan, either repeating the test in a matter of hours or even delivery. A score of 2 or 4 always calls for some action, usually delivery.

BPD: BPD is a short form of *biparietal diameter*, one of the measurements taken of the fetus to determine growth or gestation. It is the distance between one ear and the other.

Braxton-Hicks contractions: The irregular painless contractions that occur in the second half of pregnancy. Some people have called them "practice" contractions. Braxton Hicks was the person who first described them and immortalized himself on their back.

Breech: The bottom of the baby. Breech presentation therefore simply means the fetus's bottom is the leading part in the abdomen.

Candidiasis: Candida is the name of the fungus that causes vaginal thrush. *Vaginal candidiasis* therefore is the same as vaginal thrush.

Caput: The swelling that forms on the leading part of the baby's head in labour. In fact it is oedema (or swelling) of the scalp skin. It is most common in prolonged labour.

Carcinoma: Carcinoma is a type of cancer.

Cervix: Neck of the womb.

Chorionic gonadotrophin: This is the so-called "pregnancy hormone". It is produced by the placenta. The most common term for it is *HCG*, which stands for "human chorionic gonadotrophin".

Chorionic Villi Sampling: Also known in its short form of **CVS**. It is the taking of a placental biopsy for genetic or chromosomal diagnostic purposes.

Coagulation: Clotting. Used in reference to blood.

Colostrum: The protein-rich yellowish fluid produced by the breasts in the first two to three days after delivery, before milk proper is secreted.

Contraindication: Usually a medical reason why a procedure or drug should not be used.

Cordocentesis: The act of taking blood from the umbilical cord during pregnancy. It is done in specialist centres for diagnostic purposes.

Crowning: The appearance of the leading part of the head at the perineum or vaginal opening in the second stage of labour. As a rule, a crowning head does not retract back into the vagina once it has appeared.

Depo-Provera: This is a form of long-term contraception, given in the form of injection. Each injection is effective for twelve weeks, hence the term Depo.

Dilatation: The opening of, normally but not exclusively used in reference to the cervix.

Ectopic pregnancy: Pregnancy occurring outside the uterine (womb) cavity. The most common ectopic site is the fallopian tubes.

Embryo: In the early weeks after conception, before the various body structures can be identified, the fetus is called an embryo.

Endometrium: This is the lining inside the womb cavity, on which an embryo implants. This is also the lining that is shed every month if pregnancy does not occur.

Engagement of the head: When the largest diameter of the fetal head descends into the pelvis, it is said to be engaged. Normally, once this occurs, it stays there. Contrary to widespread belief, engagement of the head has no predictive value for labour onset. It could equally occur one month or one hour before the onset of labour.

Episiotomy: The incision or cut that is made on the perineum to increase the size of the opening, thereby facilitating delivery.

Erosion of the cervix: An unfortunately misleading but widely used term to describe a condition of the cervix that causes easy bleeding of the cervix. It is influenced by hormones and is therefore most common in pregnancy and with use of the combined contraceptive pill.

Expected Date of Delivery (EDD): This is the date calculated from date of the last period and which falls exactly forty weeks later (the average pregnancy duration). It is also called the Expected Date of confinement (EDC).

Fallopian tubes: Tubes which transport sperm toward the egg and to transport the fertilized egg or zygote towards the uterine cavity, where implantation ought to take place.

Fetus: The growing baby in the womb. Also spelt foetus.

Follicles: The cysts on the ovaries, which contain eggs. Normally, one follicle matures to release an egg every month.

Fontanelles: The soft areas on the baby's skull, which represent the meeting points of the various bones constituting the skull. The one to the front is called the anterior fontanelle and the one at the back the posterior fontanelle. At vaginal examination, one tries to locate these landmarks in order to determine how the baby's head is positioned in the birth canal.

Fraternal twins: Yet another term used to describe non-identical twins.

Fundus of uterus: The top of the dome of the uterus. A fundal height refers to the distance between the pubic bone and the topmost point of the uterus. It is used as a guide for the progress of the pregnancy.

Gametes: The eggs (ova) and the sperm. These are the female and male gametes respectively.

Gestation: Pregnancy.

Gestational period: The length of pregnancy, normally described in weeks.

GIFT: A short form of the assisted conception method known as *Gamete Intra-fallopian Transfer*.

Glycosuria: Sugar in the urine. This is common with diabetes, but may also occur in pregnancy without being abnormal.

Haematoma: A large blood-clot inside the body. It will normally be described by its location: hence a pelvic haematoma refers to a clot in the pelvic cavity, a vulval haematoma is when the clot is beneath the skin on the vulva, and so forth. Also spelt *hematoma*.

Haemolysis: The breaking-up or destruction of red blood-cells within the bloodstream. It can occur in a variety of conditions. Also spelt *hemolysis*.

Haemoglobin: This is the oxygen-carrying component within the blood-cells. It is also represented by a more ubiquitous term "**Hb**". When the haemoglobin count is low, the person is said to have anaemia.

Haemophilia: Genetically inherited conditions which are characterized by bleeding tendencies, low haemoglobin and sometimes the need for repeated blood transfusions.

Hydrops: A condition where the fetus is grossly oedematous, with fluid being found in practically all body cavities, including the chest and abdomen. There are various causes, but it is uncommon.

Identical twins: Twins arising from one egg, which then divides in two after fertilization.

In vitro fertilization: More popularly known as *IVF*. A process of assisted conception where an egg and sperm are harvested and fertilization facilitated outside the body. The fertilized embryo is then put back into the mother's womb.

Incompetent cervix: A condition of the cervix, which leads it to open (commonly around the halfway stage of pregnancy), thereby leading to late miscarriage.

IUCD: Stands for *Intrauterine Contraceptive Device*, which is popularly known by the misleading term "coil".

Introitus: The vaginal orifice leading into the vaginal canal.

Involution of uterus: The shrinking of the uterus, which occurs in the days and weeks following delivery.

Kick chart: A fetal movement count chart kept by the mother. It is usually instituted if there is concern about the amount of activity of the fetus, which is a loose guide to his or her well-being.

Labia: The fleshy skin-folds which enclose the clitoris and vaginal orifice.

Lactation: The production of milk in the breasts.

Liquor: see *amniotic fluid*

Lithotomy position: A position commonly used for vaginal examination, in which the woman lies on her back and her hips and knees are flexed. This allows her pelvis to tilt into a favourable position for examination. It is the opposite of being on "all-fours".

Management: Doctors and midwives may refer to the management of a condition rather than treatment.

Membranes: The bag that encloses the baby and water in the womb. The full name is amniotic membranes.

Membrane rupture: The "breaking of the waters".

Micturition: Passing water or peeing.

Monovular twins: see *binovular twins*

Moulding: The changes in the shape of the baby's head that occur in the course of labour as it negotiates its way through. It involves the coming together of the skull bones, which may sometimes slightly overlap. Moulding clears up after delivery.

Multiple pregnancy: A pregnancy with more than one fetus.

Obstetrician: A doctor who has specialized in the field of pregnancy and childbirth.

Oligohydramnios: The term used to describe reduced amniotic fluid ("waters") around the baby.

Os: The word means an opening or potential channel. It is used with a prefix; in this case it may be cervical os.

Ova: The female gametes or "eggs". One "egg" is called an *ovum*.

Ovulation: The release of ova or "eggs" by the ovaries.

Oxytocin: This is the naturally occurring hormone that stimulates the uterus to contract during labour. There is a synthetic version of the hormone, which is popularly known as Syntocinon or Pitocin. It is the same thing.

Placenta: The afterbirth.

Pelvimetry: This is the measuring of the various parameters of the pelvis. It can be done by vaginal examinations (manual pelvimetry), X-ray or CT scan.

Posterior: see *anterior*

Postnatal period: The period after delivery. It more or less means the same as the term *puerperium*.

Pruritus: Itching of the skin.

Puerperium: The period after delivery. It is generally thought to last six weeks.

Shrodikar suture: A stitch put into the neck of the womb (cervix) in a case of an incompetent cervix in a bid to prevent miscarriage.

Show: The blood-stained mucous discharge which is passed at the onset of labour. Labour may follow immediately but it may also not happen for many hours.

Superovulation: The production of many ova (eggs) in one menstrual cycle. This is usually a consequence of using fertility drugs and could lead to high-order multiple pregnancy.

Surfactant: A substance that is produced by lung cells to facilitate breathing when the baby is born. Normally it is produced over several weeks, from around the end of the second trimester. In threatened preterm delivery, steroids may be administered to stimulate production of this chemical. This reduces the breathing difficulties that many preterm babies are prone to.

Suture: This means two distinct things.
1. Putting stitches in a wound is to suture. The threads used are called suture material.
2. The potential gaps where the bones of the fetal skull meet are called sutures. For instance, the long gap running in the midline from the anterior to the posterior fontanelle is called a sagittal suture. There are several sutures on the skull.

Syntometrine: A mixture of the drugs syntocinon and ergometrine, commonly used to promote sustained uterine contraction after delivery. It is given in the form of an injection and the aim is to prevent excessive bleeding.

Trisomy: A term used to describe a set of three chromosomes. Chromosomes are supposed to be in pairs and therefore any set of three is an abnormality. Trisomy 21 is a description of Down's syndrome because set No. 21 in this condition has three chromosomes. There are a few other "trisomies", such as Edward's syndrome (Trisomy 16) and Patau's syndrome (Trisomy 13).

Uniovular twins: Yet another term for identical twins.

Ureters: The tubes that transport urine from the kidneys where it is produced, to the bladder where it is be temporarily stored before voiding.

Uterus: The womb.

Ventouse: The instrument sometimes used to assist delivery. It involves putting a rubber or metal cup on the fetal head and using a vacuum to hold it in place. It is also simply termed *vacuum*.

Vertex: This is the "highest" point on the baby's head, which then tends to be the leading part during labour and delivery.

Yolk sac: This is the ring-like structure found within the gestation sac during the first trimester. It is responsible for "feeding" the embryo in this early phase of the pregnancy.

Zygote: This is the name used for the fertilized ovum (egg). As it undergoes multiple divisions, it will be known as a *morula*, then an *embryo* and finally a *fetus*.

2. Normal pregnancy

Introduction

You conceive
You retch
You grow big
You grow bigger
You ache
You push
He or she cries
End of story?

Not a chance!

Normal pregnancy entails much more than those main predictable milestones. It is nine months (give or take) of a wide range of experiences. Even the use of the term "normal" should be preceded by a small pause for thought. There are a lot of women who will argue vigorously that their pregnancies cannot be described as normal. These protestations may range from those who claim that "I was so well and full of life and energy that it frightened me" to those who cry "there was so much sickness which went on for ever, unremitting backache that started too early, an overactive baby that kept me awake all night and a pregnancy that went on a good two weeks beyond my due date!" The truth is, these are two ends of the same spectrum.

The point emphasized in this chapter is that the experience of pregnancy is bound to differ quite enormously between one individual and another, without any of these being *abnormal*. All this is to do with constitution, environment and how each particular body responds to this momentous event. We set out here to explain – through specific answers to specific questions – what actually happens at each stage of this process.

Conception

How does natural conception take place?

Most women know that at ejaculation, a man deposits millions of spermatozoa into the vagina. The vast majority of these will not make it past the womb. Only a few thousand get to where the egg (ovum) is, which is usually at the outer end of one of the tubes. Only one of these will actually fertilize the egg. The sperm and egg fuse to form one cell, called a zygote. This cell will undergo incredible changes in the ensuing days, resulting in a mature baby about forty weeks later.

What happens soon after fertilization?

Things are happening quietly. There is absolutely no way for a woman to tell immediately whether a sexual act has resulted in conception. All those popular novels in which a woman says that *"I knew immediately after, that I had conceived"* are sheer fantasy.

Within thirty hours of fertilization, the fertilized egg undergoes the first division to form two cells. This is only the beginning of billions of divisions and changes that will take place within the first few weeks of pregnancy.

The dividing ball of cells – which is still quite tiny in size – is, meanwhile, being swept steadily along the tube towards the cavity of the womb, where it will implant.

When does implantation take place?

After the tubal journey, lasting four to five days, the ball of cells, now numbering fifty to sixty, reaches the uterine cavity. Implantation commences around seven days after fertilization and is complete by day fourteen.

Does any sign or symptom herald implantation?

In most cases, no. In a few cases, there may be light vaginal bleeding. Since this occurs about three weeks or so after the last period – and the woman is still unaware of her pregnancy – this light bleeding may be mistaken for a menstrual period. It has been known to cause confusion in dating the pregnancy. However, this problem is easily sorted out using ultrasound scan, provided the woman books for antenatal care within the first half of the pregnancy (which is the norm).

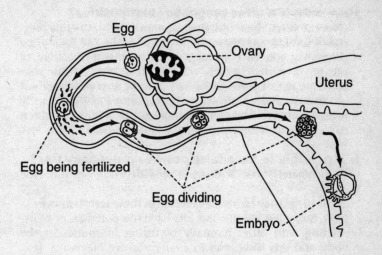

Fig 2 Thousands of sperm converge on the one egg but actually only one of them will succeed in penetrating the outer layer and fertilizing it. Immediately after, a chemical barrier is activated which prevents the rest from penetrating the egg.

What happens after the embryo has implanted?

The serious business of turning this mass of cells into a human being starts then. Even though it is still tiny in size, organs start forming at three weeks and their formation is complete by eight weeks.

From that point, only maturation and increase in size is taking place.

Even though the fetus is only about 2.3 cm in length (less than one inch) at eight weeks, the nose, ears, finger- and toe-buds are already formed.

The absolute sensitivity of this period cannot be over-emphasized. Any chemical insults – for example, in the form of drugs taken – during this particular period are likely to have the worst effect on the fetus.

Pregnancy tests

How soon is a urine pregnancy test positive?

Over the years, the sensitivity of commercially available pregnancy test kits has improved. Today, it is possible for a urine pregnancy test to confirm a pregnancy within a day of missing a period, which will be about two weeks after conception. Of course, there are still some tests which are not as sensitive and which will only be positive at significantly higher hormone levels – which may not be reached until ten to fourteen days after the date the period was due.

Is it possible to have false positive pregnancy test?

Unfortunately, yes, and again this depends on the type of test.

The pregnancy hormone detected in these tests is known as hCG. Some less specific test kits have the potential of cross-reacting with other naturally occurring hormones in the body, and this could lead to a false positive pregnancy test. Some infections may also lead to a false positive test, as may the use of some drugs, including penicillin and methadone.

Newer test kits are more specific and have greatly minimized the risk of a false positive pregnancy test.

What about a false negative pregnancy test?

It is possible, for a variety of reasons, for a pregnant woman to have a false negative test. The most common cause of this error is the use of the older test kits with low sensitivity. Because they need high hormone levels to detect a pregnancy, a test performed too early may turn out negative and probably become positive a week later, when levels are much higher.

The hormone hCG is produced in rapidly increasing quantities soon after implantation. The blood concentration of the hormone doubles roughly every two days and reaches its peak at about nine weeks after conception (eleven weeks of gestation). It gradually falls thereafter to reach its nadir at about seventeen to eighteen weeks of gestation and remains at that level for the remainder of the pregnancy.

Are there any other reasons for a false negative pregnancy test?

A faulty test kit may be one reason; wrong technique may be another and unfortunately, in some cases, a non-viable pregnancy may be the explanation. All in all, if a woman has a negative pregnancy test where she feels sure she is pregnant, she should seek prompt medical attention.

In most cases, an ultrasound scan will sort the problem out.

What proportion of tests are erroneously reported as positive or negative?

Historically, the figures quoted are 5 per cent false positive and a substantially higher 15–20 per cent false negative. These figures are certainly no longer valid, as the tests have become more refined and false positives and negatives are much rarer now.

Fetal movements

How soon does the baby start "kicking"?

As mentioned earlier, basic organ formation is complete by eight weeks of gestation.

In fact, fetal blood circulation is established three to four weeks post-conception.

Movement is detectable on the ultrasound scan even before eight weeks are complete. However, the fetus is still quite small (just over 2 cm long, at eight weeks) and the expectant mother should not expect to feel any movements for several weeks yet.

When does the mother start being aware of the fetal movements?

Some women may want to believe otherwise but it is extremely unusual for movements to be felt before sixteen weeks of gestation. In fact, in a first pregnancy, this may not take place until well into the eighteen to twenty weeks period.

Some women experience a sensation which is remarkably similar to fetal movements much earlier than sixteen weeks. In reality, this is caused by momentary spasms of muscles and even bowels, and is a result of fetal activity.

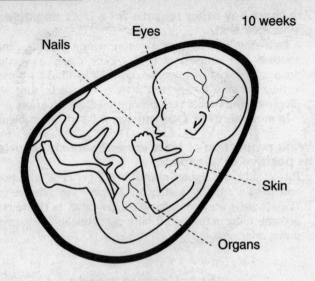

Fig. 3a Fetus at 10 weeks

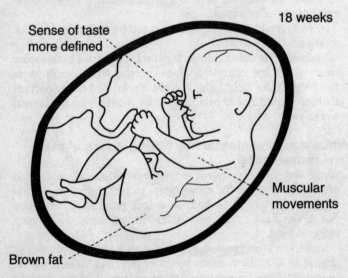

Fig 3b Fetus at 18 weeks

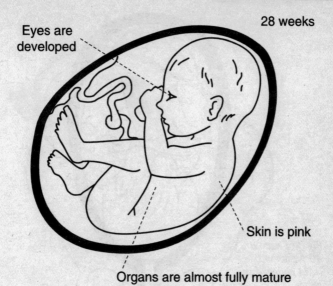

Fig 3c Fetus at 28 weeks

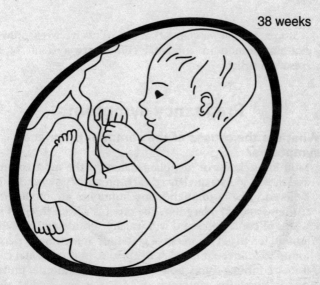

Fig 3d Fetus at 38 weeks

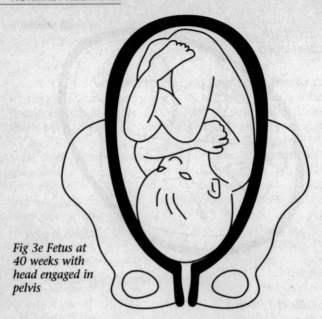

Fig 3e Fetus at 40 weeks with head engaged in pelvis

Stories of fetal movements at ten or twelve weeks, though not uncommon in antenatal clinics, are a result of this mistaken belief.

Pregnancy symptoms

What are the causes of the common pregnancy symptoms?

Morning sickness or just plain nausea is the most common and most widely experienced early pregnancy symptom. It is believed to be hormonal (many hormones are produced by the fetus and the placenta). The onset is within three to four weeks of conception and will usually subside and disappear around ten to twelve weeks of gestation. Sometimes it persists for up to fourteen or sixteen weeks and, in exceptional cases, it may continue throughout the pregnancy. Another unusual case is where the symptoms disappear as expected at about twelve weeks, only to come back towards the end of pregnancy.

Smoking exacerbates morning sickness. The severe form of pregnancy-related nausea and vomiting is regarded as pathological and is discussed in a separate chapter.

What about dizziness and bloatedness?

Dizziness normally starts later on in pregnancy. The cause is partially hormonal; progesterone, which is abundant during pregnancy, causes blood pressure to fall, especially on rising from a lying position.

The other cause of dizziness, if the mother has been lying on her back, is the pressure of the pregnant uterus on the big blood vessels in her abdominal cavity. This interferes with the blood-flow back to the heart and, on sitting or standing up, she may feel faint. In fact, this flat-on-your-back position is discouraged in pregnancy, because it also reduces the blood supply to the womb and the fetus.

Bloatedness is also a result of the high progesterone hormone levels, which causes fluid retention.

Several hormones also act to promote increased breast size, in preparation for feeding the baby. The breasts will therefore feel heavy, slightly engorged and may even feel a little tender.

What about bowel habits?

Constipation is quite common in pregnancy and again the culprit is the hormone progesterone.

Some women experience heartburn; again this is caused by progesterone. Both problems clear up after the birth and treatment of the symptoms in pregnancy is usually unsatisfactory.

It is said that presence of sugar in the urine in pregnancy is "not abnormal". Is this true?

Yes. Changes in blood-flow through the kidneys mean that loss of sugar through the urine may occur in pregnancy, without reflecting disease. Urine sugar cannot and should never be used to monitor diabetes management in pregnancy.

In the presence of other suspicious features – such as undue thirst, large fetal size and excessive amniotic fluid volume – sugar in the urine may prompt investigation for diabetes in pregnancy; but when it is found in isolation, it is of little or no significance.

In pregnancy, some areas may become darker in pigmentation.

Increased pigmentation around the nipples (areola), the navel and the perineum is common in pregnancy. Also common is the formation of a dark line extending from the navel down to the pubis, known as the linea nigra. All this is hormonal and the increased pigmentation is always temporary, clearing up within weeks of delivery.

What is carpal tunnel syndrome?

This is a condition where there is pain, numbness and even weakness of some of the fingers in one or both hands. This condition is not confined to pregnancy but may occur for the first time during pregnancy. Fluid retention is thought to be partly to blame.

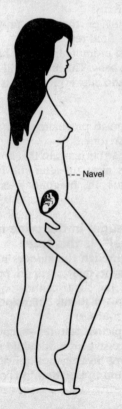

--- Navel

Fig 4a Outward appearance of pregnant woman at 10 weeks

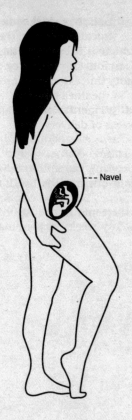

*Fig 4b Outward
appearance of pregnant
woman at 18 weeks*

- - - Navel

It can be quite debilitating, sometimes requiring surgical intervention to relieve the symptoms. In most cases, merely splinting the fingers will help. It usually disappears after delivery.

Visible signs

How does the womb accommodate the ever-increasing size of the pregnancy?

The progressive change in the size of the uterus to accommodate pregnancy is one of the wonders of nature. The uterus increases in weight almost twenty-five to thirty times from, about 30–50 g before pregnancy to about 1000 g (1 kg) at term. While the capacity of the uterine cavity when not pregnant is about 4–5 ml, this is increased almost a thousand-fold at term. The tiny structure, smaller than a woman's fist, grows to accommodate a baby, placenta and fluid with a combined weight of anything up to 8 kg or even more (such as in multiple pregnancy).

When does the pregnancy "bulge" first become visible?

To the outside world, there is no tell-tale abdominal bulge before twelve weeks of gestation. This is because, up until this point, the pregnancy is entirely pelvic. An exception is in the case of twins or multiple pregnancy, where the bulge may appear earlier.

Even in a singleton pregnancy, there may not be any visible distension before eighteen to twenty weeks, depending on

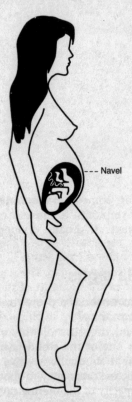

- - - Navel

Fig 4b Outward appearance of pregnant woman at 28 weeks

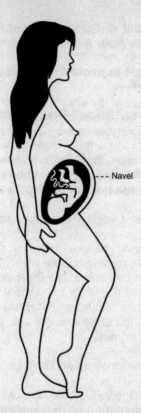

Fig 4d Outward appearance of pregnant woman at 38/40 weeks

Navel

the woman's build. After this mid-way stage, the abdomen actually distends and the increase in size is immediately apparent.

How come some women's pregnancies are hardly visible even at term while others look huge?

A combination of factors is actually at play. The size of the bulge will depend on the size of the contents of the uterus (twins will produce a bigger bulge at a comparable gestation) but this is not the only factor. The state of the abdominal muscles and their ability to rein in the growing uterus is also important. Another factor is the amount of fat deposited under the skin on the abdominal wall. This may be big enough to influence the outward impression of the size of the pregnant abdomen.

35

Contrary to popular belief, the apparent size of a pregnant abdomen is actually a poor guide to the size of the baby.

What sort of changes are expected to the lower genital tract?

There is a dramatic increase in the blood supply to the vulva and vagina. These areas become engorged and the vagina increases in length and ability to stretch, in preparation for the eventual delivery.

In some cases, this may become a problem, with development of varicose veins on the vulva. This can become extremely uncomfortable and it is not possible to cure them before delivery.

There is usually increased vaginal discharge, which may alarm some women.

Apart from the physical changes, there is significant lowering of the vaginal pH, making it more acidic. This helps prevent bacterial infections. However, the flip-side to this is that it promotes the flourishing of thrush, a problem that is quite common in pregnancy. While vaginal thrush does not endanger the pregnancy, it can be a major and protracted nuisance to the pregnant woman.

What causes stretch marks and can they be avoided?

Stretch marks are a direct result of the distension of the abdomen, which causes rupturing of the connective tissue beneath the skin. This is why stretch marks are invariably a late feature in pregnancy.

Some people are more prone than others. Obesity increases the risk of this happening. Among Caucasians, blonde women are more prone.

The stretch marks may actually become pigmented, sometimes becoming dark brown, even black. The pigmentation fades after delivery, leaving silvery-white irregular lines (known as striae).

While many types of lotions, so-called natural oils and creams have been claimed to be effective, there is no evidence that any of them can actually prevent stretch marks from appearing.

It is said contractions of the uterus start early in pregnancy. Is this true and, if so, why?

Experience of pre-labour contractions differ quite widely among pregnant women. They will also differ from one pregnancy to another for the same woman.

Painless contractions, to which the pregnant woman remains oblivious, commence as early as fourteen weeks of gestation. They will continue off and on for the remainder of the pregnancy.

At about thirty weeks, the woman may start being aware of them but they are almost always painless at this stage. They are then known as Braxton-Hicks. The placenta and the fetus produce a variety of hormones which act to promote these contractions. There are however other hormones – including progesterone – which oppose this effect, maintaining a balance which may help prevent inadvertent preterm labour.

Weight

How much weight should a pregnant woman expect to put on during pregnancy?

Again, this differs widely among individuals. The rough average is an overall gain of about 12 kg (26 lb). About 5 kg of this will be accounted for by the uterine contents (i.e. the baby, the placenta and amniotic fluid). That weight will therefore be lost immediately on delivery. The remainder of the weight gain is due to the increase in the size of the uterus itself, increase in the blood volume, fluid retention and some fat put on. Most of this weight is lost within the first few days after delivery. The fat may be a little more difficult to shift. Weight is discussed in more detail in Chapter 26, "Weight and Pregnancy".

Sex

Is sex during pregnancy a good idea?

There is nothing to prevent a pregnant woman from continuing to enjoy a normal sex life with her partner.

A problem may arise if there is vaginal spotting or bleeding in pregnancy. This may very well be the result of an innocent cervical condition. However, since penetrative sexual intercourse could provoke further bleeding, the standard advice for a woman with this problem is to avoid penetrative sex. Those women who have confirmed placenta praevia (where the placenta is too close or covering the cervix) are firmly advised to stay off penetrative sex, as this could provoke heavy and very frightening bleeding.

All the above-mentioned problems are normally confined to the latter half of pregnancy.

Work

At what stage should a working pregnant woman plan to give up work?

There is no way anybody can give a standard answer on this. Every individual's circumstances are different and it is those factors that influence a decision on how long to continue working while pregnant.

Factors such as the type of job, the woman's general health, pregnancy type (singleton or twins), and the presence or absence of potential problems (such as placenta praevia or high blood pressure) will have an influence on this decision.

For a woman who is doing an office job with low physical stress, it would be all right for her to continue working as long as possible, if that is what she wants. It certainly won't have any adverse effect on the pregnancy. The advice, therefore, is for every woman with a normal pregnancy to listen to her body.

3. Early pregnancy loss

Introduction

Early pregnancy loss is arguably the most common complication of pregnancy. Some estimates suggest that a quarter of all adult women will experience a miscarriage in their reproductive years, and this is not counting such complications as ectopic pregnancy or events such as induced abortion. Many practitioners in the field actually contend that this figure, high as it may seem, is actually a conservative estimate. All this boils down to one fact: that early pregnancy loss is depressingly common.

A matter that is highlighted in this chapter is the fact that early pregnancy loss does not necessarily take the form of spontaneous miscarriage. There are other forms of pregnancy loss such as missed abortion or blighted ovum. These are explained fully below. Most women who are unfortunate enough to experience any of these will not even have heard of them before.

Pregnancy loss, even when early, can be very distressing. It is therefore some comfort, however small, for a woman to learn that it is not a result of what she did or didn't do that led to the loss. This is virtually always the case.

It is also true that in most cases, a miscarriage is a one-off event.

It may help the woman to know that she is not alone and that her dark hour is unlikely to recur.

Note: In the last chapter of this book, there is a section on the most asked questions as compiled by some of the leading pregnancy and childbirth organizations. One of the contributors is the Miscarriage Association. There are some very interesting questions addressed there that readers of this chapter are likely to find useful.

Loss of pregnancy

How common is loss of pregnancy in the early phase?

Unfortunately, very common. It is practically impossible to know what proportion of pregnancies do not make it beyond the first trimester but conservative estimates put the rate at around 25 per cent or a quarter of all pregnancies.

If taken in the context of women who conceive, at least a quarter of them will experience a miscarriage or another form of early pregnancy loss. Some women experience more than one pregnancy loss.

Miscarriage is certainly one of the most common problems gynaecologists deal with in their day-to-day work.

Apart from spontaneous miscarriage, what are the other forms of early pregnancy loss?

Other forms of pregnancy loss include blighted ovum, missed abortion, ectopic pregnancy, molar pregnancy and induced abortion.

Blighted ovum

What is a blighted ovum?

This is a form of abnormal pregnancy development. In essence, at conception, the embryo fails to develop and the pregnancy consists of an empty sac. The pregnancy will *feel* normal to the mother. However, six to ten weeks into the pregnancy, she will experience light vaginal bleeding, which may be no more than spotting. An ultrasound scan will easily and conclusively establish the diagnosis.

What causes blighted ovum?

The causes are not known. It is thought to be a result of crucial structural or chromosomal abnormality which makes fetal development impossible. It has nothing to do with the pregnant woman's actions or lack of them.

How does a blighted ovum pregnancy affect future pregnancies?

It has no bearing whatsoever on future pregnancies. The chances of a normal pregnancy, following a blighted ovum, are not diminished in any way.

How does the hospital deal with a blighted ovum?

Most obstetric units will probably offer evacuation of the uterus (a procedure known as D&C).

It is a minor procedure performed in the operating theatre, mostly under a general anaesthetic. It usually takes about fifteen to twenty minutes and the hospital stay should not be more than a few hours.

A blighted ovum can also be dealt with medically, using drugs which facilitate the expulsion of the uterine contents. There may be a delay of possibly two or three days before this occurs. A third alternative is to await spontaneous miscarriage. It is impossible to predict how long the waiting could be: it may range from days to a few weeks, and many women find this prospect too stressful.

Missed abortion

What is missed abortion?

This is a situation where the fetus or embryo ceases to be viable in the course of the pregnancy, but is retained in the womb. Again, there is little warning in many cases. Sometimes, the warning may come in the sudden disappearance of pregnancy symptoms.

If the pregnancy is advanced into the second trimester, some women may experience some light leakage of milk.

What causes missed abortion?

The cause is not clearly known. Chromosomal or genetic abnormalities are certainly to blame in some cases, but not all.

How does the hospital deal with a missed abortion?

It depends on the stage of the pregnancy. If it is early in the first trimester, evacuation of the uterus in theatre under a general anaesthetic is preferred. Again there is the option of medical management in the form of orally administered tablets, but there is an inevitable time lag of up to three days, occasionally longer.

Another alternative is to await spontaneous miscarriage to take place. This is not popular with gynaecologists because it has an inherent risk of causing clotting abnormalities, especially if the uterine contents are retained for several weeks (which is possible). Moreover, spontaneous miscarriage may take place and surgical evacuation of the uterus may still be necessary, if some products are retained and/or there is serious bleeding.

What are the direct consequences of missed abortion on future fertility?
None.

Molar pregnancy

What is molar pregnancy?
This is an abnormal form of pregnancy where, instead of a fetus, a mass of grape-like vesicles form and proliferate in the womb. The woman will feel pregnant as usual and pregnancy symptoms such as nausea and vomiting may be greatly exaggerated. The fundus may also be bigger than suggested by the dates. An ultrasound scan will immediately confirm the diagnosis.

This condition is discussed in greater detail in Chapter 17, "Cancer and Pregnancy".

Spontaneous miscarriage

Spontaneous miscarriage is the most common form of early pregnancy loss. Do we know the causes?
This is a common problem but there is no common explanation to all of them. There is no doubt after extensive studies that *chromosomal and genetic abnormalities* account for a big proportion of spontaneous miscarriages. Some of these abnormalities are so severe that they are incompatible with life even in the womb, let alone outside.

Apart from chromosomal and genetic abnormalities, are there any other *known* causes of spontaneous miscarriage?

Yes. Abnormalities in the immune system of the mother could cause miscarriage, which could be a recurrent problem.

Abnormalities of the womb may be such that it is unable to carry a pregnancy beyond a certain time-span and this will cause early pregnancy loss.

Some infections, especially viral, may lead to miscarriage; and some diseases such as diabetes, if poorly controlled, may lead to early pregnancy failure.

Can you explain the immune system problem?

It is now well established that some women who suffer recurrent miscarriages have some abnormal antibodies, which may have a serious deleterious effect on the small blood vessels in the placenta, and therefore compromise the blood supply to the fetus. This may lead to miscarriage. In fact, the chances of miscarriage in an untreated individual is as high as 75–90 per cent. This condition is known as **anti-phospholipid syndrome**.

How is this condition diagnosed?

There is a test for the specific antibodies causing the problem. This test has yet to be perfected. It is therefore possible to have a negative result in a person who has strong clinical indicators of the syndrome. The test can also be falsely positive.

The test will usually be done if a woman has a history of recurrent early pregnancy loss.

Can anti-phospholipid syndrome be successfully treated in pregnancy?

The management of this condition continues to evolve. The current popular method is a combination of low-dose aspirin and a form of heparin. The treatment is continued throughout the course of pregnancy. This treatment has been shown to dramatically help the affected women, raising likelihood of delivering a live baby from less than 25 per cent to over 75 per cent.

How common is this syndrome?

Not common. People with conditions known as connective tissue diseases (the most common being systemic lupus erythematosus, or **SLE**) are the ones at greatest risk. These conditions are, however, uncommon. Moreover, the antibodies may be found in women with none of the known connective tissue diseases. These women will be at risk of recurrent miscarriage and will need appropriate treatment during their pregnancies.

To add to the complexity of the picture, not all individuals with SLE will have the offending antibodies causing anti-phospholipid syndrome.

Is anti-phospholipid syndrome responsible for early pregnancy loss only?

No. Fetal loss may be in mid-trimester and sometimes late, causing stillbirth. This is why it is important that treatment is maintained throughout the course of the pregnancy.

Does SLE affect the baby otherwise?

Apart from the risk of pregnancy loss, the fetus may be affected by *other* antibodies that are found in people with SLE (but not other forms of anti-phospholipid syndrome). Some babies are born with serious heart problems that could occasionally be fatal. There is no known way of preventing this from happening.

In managing SLE, steroids are used as well, and these will be continued for several weeks after delivery.

It is important that any pregnant woman affected by this condition is given as much detail about it as is practicable, so she can understand the potential problems and the possible implications and solutions.

Does the use of steroids after delivery preclude breast-feeding?

No.

Is the anti-phospholipid syndrome passed over to the baby?

No.

Going back to unexplained isolated miscarriage. Are there any factors that make this likely to happen?

Apart from those that have been mentioned already, hormonal imbalances are to blame in some cases. Women with *polycystic ovarian disease* are a case in point.

The older woman (over 35 years) is at a significantly higher risk of miscarriage, presumably because the risk of a chromosomally abnormal fetus increases with the age of the mother.

Fibroids

What about the presence of fibroids in the womb?

There is some evidence that fibroids, especially if they have grown inside the uterine cavity, may make conception difficult and if this has occurred there may be a risk of miscarriage. Fibroids which grow outside the uterine cavity (and which are commoner) do not seem to pose this risk.

If a woman has a fibroid inside the womb cavity and she is planning to conceive, should she be operated on to have the fibroid removed?

If it is obvious that the fibroid has contributed to the woman's fertility problems and that the procedure can be carried out without seriously compromising the womb's ability to carry a pregnancy, then the doctor should proceed with the operation . On the other hand, if this evidence is lacking or weak, it may be more prudent to encourage the woman to try for a baby without the operation.

It is important for the parents to be aware that the surgery may sometimes so seriously weaken the uterine wall operated on as to make future *safe* pregnancy impossible. Moreover, occasionally scarring may follow the operation, potentially reducing the ability to conceive even further. All the pros and cons should be discussed so that the prospective parents are fully in the picture.

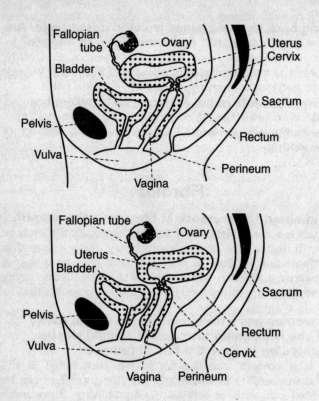

Fig 5 Tilting womb

Womb position

Some women are known to have wombs that tilt backwards. Can this cause miscarriage?

Wombs normally tilt gently towards the front. A substantial minority of women, however, do have wombs which tilt towards the back. The common term is "retroverted uterus". This does not cause miscarriage or pregnancy loss.

There is an exceedingly rare complication of this anatomical state, where a growing uterus may be trapped in the pelvis and will fail to rise into the abdominal cavity. This will cause increasing pain and an operation will easily correct the problem. This complication is very rare.

Infections

What is the role of infections in early pregnancy loss?

Any acute infection which causes the woman to have a high temperature and be generally ill has the potential to cause miscarriage.

- Urinary tract infections, especially if they affect the kidneys, frequently lead to uterine activity and miscarriage.
- Syphilis is now of largely historical interest in the western world, but is still a menace in many developing countries; it is known to cause miscarriage and stillbirth.
- Conditions such as acute hepatitis, by causing high fever may lead to miscarriage, as can the more common condition of appendicitis.
- Malaria remains a significant cause of miscarriage in tropical countries.

Infections do not have to be in the genital tract to pose a risk to the pregnancy.

Alcohol

What about alcohol and miscarriage?

There is evidence that sustained alcohol abuse can lead to pregnancy loss. Binge drinking has not been associated with this problem.

Smoking

Can smoking increase the risk of miscarriage?

Yes. The risk increases with the the number of cigarettes smoked. This is dealt with in greater detail in Chapter 20, "Smoking and alcohol use in pregnancy".

Hormone injections

Some obstetricians will recommend a course of hormone injections in the early phase of pregnancy if a woman has a history of unexplained repeated miscarriage. How useful is this?

The practice of administering progesterone injections weekly (or more frequently) throughout the first trimester, sometimes even beyond was a rather common practice in the past.

It is known that progesterone is crucial in the maintenance of pregnancy and it was assumed that somehow, for these women, this hormone was deficient and hence supplements could resolve this problem.

Evidence of this theory in *naturally conceived* pregnancies is tenuous, to say the least; and evidence to the effectiveness of this treatment is lacking. This practice is now rare.

Incompetent cervix

What is cervical incompetence?

This is a known anatomical cause of miscarriage and pregnancy loss may be recurrent.

The cervix (or neck of the womb) is normally strong enough to remain closed throughout the course of pregnancy, in spite of the ever-increasing size and weight of the womb contents. In fact, even at term, hormonal changes have to take place where specific hormones are released to act on the cervix, making it softer and thinner and allowing it to dilate in labour.

With an incompetent cervix, the cervix is anatomically weak, causing the womb to lose its contents – around mid-pregnancy. Typically, miscarriage caused by an incompetent cervix occurs between sixteen and twenty-four weeks of gestation.

What causes cervical incompetence?

The known causes of cervical incompetence include previous therapeutic dilatation of the cervix (D&C), which is done in termination of pregnancy.

Cone biopsy – a mode of diagnosis and treatment for a severely abnormal smear – is another.

Both these procedures may subsequently lead to cervical incompetence. Most gynaecologists will avoid forcibly dilating the cervix whenever possible, especially since alternatives are available, in many cases.

What happens in a miscarriage due to cervical incompetence?

In the majority of cases, it is without warning. There is a gush of fluid as the membranes of the gestational sac break. This follows a silent opening of the weakened cervix.

Once the "waters" have broken, the process is virtually irreversible. The woman will proceed to miscarry in a matter of hours.

Can cervical incompetence be remedied?

If a diagnosis of an incompetent cervix is made, following such a miscarriage, remedial action has to wait until she has conceived again. Corrective action is taken after fourteen weeks, when the possibility of spontaneous miscarriage from other causes has receded to negligible, and a scan has verified that the fetus and placenta are growing normally. Fourteen weeks is also just before entering the danger period of miscarriage caused by cervical incompetence.

What does corrective action involve?

The commonly used method is to put a special suture in the weakened cervix to close it and hold it in that closed state. The procedure is called "cervical cerclage" and, depending on how the suture is made, names for the procedure such as Shirodkar and Macdonald will be used. It is done vaginally, and the suture is subsequently removed at thirty-eight weeks of gestation, ready for labour.

The insertion of the stitch is done in theatre under a general anaesthetic. Many obstetricians will advise a subsequent hospital stay of at least a day, for complete rest and observation. There is a small risk that the action of putting the suture in could trigger a miscarriage, hence the precaution. Removal of the suture is straightforward and does not require going to theatre or an anaesthetic.

How successful is cervical cerclage?

The success rate is modest but actual figures are not clearly known. It is now being more and more accepted that probably the more difficult procedure of putting the stitch in abdominally rather than vaginally may be the better method, with a better success rate. With the abdominal method, the suture is applied to the cervix through the abdomen, hence it is a bigger and technically more difficult operation.

Ectopic pregnancy

What is an ectopic pregnancy?

This is a pregnancy that implants outside the uterine cavity. The most common ectopic site is in the fallopian tube. It could, however, occur elsewhere such as in the cervix, ovary or pelvic cavity. Our discussion here will focus on the fallopian tube ectopic pregnancy, which accounts for well over 95 per cent of all ectopic pregnancies.

How common is ectopic pregnancy?

In the UK, one in every 300 pregnancies is ectopic. In the USA, the rate is higher, at one in 100. There is evidence that rates in most of the western world are going up.

What causes a pregnancy to implant outside the womb?

Causes are not always apparent but previous infection is an important predisposing factor.

Pelvic infection, especially if there is delay in treatment, causes tubal damage. The residual scarring inside the tube may impede transportation of the fertilized egg towards the womb. This will lead to ectopic implantation. Chlamydia infection is particularly implicated, especially since it can be an entirely silent infection.

Other minor factors include surgery on the tubes (sterilization and reversal of sterilization) and some methods of assisted conception.

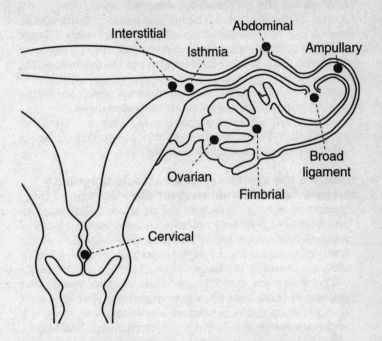

Fig 6: An ectopic pregnancy. The uterus, on the left in the picture is definitely empty. The pregnancy is outside the womb and in this case was in the tube. In most cases, the ectopic pregnancy cannot be seen on the scan.

It is a widely held belief that intra-uterine contraceptive devices may increase the risk of ectopic pregnancy. Is this true?

Strictly speaking, no. The device (or "coil", as many people call it) will not increase the risk of ectopic pregnancy. However, the family planning practitioner advising a client has to ensure this is a suitable method for her.

The "coil" is certainly unsuitable for a woman with multiple potential or real partners. This is because she is at risk of pelvic infection, which puts her at risk of ectopic pregnancy. A "coil" protects against normal intra-uterine pregnancy, so the combined oral contraceptive pill will be a better option for her.

What about the "Mirena®," device?

This is a different matter. The Mirena device or "intra-uterine system", as its manufacturers prefer to call it, is a special type of device that contains a reservoir of the progestogen hormone. This is released slowly to act on the wall of the uterus.

It is an extremely effective contraceptive, protecting against both intra-uterine and ectopic pregnancies.

It has an added bonus in that it reduces the menstrual loss to very low levels within a month of insertion, and its effectiveness may last up to five years.

What are the symptoms of an ectopic pregnancy and how can a woman suspect she might have it?

Symptoms vary quite widely. The most common symptom will be that of persistent and one-sided abdominal pain. The area will be tender to touch. This is usually – but by no means always – accompanied by vaginal spotting, light bleeding or simply a brownish discharge.

The symptoms typically start one or two weeks after missing a period. Sometimes the symptoms may start so early that the woman may be unaware she is pregnant. A woman with such symptoms should seek immediate medical help.

How is ectopic pregnancy diagnosed?

When a woman has these symptoms in early pregnancy, two essential tests (in addition to physical examination) will be done: a urine pregnancy test and an ultrasound scan.

Physical examination may reveal features that may strengthen the doctor's suspicion of an ectopic pregnancy but will not conclusively establish the diagnosis.

If the pregnancy test is positive, this is where an ultrasound scan comes in. If the scan shows the pregnancy in the uterus, then an ectopic pregnancy is virtually ruled out. If the uterus is empty, it strongly suggests an ectopic pregnancy. It is, however, not a foregone conclusion. The doctor has to look at the whole picture and decide whether or not the case he or she is dealing with is likely to be an ectopic pregnancy or not.

If a scan shows an empty uterus in the presence of a positive pregnancy test, that surely is an ectopic pregnancy?

Not really. An "empty" uterus may be because there was a pregnancy there that has since been miscarried. Alternatively, there may be a pregnancy there that is still too small to be detected on the scan. Remember, a pregnancy five weeks or less may not be visible on the scan.

Does this mean a pregnancy that is in the tube cannot be seen on the scan, so as to remove any doubts?

Unfortunately, seeing an ectopic pregnancy on the scan is an exception rather than the rule. The diagnosis is reached by exclusion and piecing the evidence together. It is not unusual to take a patient to theatre, only to find no such thing.

What happens after diagnosis of ectopic pregnancy?

The patient will be taken to theatre as an emergency. If the diagnosis is still in doubt, a diagnostic laparoscopy is performed. If the diagnosis is confirmed, the pregnancy is removed, either by opening the tube or by removing the entire affected tube with the pregnancy inside. The procedure is in many cases done entirely laparoscopically (by keyhole surgery) and the woman is able to leave hospital within twenty-four hours or so. Sometimes, this is technically not possible, which means opening the abdomen. This will mean a longer (3–5 day) hospital stay and a slightly longer recuperation period.

What are the consequences of an ectopic pregnancy?

Delay in presentation or diagnosis may lead to rupture of the fallopian tube, with potentially serious bleeding within the abdominal cavity. This will cause severe pain and occasionally fainting. The more enduring effect is that of reduced fertility. Following an ectopic pregnancy, chances of a normal pregnancy through natural conception are significantly reduced. Moreover, there is an increased risk of a further ectopic pregnancy.

Can an ectopic pregnancy occur together with a normal intra-uterine pregnancy?

Yes. This used to be rare but is now much more common, with the increases in assisted conception. Figures of one in 3000 are sometimes quoted. The ectopic pregnancy has to be removed to allow the normal pregnancy to continue.

Is surgery the only treatment available for ectopic pregnancy?

No. Chemotherapy is sometimes used as a form of treatment for ectopic pregnancy. It is not favoured by many, especially because of the potential side-effects, the inevitable delay, the intensive follow-up required to ensure cure, and occasional failure.

Can an ectopic pregnancy grow to term?

Yes, but not if it is in the tube. Tubal pregnancies inevitably cause a rupture (of the tube) in the first seven to ten weeks. Cases of abdominal pregnancies (where there is plenty of room) which went unrecognized to the late third trimester have been reported, from time to time. When recognized, delivery (inevitably by operation) is carried out immediately. Because of the environment in which they grow (which is not ideal), these babies tend to have major limb deformities. A few have managed to be delivered in a surprisingly good physical state.

Can an ectopic pregnancy diagnosed while still intact be successfully transplanted into the womb?

Obstetricians are still unable to do this and it is not for lack of trying. Watch this space!

4. Ultrasound

Introduction

Over the last two decades, ultrasound as a technology used in the practice of medicine has come on in leaps and bounds. Today, ultrasound use in pregnancy care comes as a matter of course. Attitudes towards it differ from person to person, but the overall attitude is favourable. None the less, there is always a certain amount of anxiety when it comes to the interaction of modern technology and pregnancy in particular. People rightly want to know what it actually involves, whether it is safe for them and their babies, why it is done in different ways, what the advantages are and a lot more besides.

It is always a good thing that pregnancy is allowed to be an enjoyable experience, considering what it is about. It is also important to emphasize that pregnancy is not a disease. It is a normal physiological process and the primary aim of ultrasound is to reinforce this point. In the few instances when it helps to identify something wrong, this should be looked at positively as it offers an opportunity of carrying out remedial measures, wherever possible. Here, we explain what ultrasound technology is all about.

Ultrasound – what it is

What is ultrasound?

This is a form of sound waves generated at a very high frequency. The frequency used in these machines is in the range between 3.5 to 7 million cycles per second (Megahertz). Normal sound waves audible to the ear are produced at a frequency of only a few thousand cycles per second (hertz).

How does ultrasound work?

The sound waves produced by the crystal in the probe are reflected from the various structures they encounter as they travel. The different ways in which they are reflected are translated by the scanning machine into an image that is produced on a screen. The early scanners used to produce a static picture but, for many years now, these have been superseded by the so-called "real-time" scanners, where all movements taking place are visible.

How useful is the ultrasound in pregnancy?

It is not difficult for a contemporary obstetrician to wonder how earlier obstetricians managed without the ultrasound scan. It is virtually indispensable. Ultrasound is used to confirm the pregnancy, number of fetuses and gestation age, and detect all kinds of pregnancy complications.

What ultrasound can diagnose

What pregnancy complications can the ultrasound diagnose?

Fetal demise is one. From the gestation age of six weeks, the fetal heartbeat can be clearly seen on the ultrasound. Absence of this will indicate that the fetus is dead.

Growth restriction can be objectively identified, both by a single and by serial ultrasound scans. When the gestation age of the pregnancy is known with certainty (both from the last period and an early scan), a single ultrasound scan in the late phase of the pregnancy may confirm clinically suspected poor fetal growth. Alternatively, serial scans (done at least fortnightly) could objectively show that the rate of growth is below normal.

A great many fetal abnormalities – including those of the limbs, spine, face, brain, lungs, heart, bowel, kidneys, bladder, abdominal wall etc. – can be detected by using ultrasound scanning. Other abnormalities, where the defect is very small, may not be seen.

At what gestation can the gross abnormalities be detected?

Most obstetric units operate a policy of performing scans at between eighteen and twenty weeks of gestation. (*See* Chapter 5, "Ultrasound scan at 18 to 20 weeks".) Earlier scans are likely to miss some abnormalities, as the fetus is still too small.

Even at twenty weeks, some abnormalities may not be clearly seen, and could be picked up at later scans when the fetus is bigger. To get around this problem, when one or more of the vital structures (such as the heart or spine) is not clearly seen, the mother will probably be advised to have a repeat scan in two weeks or so, to ensure everything is clearly seen.

What is the use of early (first trimester) scanning?

This may help to:

- confirm pregnancy (where there is doubt)
- confirm location of pregnancy (where there is possibility of ectopic pregnancy)
- confirm and document gestational age (where dates are uncertain)
- establish the number of fetuses
- confirm viability
- rule out or diagnose abnormal pregnancies (such as blighted ovum or hydatidform mole).

What is a blighted ovum?

This is where there is a gestation sac with fluid but no embryo (fetus). It is believed that things actually go wrong soon after conception and no embryo develops. Light vaginal bleeding at around six to ten weeks of gestation is usually the first warning. An ultrasound scan will confirm the diagnosis. (This is further discussed in Chapter 3, "Early pregnancy loss".)

Fetal anaemia

Can the ultrasound scan help in diagnosing fetal anaemia?

Not directly. If this condition is suspected and if the obstetrician sees fit to confirm the diagnosis, the scan may be used as an imaging tool while getting a blood sample from the cord for analysis.

Blood sampling can also be obtained for the purpose of making diagnosis in cases of suspected infection or chromosomal or genetic abnormalities.

What can be seen in ultrasound

Can an ultrasound scan tell whether twins are identical or not?

Only if they share the amniotic sac or placenta (in which case, they are identical).

If each twin is in a separate sac and has a separate placenta, these could be either identical or non-identical, and the scan cannot tell whether they are identical or not. Of course, if they are of different sex, then it is obvious they are non-identical.

Is it possible to tell the sex of the fetus in the first trimester by using ultrasound scanning?

No. Probably the earliest you can tell with confidence is around sixteen weeks of gestation.

What is a yolk sac?

In the first trimester, on the ultrasound picture, there appears a distinctive ring-like image within the gestational sac, adjacent to the fetus. This is the structure that is responsible for feeding the fetus until the placenta takes over, at about ten weeks of gestation. The yolk sac can be seen on the scan quite early, even before the fetal heartbeat is apparent.

At what gestation is a fetal heart visible on the ultrasound scan?

With a trans-vaginal probe, at six weeks. If a trans-abdominal probe is used, it may be up until a week later, at seven weeks, before it is seen.

What are the advantages of a trans-vaginal scan (TVS) over a trans-abdominal one?

The image with a TVS is sharper and clearer.

More detail can be discerned and some subtle things that might be missed using a trans-abdominal probe may be easily picked up. Moreover, while a trans-abdominal scan in early pregnancy requires a full bladder for a good image, a TVS does not.

A trans-vaginal scan also circumvents the problem of obesity in the mother, which tends to prevent good images – full bladder or not – if using a trans-abdominal probe.

In early pregnancy, most units use the trans-vaginal route for ultrasound scanning. However, both routes may sometimes be necessary to discern things properly. The trans-vaginal route is not necessary beyond the first trimester of pregnancy, except in special cases.

Ultrasound and the placenta and amniotic fluid

Does the ultrasound scan show anything else apart from the fetus?

Yes. Scanning in pregnancy is not confined to looking at the fetus. In the second half of the pregnancy, an ultrasound scan will be used to establish the location of the placenta, to check the amniotic fluid volume and to look at other parts of the pelvis and abdomen – especially the ovaries and kidneys.

Why is placental location important?

Because some placentas may be low-lying. This can have potential bearing on the timing as well as the method of delivery.

A condition known as *placenta praevia* – which means "low-lying placenta" – could cause vaginal bleeding during pregnancy. This is sometimes serious enough to require an emergency delivery. Even without bleeding, when the placenta is significantly low-lying, it means delivery will most likely be by caesarean section. Diagnosis by ultrasound scan allows for proper pregnancy care and planning of the time and method of delivery.

Why is amniotic fluid volume measurement important?

Abnormalities of amniotic fluid volume (either too much or too little) sometimes denote a problem with the pregnancy.

An ultrasound scan allows the doctor to make note of the fluid abnormality, its extent and its progression. More importantly, it allows for the initiation of necessary steps, either to diagnose the underlying cause or to monitor the fetal well-being.

Does a low-lying placenta at 18–20 weeks denote placenta praevia?

No. At this stage, anything between 30 and 40 per cent of placentas appear low-lying. Only around half a per cent will still be low-lying towards the end of pregnancy.

The placenta does not move. It is the pattern of growth of the womb that allows for the placenta to appear further away from the lower segment as the pregnancy advances. There is no such thing as *placenta praevia* at twenty weeks of gestation.

Ultrasound at different stages of pregnancy

How accurate is the ultrasound at estimating gestational age?

The earlier the scan is performed, the more accurate it is. In the first trimester (the first fourteen weeks), the scan will be accurate to within three days of the gestation. In the middle of the second trimester (at about 20–22 weeks), the accuracy drops to about a week. If the scan is performed in the third trimester, it may miss the gestation by up to three or even four weeks. The bigger the fetus, the more inaccurate the scan tends to be.

Generally speaking, scans performed in the last ten to twelve weeks of pregnancy cannot be used to date a pregnancy because their margin of error is considered too wide.

If I had an ultrasound scan in the early part of the pregnancy which established the gestational age, then a repeat scan several weeks later showed a different "gestation", isn't this confusing?

It should not be. Your earliest scan is the most accurate one. A subsequent scan should not prompt a recalculation of the gestation age. Once this is established, it does not change.

Why would there be a discrepancy between scans of the same fetus performed at different phases of the pregnancy?

Because of the inherent weakness of the ultrasound in dating late pregnancies, the differing growth rates of babies and, not least, human error. The emphasis here is that if a scan is to be useful in dating a pregnancy, this has to be done as early as possible, preferably below twelve weeks and certainly before twenty weeks.

What if the woman for some reason was unaware that she was pregnant until very late, let's say after seven months of pregnancy?

Then she has to accept that the date she will be given has a potential error of up to three weeks, even more. The obstetrician will monitor the remainder of the pregnancy with this factor in mind.

How is the ultrasound scan used to monitor fetal well-being?

If there is any cause for concern on the fetal well-being, the attending obstetrician may request tests which may be repeated every few days to monitor the fetal condition. Most tests require the use of ultrasound. This may be to observe the rate of movements, the tone of the muscles, breathing movements, the amniotic fluid volume and (*in some cases*) to check the pattern of blood-flow in the umbilical cord.

Safety of ultrasound

How safe is ultrasound?

Vast and extensive studies have been carried out since ultrasound came into widespread use in obstetrics in the mid-1970s. None has shown adverse effects to mothers or children involved. We are taking millions of people and a time-scale of decades into account here.

5. Ultrasound scan at 18 to 20 weeks

Introduction

In the UK, as in many industrialized countries, the majority of hospitals offer a routine mid-trimester ultrasound scan to all pregnant woman. It is normally termed a "detailed anatomy scan", because this is the principal purpose of the scan: to do a detailed surveillance of the anatomy of the fetus, with the aim of detecting any major anatomical anomalies.

Is this routine scan beneficial or even desirable? This is not as easy to answer as one may be tempted to believe. None the less, there is strong evidence that most mothers desire it and actually look forward to it.

The fact that this examination is widely termed an "anatomy scan" does create a few problems, however. It may create an impression in the parents' minds that their baby is definitely getting an absolute all-clear at this stage. When, in the end, this turns out not to be the case, this innocent fact may unleash anxiety and a suspicion that something was held back from them. Unfounded as this might be, it can and has occasionally caused considerable distress to some parents.

It is therefore important that all obstetric units offering this service should ensure that pre-scan information and counselling is not cursory but detailed, so that every single woman has realistic expectations.

The potential benefits and limitations of this examination are spelt out in detail in this chapter. Most obstetric units have a set-up which ensures the comfort and the interaction of the parents-to-be in the examination using highly skilled technicians who are able to explain things as the examination is in progress. It is this element which most parents appreciate the most. In effect, it is the first virtual bonding session between the unborn baby and his or her parents.

A few units have opted not to offer this particular scan to all women and instead offer a less detailed scan at an earlier gestation. This is normally confined to confirming viability, the number of fetuses and the gestational age. Women deemed to be at risk by virtue of their family history, previous obstetric history or other reasons – and those who make a specific request, judged to be valid – are offered the detailed anatomy scan.

In this chapter, we explain what the detailed mid-trimester (eighteen to twenty weeks) scan entails.

The benefits of scanning

Is an ultrasound scan necessary for every pregnant woman at this gestation?

No. It is not necessary. It is, however, almost universally accepted that this is an extremely useful measure which benefits the expectant mother, her family, the caregivers and in some cases, the unborn baby.

What are the potential benefits of a twenty-weeks ultrasound scan?

- *It confirms the number of fetuses*. Many twin pregnancies are established for the first time at this scan.
- *It confirms viability*. In a few cases, the fetus may die in the womb and the expectant mother may get no warning whatsoever. This is called *"missed abortion"*. An ultrasound scan arranged routinely at this stage may be the first opportunity to discover this unfortunate turn of events. This is an uncommon finding.
- *It confirms gestation*. Very often, an ultrasound scan may show that the pregnancy is far more or less advanced than suggested by the mother's dates. This has important implications, as we shall see shortly.
- *It identifies high-risk pregnancies*. Potential problems may be identified for the first time at the twenty-weeks ultrasound scan. This will allow for the necessary input at the appropriate time.
- *It identifies gross anomalies*. This scan is used to do a detailed anatomy assessment. Most major malformations will be identified. This allows for proper analysis and action.

Occasionally, fetal malformations where the baby has no chance of surviving outside the womb are discovered. This enables the mother, her family and the caregivers to reach a decision on what needs to be done. Some non-lethal problems, which can be treated either in the womb or after delivery, may also be identified.

● *It establishes the location of the placenta (afterbirth) and its structure.* In a few cases, the placenta may overlay the cervix, slightly increasing the risk of bleeding in pregnancy or a later diagnosis of **placenta praevia** (where the placenta is abnormally low). This discovery allows for proper advice to the expectant mother. A low-lying placenta at a twenty-weeks scan report is not in itself considered to be a risk factor and the mother should not be unduly worried.

● *Early bonding.* The expectant mother (and her partner if he accompanies her) can see the fetus clearly on the screen. At this stage of the pregnancy, the fetus is a miniature baby with all structures formed. It is also quite active, moving its limbs, kicking and sucking its thumb. Observing all these is believed to have a powerful bonding effect and is considered very important. This is why the whole exercise is fully interactive, with the parents encouraged to ask questions and make comments whenever they feel like it.

Why is precise dating important? After all, "baby comes when it is ready".

This may indeed be so but is not always the case.

When there is an apparent prolongation of a pregnancy, it is too late to verify the dates at the end of pregnancy. An ultrasound scan cannot accurately estimate the gestation if it is performed beyond the second trimester. Such a situation makes the decision of whether to intervene or not very difficult. A post-term pregnancy may be a risk situation, in some circumstances. Having precise dates goes a long way in helping to make the right decisions.

Another situation is when there is a factor that may necessitate premature delivery. The decision in such a situation hinges on knowing the gestation precisely, because fetal survival outside the womb is at stake. If the dates are erroneous and the pregnancy wrongly believed to be more advanced than it actually is, delivery may have disastrous results. An ultrasound scan at twenty weeks will remove this potential problem.

There are a few other scenarios where dating by an early scan comes in useful.

Why is it essential for everybody to be scanned? Can the test not be confined to those "at risk"?

The whole essence of screening is that the test is available to everybody.

Experience shows that problems are usually identified mostly among those where they are least expected, where there is no apparent risk factor. If the scan was offered to only those who are regarded to be at risk, most problems such as fetal abnormalities will be missed.

It should be emphasized here that the vast majority (over 85 per cent) of scanned pregnancies are found to be perfectly normal. Absence of a detectable problem does not imply wasted effort or resources, however, as it allows for provision of appropriate minimal intervention antenatal care. Nor should one ignore the bonding engendered by this test. Most mothers find the experience positively uplifting.

Does the expectant mother have a choice regarding having the scan?

Of course she has. Like any other antenatal test, the ultrasound scan is voluntary. It is, however, imperative that that caregivers ensure that any mother who declines the test is well informed and is not making this decision based on patchy information and half-truths.

Targeted scans

What is meant by a "targeted scan"?

In some cases, there is an identifiable risk factor for specific fetal abnormalities. This may be in cases of:

- previous malformations
- known carriers of genetic or chromosomal defects
- mothers on certain medication (such as anticonvulsants)
- a diabetic or epileptic mother.

In others, the earlier blood tests such as the Down's syndrome screening test (also known as the "triple test" or "double test") may have given results that show an increased likelihood of presence of abnormalities. A component of this test may also indicate increased likelihood of neural tube defects such as spina bifida. In all such cases, the scan is targeted to look very closely for specific potential abnormalities and confirm or rule them out. As a general rule, scans in the older mother (i.e. those in their late thirties or their forties) will be "targeted" because of increased incidence of fetal abnormalities in this age group.

Can a targeted scan miss an abnormality that is actually there?

This is rare but possible. Most gross abnormalities will almost certainly be detected. However, some abnormalities of the heart, genitalia and even the upper lip can be missed at twenty weeks. The heart has four chambers. If the heart view is not clear for some reason at twenty weeks, it is normally recommended repeating the scan at twenty-four weeks. when the views are better. The same may apply for cleft lip. Poorly visualized genitalia is not an indication to repeat the scan, unless there was an identified risk of having a problem in this area. In addition, if the parents are carriers of a condition that is sex-linked (i.e. affects children of one sex only, usually boys), then it may be imperative to clearly identify the sex of the fetus, so as to appropriately advise the parents.

Performance of the scan

Who performs the scan?

In most obstetric units, experienced ultrasonographers perform the scans. Occasionally, obstetric specialist trainees may perform the scan under direct supervision. A mother can expect to have one or two people in the room with her. Many units encourage the partner to accompany the mother and be with her during the test.

How much interaction should the expectant mother expect during the performing of the scan?

The person performing the scan, be they a radiographer or a doctor, will in most cases ensure that the mother has an uninterrupted view of the screen. He or she will, in most cases, give a running commentary of what he or she is seeing and doing. The mother will be allowed time to appreciate all that is going on "on the screen" – in effect, in her womb. If there are any significant findings which need explaining or further action, the person scanning will leave this task to the obstetrician, who will normally see the mother soon after the test, with the report.

The test normally takes around thirty minutes. The parents should expect to see a baby that is in perpetual activity in the entire period. Prepare to be dazzled.

Should there be a repeat scan after the 18–20 weeks scan?

Except where another scan is specifically called for, no repeat scan is indicated.

As mentioned earlier, in some cases, not everything that one needs to see is seen at the twenty-weeks scan. In such circumstances, it is not possible to give a clean bill to the parents regarding their unborn baby. If the areas which have not been sufficiently seen are such vital structures as the heart or spine, most obstetricians will recommend a repeat scan, usually about four weeks later. Factors which may preclude an adequate scan include maternal obesity and an unfavourable fetal position in the womb.

Why is twenty weeks the chosen gestation for the detailed scan?

This scan is performed at anything between eighteen and twenty weeks. This is considered optimal for a number of reasons. Firstly, the fetus is of such a size that virtually all the organs and structures can be seen. It also still fits on the screen, which is good for the parents – who are seeing their unborn baby. Secondly, the antenatal screening test results are usually available at this stage and, where indicated, a "targeted scan" can be performed. Another reason is that those conditions that may affect fetal growth – such as gestational diabetes or pre-eclampsia – will not have appeared or taken hold at this stage and hence everything is still "normal", the way it should be.

On a less pleasant note, when a fatal condition is discovered at this stage of pregnancy, where termination of pregnancy is considered to be the inevitable course of action, this is relatively less traumatic (both physically and emotionally) than if this was done much later, with a more advanced pregnancy.

What are the benefits of an early scan?

Occasionally, an ultrasound scan may have to be performed early in pregnancy, probably within the first twelve weeks. This is usually in situations where the woman wants to confirm that she is pregnant. This may arise for a variety of reasons.

Other indications for an early scan may be:

- *Confirming the viability of the pregnancy* e.g. in instances where there has been vaginal bleeding in early pregnancy.
- *Identifying the location of the pregnancy*. This is in cases where there is increased possibility of ectopic pregnancy, such as in women with a history of previous ectopic pregnancy, a history of pelvic infection or those suffering localized lower abdominal pain in pregnancy.
- *Excessive morning sickness*, which may be a sign of multiple pregnancy or even an abnormal pregnancy (molar pregnancy). An early scan will establish this.
- *Sudden disappearance of pregnancy symptoms* or unexplained production of milk in early pregnancy. This may be a sign that the pregnancy is no longer viable. A scan should establish whether this is the case.
- *In assisted conception (IVF)*. An early scan is important to confirm the viability, the number of implanted embryos and establish whether the pregnancy is ectopic (there is increased risk of this in some forms of assisted conception).

When is a *late* scan of benefit?

Some pregnancies, by their very nature, are regarded as high risk. Multiple (twins, triplets etc.) pregnancies come immediately to mind. Other pregnancies are apparently normal at twenty weeks but problems occur later in the course of the pregnancy. These will usually be detected through clinical monitoring of the progress of the pregnancy. In some cases, the midwife or doctor may notice that the growth is lagging behind or is excessive.

Also, it may be noted that there is too much or too little fluid around the baby. In other cases, the mother may be concerned by the rate of activity of the fetus (usually too little). All these and several other factors may be indications for performing a scan in the later phase of pregnancy. In some cases, usually when there is concern at the rate of growth of the fetus, serial scans may be performed to closely and accurately monitor the progress. (*See* chapter 4, "Ultrasound".)

Different types of scan

How does an abdominal scan differ from a vaginal scan?

A vaginal scan will normally be performed in early pregnancy. This is because it gives quite significantly better views of the womb and its content at this early stage, compared to the abdominal scan. Consequently, the information obtained is better and more detailed.

After about ten weeks, the abdominal route may be just as good, for most mothers. For mothers who are very obese, a vaginal route may continue to be ideal for several weeks more. In late pregnancy, a vaginal route may be used only occasionally, especially when there is difficulty in establishing how close the placenta is to the cervix. Again, this may occur in women who are overweight, where views through the abdominal route are not as good.

Is the vaginal scan safe?

Like the abdominal scan, the vaginal scan has not been shown to have any adverse effect on either the mother or baby. Remember that sound waves are used in this technology. There is no radiation.

Accuracy of scans

How accurate is the scan at estimating the gestation?

In the first trimester (the first fourteen weeks), ultrasound scan is very accurate, with a margin of error of only about three or four days either way. The accuracy reduces as the pregnancy advances and may be out by as much as one week at eighteen to twenty weeks.

For a scan performed around twenty weeks, if the discrepancy between the mother's dates and the scan is less than ten days, the mother's date is usually given the benefit of the doubt. If it is more than ten days, she will be advised that the estimation from her date is very likely wrong and therefore the expected date of delivery is revised, using the scan estimate as the basis. It is usually a point of contention because dates are, in most cases, reviewed backwards, putting the expected date of delivery further ahead. Nobody wants to carry a pregnancy for a day longer, if this can be helped! However, this may be crucial, for reasons discussed earlier.

Can a twenty-weeks scan predict the eventual weight of the baby at birth?

No. It is impossible at twenty weeks to predict whether there will be restricted or excessive growth. If the fetus is found to be abnormally small at this gestation, and if there is no reason to doubt the accuracy of the gestation, this signifies a more profound problem and not simple growth restriction. Such a finding calls for further tests. If the fetus appears larger than it should be at twenty weeks, as a rule, it means the gestation is wrong. It does not mean the fetus is growing into a big baby.

Occasionally there is a big discrepancy between the gestation as estimated by abdominal examination and that estimated by ultrasound scan. Which one should be trusted?

This problem is uncommon but by no means rare. In such a case, the scan is the one which should be taken to be accurate. This is because the scan measures the fetus itself, while abdominal examination depends on the size of the womb (fundal height). The latter may be influenced by several unrelated factors such as a full bladder, pelvic tumour or maternal obesity.

Scan accuracy holds true only in the first half of the pregnancy. This is why it is essential to establish the accurate date in this phase of the pregnancy. Both the scan and abdominal examination could be grossly inaccurate and wildly off the mark in late pregnancy.

For late-bookers, there are occasions when it is actually impossible to accurately date a pregnancy.

How much of the scan findings at an ultrasound scan are documented?

Normally the person performing the scan will produce a report that highlights all the significant findings. Whenever it is seen fit, still pictures may be taken for future reference. Rarely, a video recording is made, sometimes to allow for consultation with colleagues who may not be immediately available during the test but also for training purposes. A verbal consent is usually obtained from the mother for this. Some fringe "rights" groups, especially in the USA, have called for all scans to be similarly documented for possible "future evidence". This is a classic case of defensive medicine gone mad. It is not only financially nightmarish for the unit (in the UK, read "taxpayer"), it is probably rarely useful.

Comfort of the scan

How comfortable is the test?

Probably the only discomfort encountered by the mother is the full bladder that she is asked to maintain for the test in early pregnancy. A full bladder is really important because it facilitates the lifting of the womb out of the pelvis into the abdominal cavity. This allows for optimal scanning. If the bladder is empty, scanning is possible but may be incomplete, because some parts of the fetus may be deep in the pelvis and it may not be possible to see them properly or take measurements. Also, a full bladder facilitates good scan views that are helped by the water in the bladder directly overlying the uterus.

A full bladder is not required for a vaginal scan; the mother will be asked to empty her bladder *before* the procedure.

The expectant mother at a routine eighteen to twenty weeks scan should be assured that she will lie on a comfortable couch or bed, well propped up to see the screen, and she won't have to take her clothes off. The test lasts twenty to thirty minutes only, unless there is an unforeseen problem.

Findings of the scan

What exactly will the examiner be looking for during scanning?

In summary, the number of fetuses will be confirmed, the viability of the fetus, anatomy of the fetus, placental anatomy and its location, fluid volume, the size of the fetus and a specific search for particular abnormalities.

The report for every scan will mention the presence or absence of gross abnormalities, adequacy (or otherwise) of fluid volume, the placenta (location and any abnormality) and the size of the fetus. The opportunity is used to assess the other pelvic structures, especially the ovaries. Any significant finding will be documented.

How is gestation determined on the scan?

This is by taking various measurements of the head, body (abdomen), thigh-bone (femur) and occasionally (only when necessary), the size of part of the brain (cerebellum) or even the length of the foot.

Can a twin be missed at a twenty-weeks scan?

This is virtually impossible. If a mother is told she is carrying one baby at twenty weeks, she should expect no surprises later on. Likewise, if the count is two at this stage, there is no chance it is going to mysteriously be three later on.

How often is a major fetal abnormality discovered at a twenty-weeks scan?

In about 2–3 per cent of cases. Most would not require any intervention. Sadly a few are incompatible with life. The latter scenario – which is mercifully rare – sets into motion a course of information, counselling and, in most cases, pregnancy termination. Occasionally the suspected diagnosis will require a confirmatory test, involving amniocentesis (the sampling of the amniotic fluid) or taking a placental or blood sample. This will entail an inevitable delay of some days before the results are obtained to allow for decision on the definitive action.

There have been cases where, even in the presence of incontrovertible evidence as to the hopelessness of the situation, mothers have refused to have their pregnancies terminated. Full support in the antenatal care is still given in such cases, and appropriate counselling is given regarding the expected delivery of a baby that will not live.

What kind of abnormalities will inevitably lead to recommendation of pregnancy termination?

Conditions which are incompatible with life outside the womb, such as absence of the brain or kidneys.

There are several other rarer conditions. Other conditions such as Edward's syndrome (a chromosomal disorder) may be suspected but will require a confirmatory test. In a confirmed case of Edward's syndrome, termination will be advised because such babies survive for days or at most, a few weeks only.

What conditions which are serious but not necessarily lethal could be missed at twenty weeks?

Occasionally, a diaphragmatic hernia affecting the fetus may be missed. Conditions such as fetal ovarian cysts may not have developed at this stage and will therefore be missed by default. These conditions are rare.

Can a twenty-week scan fail to establish the sex of the fetus?

Most definitely yes. Sometimes the fetal position does not allow for clear visualization of the fetal genitalia. This means one cannot say with certainty what sex the fetus is. This is, however, uncommon.

Is every unexplained abnormal finding ominous?

Certainly not. Commonly, shadows that are unexplained are clearly seen, especially in the abdomen. The baby is usually born healthy with no problems whatsoever. The assumption is that this may result from a self-limited viral infection. In the absence of any compelling reasons, such findings only call for observation of the progress of the pregnancy and nothing invasive.

Can spina bifida be missed at twenty weeks of gestation?

This is extremely unlikely. If for any reason the spine is not clearly seen at this stage, a repeat scan will be recommended, usually within four weeks. The resolution is of such high quality that a report of a normal spine means exactly that. *See* Chapter 18, "Spina bifida and related problems".

Can one tell what colour the baby's hair is likely to be?

No. At this gestation, no hair or even nails can be seen; the image is only in grey-scale, giving the picture in black and white.

In case of previous loss of pregnancies through stillbirth, should the mother expect blood-flow to be measured at this stage?

Measuring blood-flow (usually using Doppler ultrasound) has no useful purpose at this stage of pregnancy, and absence of this test should be no cause for panic.

If the placenta is reported to be low at twenty weeks, should a repeat scan be offered; and, if so, at what gestation?

There is really no need to repeat a scan for this indication only. Exceptions will be made in special situations. These will include:

- where the placenta is actually overlying the cervix, so the risk of placenta praevia later in pregnancy is probably significant
- history of previous placenta praevia, as the expectant mother will be understandably anxious and because of the tendency of this condition to occasionally recur.

Repeat scans could also be considered in cases of multiple pregnancy (twins, triplets etc.), smoking and drug abuse and previous caesarean section. Even here, the usefulness is debatable. The most important thing to remember is that, for the vast majority of women reported to have a low-lying placenta at twenty weeks, this finding is of no consequence, as the placenta will be in a normal position within weeks. If a repeat is to be done, most units perform this at about thirty-two to thirty-four weeks, unless there are clinical indications to do it earlier. Vaginal bleeding is normally the indication for an unscheduled repeat scan.

Drawbacks of scanning

Are there any drawbacks from routine scans at twenty weeks?

Unfortunately, yes. As mentioned earlier, sometimes there are findings that are clearly abnormal but whose significance cannot be established until delivery. Such findings include abnormal abdominal shadows; cysts in the brain; "low-lying" placenta; and increased or reduced fluid volume. Such findings quite understandably cause anxiety, not least because the causes remain unexplained.

Such mothers should draw comfort from the fact most of them will have perfectly normal babies at the end of the day. Unfortunately, there has to be closer monitoring of the pregnancy, in an effort to identify those pregnancies which might require specific action or intervention.

The final word?

Most mothers will have a perfectly normal scan with normal findings all round. A few will have some great surprises, such as unexpected twins; fewer still will have devastating findings such as a non-viable pregnancy or a fetus that has a condition incompatible with life. One in fifty will find that their baby has a gross abnormality that may require surgical correction soon (or later) after birth.

The puritan will point to the fact that we have to scan ten women to detect anything useful in one. This is ignoring the fact that the other nine will have got to see and know their baby for the first time – not a fact to be sniffed at.

6. Exposure to infection during pregnancy

Introduction

There are a good number of viruses which infect children and adults alike. To the majority of these, the body's immune system responds promptly and the infection is literally shrugged off in a matter of days. In a number of instances, the individual may be unaware that he or she has been suffering from an infection. Some types of viral infections have specific signs and symptoms and are easily identifiable. These include such infections as measles and chicken-pox.

The differences in the behaviour and course of viral infections do not end there. Significantly, some infections render the individual immune to them for the remainder of his or her life, including infections such as Rubella. Other viral infections may stay there for life, with occasional or sometimes frequent flare-ups; a typical example is genital herpes. Yet others may cause a chronic condition, which may be progressive and even fatal in the long-term; HIV infection is a case in point.

Just to add to the complexity of the picture is another subset of viral infections where the outcome is not immediately predictable. An example is Hepatitis B. If one is infected with Hepatitis B, rapidly progressive liver disease may ensue or the individual may develop a chronic condition with a capacity of passing on the disease to others, while remaining outwardly healthy for many years. Conversely, the infection may be completely cleared from the body by the immune system, leaving the individual immune for life. All these examples show how varied viral infections are and why doctors cannot possibly give standard advice to cover all of them.

While most viral infections are relatively inconsequential in non-pregnant individuals, pregnancy is a unique condition because of the developing fetus. The fetus is vulnerable and the vulnerability differs according to the stage of gestation. An infection such as Rubella, relatively innocuous at other times, could have devastating effects when contracted in the first few weeks of pregnancy. Chicken-pox, which might be shrugged off if contracted at twenty weeks, might cause very serious problems if it bursts on the scene at term on the eve of labour.

All these are extensively explored and explained in detail in this chapter. It is important for the reader not to lose sight of the fact that complications of pregnancy due to infection are uncommon. However, if it occurs, it is important to know what that might mean and what needs to be done. On the bacterial front, the relatively common and relevant areas of interest such as urinary tract infection, sexually transmitted diseases and ascending infection (infection affecting the "waters") are discussed in detail.

Measles

If I am exposed to measles during pregnancy, what should I do?

Don't panic. That is the first thing. Most adults of child-bearing age will either have been vaccinated sometime in their childhood or would have had the infection. The immunity acquired from either is life-long and 95 per cent of all those who are vaccinated acquire this immunity.

This leaves only a small minority who may be susceptible during pregnancy. If you are unsure whether you have had the infection or been immunized, then you should contact your doctor promptly after exposure to have your status checked. If no records are available, then a simple blood test may establish whether you are immune or not.

If you are susceptible, an injection of a protective protein (immunoglobulin) may be administered to give you passive immunity. The protection from this is not total, but even if you go on to get the infection, it will be attenuated and therefore mild.

What if I am exposed to measles without being aware of it, only to discover that I have got the infection?

Again, this is a rare occurrence, for the reasons explained above. However, when this happens, the infection can be serious, needing hospital admission and isolated nursing. Measles pneumonia, which may be complicated by secondary bacterial pneumonia, is the most likely problem. The potential complication of measles infection in pregnancy is that it could provoke labour and lead to premature delivery. If this happens, attempts may be made to suppress the contractions, provided the mother is not too ill and there are no features of fetal distress. These efforts are not always successful.

If I know I am not immune to measles, can I be vaccinated during pregnancy?

No. Vaccination for measles employs a live virus and no such vaccination can be given during pregnancy.

If I was vaccinated for measles during pregnancy, before I discovered that I was pregnant, what should I do?

Most doctors will check your menstrual history before vaccinating a woman against measles. Some will go so far as to perform a pregnancy test, to avoid any mishap. However, cases of vaccination during pregnancy have been frequently reported. No adverse effect to the babies have been observed and therefore, even in such an accident, there is really no question of recommending termination of pregnancy.

Rubella (German measles)

If I am exposed to Rubella (German measles) in pregnancy, what should I do?

Most mothers born after the mid-1960s will have been immunized and over 90 per cent of these will have acquired long-term immunity. A fair proportion of the rest will have had the infection and acquired immunity that way.

If you are unsure whether you are immune or not, you should see your doctor promptly to have a blood test to establish your immune status.

If I am immune to Rubella, can my baby be affected by my exposure to the infection during pregnancy?

No. You are immune, so you cannot acquire the infection and therefore cannot pass it on to the fetus.

If I am found not to be immune, is there anything that can be done to help the fetus?

If you acquire the infection during pregnancy, there is nothing that can be done to influence what happens to the baby. Since most Rubella infections are unrevealed, if you have been exposed, blood tests will be required to confirm whether the infection has indeed been passed on to you.

What are the effects on the fetus?

Rubella causes what is called *"Congenital Rubella Syndrome"*. The earlier in pregnancy the infection is acquired, the more severe the features of the syndrome. They may include some or all of the following:

- jaundice
- enlargement of the spleen
- cataracts
- deafness
- heart disease
- a small head, accompanied with mental retardation
- thyroid dysfunction.

The syndrome could be so severe as to make the quality of life of the child questionable. Most (*over 70 per cent* of) babies will be affected, to varying degrees, if the mother acquires the infection in the first twelve weeks of pregnancy.

As there appears to be a window for a few babies to escape infection, is there any test that can identify babies that have been affected and those who have escaped?

Yes, but unfortunately this can only be done *and is only reliable* after twenty weeks of gestation. A cord blood sample is taken and analysed to establish whether the infection was passed to the fetus. This procedure does carry a small but significant risk of killing the fetus or provoking a miscarriage.

What are the options for the mother who has been exposed to Rubella in the early part of the pregnancy?

It is important to confirm (by doing the appropriate test) whether what she has been exposed to is indeed Rubella. This is because a few other infections do have symptoms similar to Rubella. If it is established that she was exposed to Rubella and that she has acquired the infection, the mother is faced with the difficult decision of terminating the pregnancy or taking chances with it. Unfortunately, most babies exposed at this stage of pregnancy will be affected.

Suppose the exposure is late in pregnancy?

The proportion of babies affected if exposure is in late pregnancy is reduced and so is the severity. None the less, infection should be confirmed, using a blood test. The obstetrician should then discuss with the mother whether she wants to have an invasive test to check whether the baby has been affected as well. Many probably wait to have this done after delivery. If infection of the baby is confirmed, monitoring of the growth and general health of the child are all that is required.

Some features of congenital rubella syndrome appear late. These may include:

- thyroid dysfunction
- diabetes
- abnormally early puberty (precocious puberty).

What is the advice if rubella vaccination is inadvertently given during pregnancy?

Nothing really needs to be done. There has been no recorded adverse effect as a result of vaccination in pregnancy. However, no deliberate vaccination should be carried out in pregnancy.

Is there anything else that can be done to reduce the effect of rubella infection during pregnancy?

Nothing really. Even though there is an immunoglobulin preparation to confer passive immunity to exposed individuals, this is *not* recommended for administration in pregnancy. This is because it is known *not* to prevent fetal infection and there is no evidence that it could reduce the severity of the effects of the infection to the fetus.

Chicken-pox and shingles

What should I do if I am exposed to chicken-pox during pregnancy?

You need to have your immunity checked. You will probably know whether you have had chicken-pox earlier in life. If that is the case, then you are in the clear. Ninety per cent of all women of child-bearing age are immune, by virtue of previous infection, and therefore exposure during pregnancy poses no risk to their babies. This of course leaves one in ten who are susceptible.

If, on checking immunity, one is found to be susceptible, what then?

The potential effects on the fetus depend on the gestation.

The known effects to the baby will occur in about 10 per cent of babies if the infection is in the first twelve weeks of gestation. The potential damage is less if the infection occurs later. The exception to this is if the baby is born within the period when the infection is still active.

What effects do infected fetuses suffer from?

It could be a few or more of these:
- large patches of skin scarring
- small head
- eye complications, including cataracts and scarring inside the eye
- paralysis of limbs
- deformed, even absent fingers and/or toes
- convulsions.

It is important to remember that only a small proportion of babies whose mothers acquired the infection in pregnancy will be affected. It is also true that the later the infection in pregnancy, the milder the fetal effect. In some cases, babies are found to have no identifiable effect and may only suffer shingles later on in infancy or early childhood.

Why is delivery during active chicken-pox infection uniquely significant?

Babies born in such a situation are susceptible to develop a severe and generalized infection in less than a week post-delivery.

Up to a third of babies are affected. This is because the baby has not had time to acquire protective antibodies normally passed to him or her from the mother across the placenta.

To try to prevent or at least moderate the effects, paediatric specialists will evaluate the situation and will put in place management measures, which may include a combination of vaccination, passive immunization and antiviral medication.

Is there anything that can be done if a pregnant woman develops chicken-pox in pregnancy?

If the infection has already developed, nothing can be done.

What if on doing the blood tests, a person who has been exposed is found to have no immunity against chicken-pox?

The incubation period of chicken-pox is ten to twenty days. If the investigations to establish the immune status are carried out promptly, there is enough time to intervene before the manifestation of the infection. Passive immunity in the form of injection might be considered. This is meant to moderate the effects of the infection in the mother (and therefore the baby). It rarely prevents it altogether.

There is really no consensus on the necessity of this and some experts argue that if the infection exposure is beyond the first twelve to fourteen weeks of gestation, the risk to the baby is very small and passive immunity is unnecessary. An exception to this is those mothers who, for some reason, have low immunity in general.

What is the relationship between chicken-pox and shingles?

Shingles can be described as a later manifestation of chicken-pox. The two are really one and the same thing.

The virus that causes chicken-pox usually stays in the body life-long. This means that even though the individual has life-long immunity against chicken-pox, he or she is still susceptible to developing shingles, which is in fact a reactivation of the same virus. Shingles is usually provoked by a fall in general body immunity.

Shingles is also known by the name *herpes zoster* or simply as "zoster". This is because the virus which causes chicken-pox and shingles is called *Varicella zoster*, which belongs to the herpes family.

What are the consequences of developing shingles in pregnancy?

The fetus is *not* at risk. Any mother who develops shingles in pregnancy would have had chicken-pox in the past. This means she is carrying protective antibodies in her circulation, and these are continually passed to the growing fetus, which is thus protected.

Is there any medication that can be used in the event of chicken-pox or shingles in pregnancy?

Normally only symptomatic relief is aimed for in chicken-pox, because this is a self-limiting condition. However, if there is any hint of an abnormally severe disease – such as lung involvement – antiviral medication can be used. The standard drug acyclovir has been used in thousands of cases all over the world without any report of untoward effect to mother or baby. However, its absolute safety cannot be guaranteed and it should only be used where the benefits outweigh potential untoward effects.

Can chicken-pox infection cause miscarriage or preterm labour?

Yes. This is uncommon but, if severe, this infection can provoke uterine activity, which may subsequently end in miscarriage or preterm labour, depending on the gestation.

Herpes

What should a mother do if genital herpes infection occurs for the first time during pregnancy?

It is important to keep a close eye on the infection. There is no specific treatment for herpes and treatment to reduce the severity of the symptoms is all that is normally given. If there is evidence of the infection involving other organs, then the antiviral medication acyclovir may have to be administered, to moderate the course of the disease.

What if there is a recurrence of genital herpes in pregnancy?

Herpes infection will remain for life. If herpetic genital lesions reappear during pregnancy, it is just a repeat manifestation of the old infection and no specific measures are called for. Only symptomatic treatment will be required.

Can genital herpes causes miscarriage or preterm labour?

Yes. If it is a primary infection, and if it affects the rest of the body, it could provoke uterine activity. This may lead to miscarriage or preterm delivery. Attempts will be made to prevent preterm delivery if uterine activity is noted, as long as there are no contraindications to this.

Does the fact that a pregnant woman has genital herpes influence the method of delivery?

Only if there active lesions at the time.

If there are no active lesions when she goes into labour, then the aim will be for a vaginal delivery – unless this is not possible for some other reason.

If there are active lesions, then delivery is made by caesarean section, the aim being to protect the baby.

Hepatitis

How can a mother know if she has been exposed to Hepatitis B?

It is very difficult, unless there is a specific risk factor. Known risk factors include injecting drugs (with sharing of needles) and unprotected sexual encounters with multiple partners.

Blood transfusion is no longer regarded as a risk factor, because all blood and blood products are screened for viral infections, including Hepatitis.

Because it is now recognized that dependency on known risk factors is really not an efficient way of identifying mothers carrying this infection, in the UK, every expectant mother will be offered the test. Those identified to be carrying the infection can then have protective injections given to their babies at birth. This service should be available nationwide by spring of the year 2000.

What are the symptoms of Hepatitis B?

This is where the difficulty arises. For the majority of patients, it appears like mild flu and they may have no symptoms at all. There may be a little nausea and vomiting, occasionally with abdominal pain – just under the right ribcage, where the liver is situated.

Surely a person with Hepatitis B infection will have jaundice?

Not really. Probably up to half of patients with the acute infection will have no jaundice at all. Even those who have jaundice may have mild symptoms that can easily be missed. This is compounded by the fact that the symptoms are non-specific.

So once one is infected with Hepatitis B, it is there for life?

No. Nine out of ten people infected with Hepatitis B will be clear of the infection within a few months. What they are left with is immunity against it for life. The remaining 10 per cent, however, carry the infection for life and could pass it on to others, including a baby in the womb.

So, if a pregnant woman acquires Hepatitis B infection or is a carrier before conception, the baby is at risk?

Yes. In fact babies, do not do nearly as well from the infection (compared to adults) and the majority of those who have the infection passed on by their mothers go on to develop chronic hepatitis. This may lead to chronic liver failure or even cancer of the liver.

Can Hepatitis B infection lead to miscarriage or stillbirth?

There is no evidence that Hepatitis B leads to miscarriage, preterm labour or even stillbirth. The devastating effects are to the newborn. If miscarriage, preterm labour or stillbirth happens to a Hepatitis B carrier mother, hepatitis is unlikely to be the cause. Very rarely, if infection is acquired during pregnancy and if symptoms are severe, uterine activity may be provoked.

So how can the baby of a mother with Hepatitis B be protected?

Soon after birth, the baby is given an injection of HBIG. This is a protein that confers passive but temporary protection. To be effective it should be given within twelve hours of birth. This is combined or followed soon after with vaccination against Hepatitis B (this may be given the same day, but not on the same site). The vaccination will be repeated one or two more times in the next few months. Of course, the parents would have been thoroughly counselled about all this in the time leading to delivery, once the Hepatitis B carrier status has been established.

Do these measures protect all newborns?

No, but up to 90 per cent will be protected. It is assumed that the small proportion who do not benefit from the vaccination are those who acquired the infection from the mother long before delivery and it had plenty of time to establish itself.

Since there is a small risk of vaccination at birth not being effective, can this not be given to the mother during pregnancy, to cover this prospect?

No. It will not be effective at all.

We have discussed Hepatitis B; what about Hepatitis A and its risk to the unborn child?

Hepatitis A is not transmitted through body fluids but through eating contaminated foodstuffs. Infection acquired by the mother during pregnancy poses no risks to the baby and cannot be passed on to her or him. As in all such cases, if symptoms are severe, they may lead to uterine activity and threatened preterm labour, but the infection itself poses no direct risk. The infection is always self-limiting and there is no chronic carrier status.

HIV

If an expectant mother suspects that she has been exposed to the HIV virus, what should she do?

It is important that her doctor is informed at once, and she will be given thorough counselling. This will normally lead to an offer for a test to check whether the infection has been passed on to her.

What is the importance of screening for the HIV infection?

Apart from the obvious longer-term benefit of the mother knowing whether she has the infection or not, there is the immediate issue of the newborn baby. Some mothers, on learning that they are HIV positive, opt for termination of pregnancy. Those who opt to continue will need to explore the options available.

What are the options available to an HIV positive expectant mother who wishes to carry on with the pregnancy?

The mother will carry on with normal antenatal care until delivery. Or she may be put on medication which has been shown to significantly reduce the chances of the baby acquiring the infection from the mother. For obvious reasons, the short- and long-term effects of these drugs to the baby are not fully understood, even though so far children exposed to them in the womb have shown no ill effects. There is a lot of research going on in this area and new management strategies are being developed all the time.

What percentage of babies acquire the infection from their mothers?

Figures differ from different centres but roughly a third of all babies will be infected when they are born. Antiviral medication is estimated to cut this risk by almost two-thirds.

Does HIV infection lead to miscarriage or stillbirth?

There is no evidence that HIV infection could lead to either of these directly. If the infection was acquired a few years back, it may have advanced to full-blown AIDS which is, of course, characterized by recurrent infections, some of which may lead to miscarriage or preterm labour.

Can caesarean section reduce the rate of transmission of the virus from the mother to the baby?

There is no evidence that caesarean delivery confers any such advantage and HIV infection is not an indication for caesarean section.

What is the effect of pregnancy on the disease itself?

A number of early studies did suggest that pregnancy may accelerate the progression of the disease to full-blown AIDS. Better-controlled subsequent studies have failed to support this claim.

What is the advice regarding breast-feeding?

In developed countries, the advice is to avoid breast-feeding. This is because there is a small but real risk of transmitting the virus to the baby via breast-milk. In the presence of good substitutes, the risk is not considered worth taking.

Toxoplasmosis

What is toxoplasmosis?

This is an infection caused by a parasite called toxoplasma. It is not a virus and transmission is through eating contaminated food – especially meat products.

Who is at risk of acquiring toxoplasmosis?

Everybody; but some people are at more risk than others. Eggs of toxoplasma are found in cat faeces and therefore cat keepers and those whose food is exposed to contamination by cat faeces will be at increased risk.

Likewise, eating undercooked (or raw!) meat may also lead to infection, as a small percentage of lamb, pork and beef samples are found to contain the cysts. These can be found in milk and eggs as well. All are destroyed by cooking. In theory, blood transfusion is also a risk factor; but in practice, this is exceedingly unlikely as a source, since all blood and blood products are screened.

How can a mother know or suspect if she has the infection?

It is very difficult. Most people will have no symptoms at all. A few may have a mild flu-like illness, usually ignored. This may be accompanied by slight swelling of the lymph glands in the neck. All these clear up by themselves without treatment in days or weeks. The exception to this pattern is in patients with low immunity, e.g. following transplants, or those with AIDS, where the infection may be quite dramatic, even fatal.

Anything between 25 to 50 per cent of women of child-bearing age have evidence of having had the infection in the past.

What are the consequences of acquiring toxoplasmosis during pregnancy?

If the infection is acquired for the first time in pregnancy (primary infection), the risk of transmission to the fetus depends on the stage of pregnancy. This risk is higher, the more advanced the pregnancy is. It is roughly estimated to be about 17 per cent in the first twelve weeks of pregnancy, rising to over 60 per cent in the last twelve weeks. Of all the babies who acquire the infection in the womb, about a third will have a variable degree of damage. The remainder will be completely normal.

What kind of damage do toxoplasma-infected infants have?

There could be combination of features including damage to the eyes (chorioretinitis), a small or big fluid-filled head and/or brain damage. As mentioned before, the clinical picture tends to be variable, ranging from mild and almost unrecognizable, to very severe, bordering on incompatibility with life.

Other features may include enlargement of the liver and spleen, jaundice and seizures. Later on, the child may be found to be deaf and mentally retarded.

Even though incidence of infection to the fetus is highest in the later phase of pregnancy, the fetus infected in the earlier phase has the highest risk of severe damage.

Can toxoplasmosis lead to miscarriage or stillbirth?

Yes. Again, infection in the earlier phase of pregnancy increases a risk of such an outcome. It is less likely, the more advanced the pregnancy is.

Since not every fetus is affected by the infection, what is the advice to an expectant mother confirmed to have the infection?

The risk to the fetus will be assessed, normally using ultrasound. If features suggestive of congenital infection are there, advice may be given to perform a fetal blood sampling, which will confirm or exclude the diagnosis in most (not all) cases. Since the extent of damage and resultant disability is difficult to quantify before delivery, it is normally up to the parents to decide whether to proceed with the pregnancy or not. Unfortunately, termination is never an easy option after the tests, because they can only be carried out rather late in pregnancy, certainly not before twenty weeks of gestation.

Is there any treatment if the fetus is infected and parents want to continue with the pregnancy?

Yes. There are a few treatment options that may be used by any mother with primary infection, even in the absence of documented fetal infection. This is because, in theory, the treatment may reduce the risk of fetal infection or at least moderate it. The doctor should fully explain the potential side-effects of the chosen drug and how long it needs to be used to confer the required benefit.

One of the options, spiramycin, is claimed to reduce the risk of fetal infection by half. The other, which is a combination of pyrimethamine and a sulphonamide, is similarly – if not more – protective.

Does secondary infection to the mother pose a similar amount of risk?

No. Secondary infection is probably an inappropriate term. Some people with toxoplasmosis have unusual manifestations, such as eye lesions. In such cases, the eye lesions may flare up months or years after the primary infection. There is no evidence that specific action is required, as far as the pregnancy is concerned.

For somebody with primary infection, are there any special measures regarding delivery?

Not normally. Of course, the method of delivery will depend on all the usual obstetric variables. If the fetus is affected and one of the features is an abnormally large head (*hydrocephalus*), a caesarean section may be opted for, as long as the baby is viable.

Paediatricians will be on hand at delivery to give the required immediate treatment, if any.

Will infection in one pregnancy have any bearing on further pregnancies?

No. Fetuses in subsequent pregnancies will not be affected.

Surely all this risk calls for universal screening for toxoplasmosis in earlier pregnancy?

As mentioned before, different population groups have varying degrees of risk, depending on life-style. Moreover, there is evidence that 25 to 50 per cent will have had the infection in the past and are therefore not at risk. Some countries, such as France, offer the screen test to all mothers, because the prevalence of the disease there is relatively high. Most other countries do not and instead target those expectant mothers at risk. These will include those keeping cats and those whose occupations involve frequent handling of raw meat or cat litter.

What is the general advice against toxoplasmosis?

- Avoid eating raw meat and eggs
- Ensure meat is properly cooked, or at least frozen to minus 20°C prior to cooking, if it is to be done rare.
- Use milk which has been pasteurized.
- Avoid cat litter or, if this is not possible, ensure protective gloves are used each time.
- Use gloves when gardening.
- Wash vegetables thoroughly before consumption

7. Asthma and cystic fibrosis in pregnancy

Introduction

A prospective mother with asthma, which is a chronic condition characterized by breathlessness and attacks of wheezing, will inevitably worry about the effect of the condition on the pregnancy and vice versa. This is particularly so in the first pregnancy. The questions and answers here are bound to clarify the situation for most asthma sufferers. The bottom line remains good control of the condition, which in turn hinges on taking medication and other prevention and treatment measures.

There are usually no additional or special measures required during pregnancy and exceptions to this general rule are few.

Labour is a time that may conceivably require special measures, both in ensuring certain ideal conditions and avoiding administration of certain types of medication commonly given to other delivering mothers. All these are clearly explained here.

Cystic fibrosis is another chronic condition, charaterized by a tendency to chronic lung infections; pregnancy may pose special problems, which may be formidable and difficult to deal with. As it is a genetic disease, passed from parents to children, anxiety about this aspect is inevitable.

Not every young woman with cystic fibrosis can safely carry a pregnancy. Questions surrounding all these problems are answered in this chapter.

Asthma

If an asthmatic is planning to become pregnant, what is she advised to do?

Neither asthma nor the attack-preventing medication in common use has any direct adverse effect on the pregnancy or the baby. The advice is to optimize treatment to ensure good control of asthma before trying to conceive.

What are the drugs used to prevent asthma attacks?

Commonly used is an inhalant steroid called beclomethasone, usually prescribed under the trade name Becotide. This is certainly safe for use in pregnancy and there is only minimal absorption from the airway.

Other steroids used similarly include budesonide and fluticasone, prescribed under the popular trade names Pulmicort and Flixotide. These steroids are also known to be safe.

Are there any other preventative drugs for asthma attacks?

Sodium cromoglycate, popularly known as Intal, is used to prevent attacks. It is safe to use in pregnancy.

Also used for preventing attacks is ipratropium (Atrovent). It has no known adverse effect on the pregnancy or the fetus.

Drugs such as salmeterol (Serevent) have been in use only in the last few years and even though there has been no report or any indication of any ill-effect on pregnancy, the data is considered to be insufficient to advise on their safety.

What happens to asthma itself during pregnancy?

It does *not* get worse and, in some cases, the attacks may lessen or be less severe. However, this is by no means standard and the active advice is to optimize prevention of attacks and treatment.

For anybody who has been on regular medication to prevent attacks, stopping this during pregnancy is a mistake.

What role is there for other steroids, such as prednisolone or hydrocortisone, which are taken orally for asthma?

They do have a role in some cases of asthma in pregnancy as maintenance therapy. Regarding safety, if prescribed, they should be used. In fact, in normal dosage, these steroids do not cross the placenta and therefore do not reach the fetus. In very high doses, minimal amounts may cross the placenta, but there is no undue adverse effect on the fetus.

What about the safety of medicines such as salbutamol (*Ventolin*, *Volmax*) used to treat attacks?

Salbutamol is safe to use in pregnancy. So are the other related preparations such as terbutaline (Bricanyl).

If somebody has been using theophylline to treat attacks of asthma, is there any need to switch to anything else if she becomes pregnant?

No. Theophylline and the related drug aminophylline are known to be safe for use in pregnancy. In fact, they are the more widely used anti-asthma drugs in the United States. However, sometimes pregnancy may necessitate adjusting the dose upwards.

In all cases of an asthmatic pregnant woman, a specialist physician (for respiratory conditions) will be involved in her care.

Should an asthmatic expect to be delivered early?

Asthma is not in itself an indication to induce labour. If intervention becomes necessary, it will be for the usual obstetric reasons.

Are there any potential problems in labour for an asthmatic?

If labour is being induced, prostaglandins may be used, provided the doctor ensures it is not Prostaglandin F, which could provoke an asthmatic attack. Prostaglandin E, which is perfectly safe, is the type in widespread use for induction.

Labour itself has no direct bearing on asthma and oxytocin (Syntocinon) to augment labour may be used without fear. It is safe.

Ergometrine is a drug usually administered to facilitate delivery of the placenta and minimize bleeding after delivery. It will not be used in asthmatics; this is because it has the potential of provoking an attack. Oxytocin is normally an adequate substitute.

What about after delivery?

There is no increase in the risk of an attack following delivery but preventative treatment (if the woman has been on this) should be maintained. The usual advice regarding physical activity in this period applies equally to asthmatics as to any woman who has just given birth. *See* Chapter 27, "Sport and exercise in pregnancy".

What is the advice regarding breast-feeding?

An asthmatic who is on standard medication of any kind should not worry with regard to breast-feeding. This is perfectly safe.

Cystic fibrosis

What advice will be given to a cystic fibrosis patient who wants to conceive?

There is no standard advice. In short, she must be in a satisfactory physical shape without any serious complications of cystic fibrosis. The one important contraindication to pregnancy is if she has developed pulmonary hypertension, where the blood pressure in the arteries in the lungs is abnormally high. Pregnancy in such a situation could cause heart failure, which many necessitate terminating the pregnancy as a life-saving measure.

The physician looking after the woman will carefully assess the effect of the disease, including on her lungs, the gut, pancreas (risk of diabetes) and heart, before giving his or her "blessing" for the planned pregnancy.

What is the advice regarding the prospects of the offspring?

This is a difficult area. One consideration is the inevitably limited life-span of the mother. This should be looked at critically by the prospective parents.

The second issue is the possibility of the child being affected. The mother will definitely pass on the rogue gene. It may be important to check whether the partner carries the gene. About 5 per cent of the Caucasian population carry the gene, so the chances among them is relatively high. The rate among those of African or Oriental descent is much lower.

A test to check the status of her partner is available but it detects only about 70 per cent of the carriers, and therefore there is still a risk of a carrier being missed.

Can pregnancy worsen the condition of the patient?

This is possible. A careful eye will be kept on the pregnant woman through the course of the pregnancy.

Will physiotherapy and antibiotics continue to be necessary during pregnancy?

Yes, and more so. Penicillin or a form of cephalosporin commonly used to prevent infection are safe.

Also inhalational drugs to help dilate the lungs will almost certainly be required on a regular basis. All these are known to be safe.

Is the baby at any kind of risk?

By virtue of the respiratory and nutritional problems cystic fibrosis patients encounter, the risk of growth restriction in the womb is quite considerable. Sometimes it gets so bad that preterm delivery becomes inevitable. Other maternal complications such as respiratory or heart failure may also prompt preterm delivery.

Is induction of labour any different if the woman is a cystic fibrosis sufferer?

No. Prostaglandin E – which is the most popular induction agent – is safe to use in cystic fibrosis sufferers. Oxytocin (Syntocinon) is also used, when necessary, to augment labour.

What about pain relief in labour?

In cystic fibrosis, there is a slight worry about the effects of opiates such as morphine or pethidine, because of their depressive effect on respiration. Because of this, epidural analgesia is strongly encouraged among these patients.

This has additional advantages in the sense that it prevents unnecessary exertion in the late stages of labour, something a cystic fibrosis patient can ill-afford. In addition, if a caesarean section becomes necessary, this may be the only form of anaesthesia required, avoiding a general anaesthetic. An epidural is, by far, the most effective form of pain relief in labour.

Are there any additional measures required in labour?

Sometimes it may be necessary to give oxygen supplement to a cystic fibrosis sufferer in labour. Epidural analgesia reduces the requirement for this.

Are other methods of intervention used?

Yes. To avoid undue exertion in the second stage of labour, assistance in the form of forceps or ventouse is often advised for delivery.

What is the advice regarding breast-feeding?

As long as the mother's general health and nutritional status is satisfactory, breast-feeding, if desired, should be encouraged.

If the mother's nutritional status is poor and she is very weak, attempts at breast-feeding will be counterproductive for both mother and baby. Bottle-feeding will be better in such a case because it will have the additional benefit of allowing her more rest, where her partner or somebody else may feed the baby.

There is concern that breast-milk from cystic fibrosis sufferers may have an excess of some minerals. Is this true?

Not at all. In the past there was some concern that there might be an excess of sodium in these patients' breast-milk (as is the case with their sweat). Scientific analysis has disproved this.

8. *Anaemia*

Introduction

Anaemia – a condition where the concentration of the haemo-globin (which transports oxygen from the lungs to the tissues) in the blood is below normal – is one of the most common medical problems. In its milder form, many people go about their daily activities, unaware that there is anything amiss. In pregnancy, anaemia is likely to be discovered. Many women are surprised and some a little irritated when they are told that they are anaemic. They don't take too kindly to the seemingly overbearing attitude of the midwife or doctor who stresses that they need their iron tablets and that they are going to continue needing these for the remainder of the pregnancy. Such reactions are understandable and readily forgivable. These women are feeling well and are not keen on taking tablets for such a long period.

The truth is, anaemia is a potentially serious condition, and mothers-to-be should be aware of this. Pregnancy puts an added demand on the woman's resources and, if these are already precarious, there is a potential for things to go seriously wrong.

Contrary to popular belief, iron deficiency is not the only cause of anaemia: though it is, admittedly, the most common. Sometimes there is a combination of deficiencies where multiple supplements are required to correct the problem. This is usually associated with eating disorders. Some people end up being anaemic, not because of a poor diet but because they suffer from diseases that make it difficult for iron to be absorbed from the stomach. Then there are those people who have an iron overload in their bodies but are still anaemic and chronically so. The prime examples are people with sickle cell disease or thalassaemia. All the various conditions associated with anaemia are discussed below.

Finally, many people are aware of the fact that folic acid is good for reducing the risk of neural tube defects, such as spina bifida, when taken at the right time. Not so many know that folic acid is a significant player in the prevention of anaemia. It is not a substitute for iron; rather, these two "elements" play distinct but complementary roles in a lot of physiological functions, including prevention of anaemia.

Anaemia and its causes

What is anaemia?

Haemoglobin (Hb) is the oxygen-carrying component of red blood-cells. Its normal range is around 12–16 g/dl. In pregnancy, many experts agree that the normal range can and should be extended to be 11–16 g/dl. When the level of this component falls below 11 g/dl, that is anaemia.

The short form 'Hb' is almost universally used to describe haemoglobin. So, if you encounter a tired junior doctor and he blurts out that, "You have a low Hb," what the poor chap means is that you are anaemic.

The abbreviation "g/dl" that appears in front of the numbers is the form of measurement used for the haemoglobin level. It simply stands for grams per decilitre.

What causes anaemia in pregnancy?

The production of haemoglobin and that of red blood-cells (the latter by the bone marrow) is dependent upon the adequate supply of several "raw materials". The most important of these is iron.

Over 90 per cent of those found to have anaemia in pregnancy will have the problem because of iron deficiency.

What are the other possible causes of anaemia in pregnancy?

Vitamin B12 and/or folic acid deficiency could lead to anaemia. They are a relatively uncommon cause in pregnancy but, when evidence of iron deficiency is lacking, these possible causes will be investigated.

Are there any other causes?

There are conditions which are collectively called "haemoglobinopathies". Affected people tend to have chronic anaemia and pregnancy will tend to make this worse. The most common among these are sickle cell disease and thalassaemia. These conditions are discussed in detail in

Chapter 10, "Thalassaemia and sickle cell disease". Iron deficiency is hardly ever a cause of anaemia in these conditions. In fact, the tendency is to have iron overload. This is a direct result of multiple repeated transfusions, which are inevitable in most of these conditions. The transfusions will have started in childhood. These conditions are hereditary.

Why does pregnancy make a woman prone to anaemia?

The demand for iron goes up quite markedly in pregnancy. This is because there is an expansion of the blood volume to meet the new demands of pregnancy. The red cell mass may go up by as much as 25 per cent. In addition to this, the fetus also takes its share. The fetus is totally dependent on the mother for everything, including iron.

Iron-deficiency anaemia

What role does diet play in preventing iron-deficiency anaemia?

The requirements for iron that is absorbed from the diet roughly doubles in pregnancy. In fact, the more advanced the pregnancy gets, the higher the requirements for iron. If the diet has poor iron supplies, the iron stores in the body will be mobilized but will not be adequately replenished from the diet. Eventually, the stores run empty and the haemoglobin levels start to fall. Some people conceive while already mildly anaemic, with hardly any iron stores. Such mothers will quickly become anaemic relatively early on in pregnancy.

Without remedial action, the degree of anaemia continues to worsen with advancing pregnancy. The fetus will continue to extract all its required quantities from an already deficient mother and the Hb level gallops along downwards.

What sort of diet will be unfavourable for supplying dietary iron?

Vegetarians are at a particular disadvantage in this respect. This is simply because they don't get the so-called "heme" iron which is found in meat and other animal products only. "Heme" iron is much more easily absorbed and actually promotes absorption of non-heme iron as well from the gut. Vegans are therefore at a double disadvantage in this regard. They don't get to eat products with heme iron and the iron they get from plant products is not so efficiently absorbed.

Any special advice for vegetarians?

As far as preventing iron-deficiency anaemia is concerned, the advice to take oral iron supplements, even before there is detectable anaemia, is specially relevant for vegetarians.

What are the consequences of iron deficiency?

With the fall in haemoglobin (Hb) concentration, the capacity to carry oxygen is reduced. This is not the only problem, though.

Iron is crucial in the production of a variety of critical enzymes in the body. The production of these will be affected, too. As a result, various body systems may be affected. These may include the brain and nerves, muscles, the gut and the skin. There is reduced exercise tolerance and even the common chores that you may be used to doing without a second thought become increasingly hard to cope with. There is general and almost constant lethargy and fatigue.

Can iron deficiency affect the pregnancy directly?

Yes. There is fairly strong evidence that iron deficiency can lead to preterm labour.

What about the effect of iron deficiency on labour?

Iron deficiency has no direct effect on labour as such. However, a woman who is anaemic when going into labour will tolerate badly any blood loss, an inevitable occurrence at delivery. Normally, a mother can take blood loss of up to 1000 ml (one litre) in her stride. A markedly anaemic woman may find this to be a tall order and it could create a life-and-death crisis.

There is also evidence, though not very strong, that iron-deficient women are more prone to heavy bleeding at delivery (postpartum haemorrhage), the very complication they are ill-equipped to deal with.

Anaemia in pregnancy does also rob the affected women of options that, like everybody else, they might be interested in:

options like home delivery or, where available, maternity homes and cottage hospitals for delivery. These will no longer be options because of the potential risks, which such places cannot deal with.

Is the fetus affected in any way by iron-deficiency?

Yes. When maternal iron stores are depleted, the levels of iron in the fetus will also end up being lower than normal, for obvious reasons. It follows that these babies will be more prone to develop anaemia within the first year of life. Other collateral effects include the child's increased susceptibility to infections.

Is it possible to know the levels of iron *stores* in the body?

This is easily done by estimating the levels of a certain blood protein called *Ferritin*. This protein accurately reflects the long-term iron store levels.

Is the message, therefore, that every pregnant woman should take oral iron supplements?

Except for those women who have specific conditions that contraindicate use of iron supplements, everybody else will benefit from oral iron supplements in pregnancy, some more so than others. For those who embark on pregnancy with a good haemoglobin level and with good iron stores, the iron supplements may not give any clinically apparent benefit. They will, none the less, allow for maintenance of healthy iron stores, allowing for optimal production and function of various essential enzymes in all body systems. That state will also mean a continued general well-being. Such a woman can and will tolerate unduly heavy blood loss much better. She will also go into the postnatal period a healthier person, better placed to face the challenges of new motherhood.

For women who are total vegans and those who embark on pregnancy while already anaemic or with low iron stores, the taking of oral iron supplements is imperative.

But some people cannot tolerate oral iron!

For most, it is a question of getting the right brand. The doctor will strive to help the expectant mother to identify the right one for her. There are quite a few on the market and some women tolerate one brand and not others. Ultimately, they all deliver the same ingredient, iron. She should be encouraged to persevere because this is for her and her baby's own good. It is not simply a ritual.

Some women find it easier to tolerate liquid preparations.

When all these avenues fail, doctors have to assess the situation and decide whether the degree of deficiency and anaemia warrants giving iron in the form of injections.

Why is the "injections" option a near-last resort?

Even though this route replenishes iron stores more efficiently and usually more quickly, it is associated with potential problems and is therefore not a suitable first choice. Some people develop an allergic reaction to it (and therefore a test dose in hospital is an absolute prerequisite). Also, the injections have to be given deep in the muscle and are fairly painful. Moreover, there is a small risk of developing abscesses at the site of the injection. There is also the fact that each course will consist of many injections (at least ten) which have to be administered either daily or on alternate days. This is certainly not everybody's cup of tea and it is evident that the oral route is, in many respects, a great deal better.

Does a newly delivered mother need to continue taking iron?

The degree of need for this is dependent on a few factors:

If the mother was taking iron during pregnancy because she was found to be iron-deficient, then it is advisable that she continues to take iron for several weeks (six to eight) after delivery.

- If the blood loss at delivery was heavy, even if she was not particularly anaemic during pregnancy, the advice will be to start or continue taking iron, again, for several weeks at least.
- If she is breast-feeding, the need for iron supplements is increased.
- If she is a total vegetarian, where the diet may not supply adequate iron, supplements are strongly advised.

Every individual woman's needs should be assessed and advice given accordingly. As a general statement, haemoglobin levels will tend to rise in the days and weeks after delivery. However, this does not mean that the need for iron is diminished or eliminated.

Folic acid-deficiency anaemia

How common is folic acid-deficiency anaemia?
It is uncommon.

What is the natural source of folic acid?
Practically all foodstuffs contain folic acid. This includes grains (such as corn and rice) as well as vegetables. Unfortunately, folic acid is very susceptible to heat and is rapidly destroyed by cooking. Boiling vegetables for five minutes will destroy about 90 per cent of their folic acid content. A proper balance and preparation of food generally provides adequate folic acid, in normal circumstances.

What are the special circumstances in which folic acid supplements are necessary?
Women who suffer from conditions in which there is chronic destruction of red blood-cells need to take increased folic acid supplements. This is more so during pregnancy. Such conditions include sickle cell disease, thalassaemia and hereditary spherocytosis. Women with these conditions will almost always be aware of this well before they conceive, because these are chronic conditions that they live with from childhood.

The recommended daily dose of folic acid in such circumstances is 5 mg. A higher dose of 10 mg or thereabouts is occasionally recommended when the problem is particularly serious. This is uncommon. In any case, many of these women will be taking folic acid even before conception and it will be a matter of checking whether the dose needs to be adjusted.

Women who suffer from epilepsy and who are taking anti-convulsant medication are also strongly advised to take folic acid supplements preferably at a dose of 5 mg daily.

Multiple pregnancy is another indication for folic acid supplements, because of the increased demand and therefore an increased risk of deficiency.

The mother's possible anaemia apart, how will folic acid deficiency affect the fetus?

If the mother was folic acid deficient before conception, the risk of neural tube defects – especially spina bifida – is increased. There is irrefutable evidence that folic acid supplements taken in the period leading up to conception and in the days immediately after will reduce the risk of spina bifida quite considerably. It is particularly crucial for mothers who have had an affected baby in the past.

Other anomalies that have been associated with folic acid deficiency pre-conceptually include cleft lip ("hare-lip") and cleft palate.

Can the fetus become folic acid deficient as a result of maternal deficiency?

Not the fetus. Even when the mother is deficient of folic acid, the placenta will actively transport folic acid to the fetus to meet its needs. However, since the stores are likely to be tenuous, the newborn is at risk of developing anaemia as a result of folic acid deficiency within a few weeks of birth.

Can folic acid deficiency lead to preterm labour?

Folic acid deficiency has not been linked with preterm labour or delivery.

What is "megaloblastic" anaemia?

This is a descriptive term used for the type of anaemia brought about by folic acid deficiency. The term "megaloblastic" is purely descriptive. It reflects the fact that in this type of anaemia, the blood-cells are larger than normal ("mega").

It is also important to emphasize that folic acid deficiency is not the only cause of megaloblastic anaemia. Deficiency of vitamin B12 will also cause this.

Are there any particular precautionary measures required during labour if the mother is folic acid-deficient?

If a woman gets to term and into labour still having folic acid deficiency anaemia, this should be regarded as some kind of failure of management. It is such an easy problem to correct.

No specific measures are required or called for in a case of folic acid deficiency anaemia in labour. The usual precautions for anaemia (regardless of type) will, of course, be taken. These may include cross-matching blood to have it ready in case transfusion becomes necessary, especially post-delivery.

Does breast-feeding increase folic acid requirement?

Yes, to some degree. A breast-fed baby will be completely dependent on the milk for his or her folic acid requirements, among other things. It follows, therefore, that for a mother who was noted to be folic acid-deficient antenatally, supplements will be advisable. For the majority, however, this is not necessary as long as she is getting the right diet. Normal diet supplies more than adequate folic acid, even for a breast-feeding mother.

Vitamin B12-deficiency anaemia

How common is vitamin B12-deficiency anaemia in pregnancy?

Pretty rare. Of the three types of deficiency anaemias (iron, folic acid and vitamin B12), this is the least common by a long way.

Can vitamin B12 deficiency affect ability to conceive?

Yes. Uncorrected vitamin B12 deficiency will make it extremely difficult to conceive. It is a cause of reduced fertility, albeit a rare one.

What is the natural source of vitamin B12?

An average diet will supply more than adequate vitamin B12. Animal products are undoubtedly the best source of this vitamin. Strict vegetarians may therefore be at some disadvantage in this regard and supplements may be required. Many processed food manufacturers add vitamin supplements, which may include B12.

Are there any conditions that make one prone to vitamin B12 deficiency?

Pernicious anaemia is a condition with which it is difficult to absorb vitamin B12 from the gut. The vitamin contained in food simply goes through unabsorbed to end up in the faeces. This leads to vitamin B12 deficiency and anaemia, hence its name. This may not be relevant as far as pregnancy is concerned, because it is unusual for this condition to occur during the reproductive years.

Another condition, called *Tropical sprue*, does cause vitamin B12 deficiency and this can occur at any age. It can therefore cause vitamin B12 deficiency in pregnancy.

Remedial action for these conditions is simple and entails giving injectable vitamin B12. These conditions are rare.

Is it possible for anaemia in pregnancy to be due to a combination of causes?

This is not unusual. Since iron-deficiency anaemia is the most common, treatment of anaemia with iron could unmask a co-existing folic acid deficiency. That will also have to be treated because the two play completely different roles; one cannot substitute for the other.

As mentioned before, vitamin B12 deficiency is rare but, in some extreme cases of eating disorders, this may be encountered.

A combination of all three deficiencies is probably extremely unlikely to be seen in pregnancy because such a person is unlikely to conceive in the first place. However, in medicine, never say never.

To cater for those who may have a combination of deficiencies, there are oral preparations available in which iron and folic acid have been combined. They are probably suitable for people who are taking supplements to prevent deficiency from developing. Generally, they are not as good for treatment where deficiency is already established.

9. Clotting disorders (thrombosis) in pregnancy

Introduction

Thrombosis, which is the clotting of blood within the blood vessels, is a serious but fortunately uncommon complication in pregnancy.

When thrombosis occurs, treatment is necessary and will need to be continued for the remainder of the pregnancy and for several weeks beyond.

Apart from being a painful condition, deep vein thrombosis – or DVT, as it is known in the short form – requires treatment in the form of injections during pregnancy. These have to be administered at least once a day, every day. Though clearly unpleasant, this is necessary. When a clot is dislodged, it is transported via the bloodstream to the heart and ultimately to the lungs. At that point, the matter is deadly serious. This is what is known as pulmonary embolism, a highly dangerous complication.

Pulmonary embolism has remained one of the three leading causes of maternal death in the developed world for many years now.

Even without the potentially fatal complication of pulmonary embolism, deep vein thrombosis can cause chronic problems, as we shall discuss shortly. With proper information, most affected mothers are adequately motivated to continue with treatment.

Risk factors for deep vein thrombosis

Where does thrombosis commonly take place?

In the deep-lying veins. The veins in the calves, as well as the inside upper part of the thighs, are particularly prone.

There are two major types of blood vessels in the body. These are veins and arteries. The function of veins is to take blood from all parts of the body back to the heart. The arteries take freshly oxygenated blood from the heart to all parts of the body. Thrombosis in the arteries is extremely rare and occurs only in special circumstances, as we shall see later.

Are there any factors that increase the likelihood of deep vein thrombosis (DVT)?

Yes. Some factors are known to increase susceptibility to this problem. Among the leading factors are:

- *High parity*: The higher the number of deliveries in the past, the higher the risk. It means, all other things being equal, a mother in her fifth pregnancy is at a higher risk of DVT compared to in the first pregnancy.
- *Obesity*: An expectant mother who is overweight is at an increased risk of DVT. The increase in risk is roughly in a linear fashion: the higher the weight, the higher the risk.
- *Immobilization*: Prolonged lack of physical activity during pregnancy (which may range from enforced confinement to bed or lounging about in front of the television interminably, to long-haul air travel) are recognized risk factors especially in late pregnancy.
- *Caucasian race*: There is a clear ethnic difference in suscept-ibility to thrombosis. Women of Asian and African ancestry are less susceptible when compared to Caucasian women.
- *The older mother*: Pregnancy in the late thirties and afterwards is associated with increased risk of thrombosis.
- *Dehydration*: Inadequate fluid intake in the face of excessive fluid loss, be it through vomiting, diarrhoea, vigorous exercise etc. leads to dehydration. This increases the risk of thrombosis.
- *Previous history*: A pregnant mother with a past history of thrombosis or thrombo-embolism, even if this was not during pregnancy, is at a higher than average risk of thrombosis complicating her pregnancy.

Of course, these factors may not appear in isolation. As such, if a mother in early pregnancy is at a weight of 95 kg, age 37, in her sixth pregnancy and complains of a backache which is confining her to the settee most of the day, even in the absence of a previous history of thrombosis, she is clearly high risk.

Sickle cell disease is said to be a risk factor for thrombosis. Is this true?

Yes. The very nature of the condition makes clot formation within the vessels more likely. People suffering from this condition will almost always be aware of the fact that they have to avoid dehydration, which increases the risk of a "sickling" crisis, which in itself may lead to thrombosis. (*See* Chapter 10, "Thalassaemia and sickle cell disease".)

Are there any other risk factors?

The other two significant risk factors are malignancy and conditions collectively known as "Thrombophilia syndrome".

A malignant disease (such as cancer) during pregnancy will tend to increase risk of thrombosis.

What is thrombophilia syndrome?

There are several chemicals and enzymes in the body, an interplay of which keep the perfect balance in the clotting mechanism. This is a finely tuned system, which prevents undue clotting of blood and allows and promotes this when the need arises. This may happen when there is an injury and a clot is required to prevent excessive blood loss.

If this balance of the clotting factors is upset, there will either be a risk of excessive bleeding or undue clotting. In the thrombophilia syndrome, there is undue clotting and therefore susceptibility to deep vein thrombosis (DVT).

What causes thrombophilia syndrome?

There are many factors involved in the clotting mechanism. Some of the factors' specific function is to prevent undue clotting. Others promote clotting. When the former (which prevent clotting) are deficient, the risk of thrombosis is increased.

The factors that are looked for when the syndrome is suspected are:

- Protein C
- Protein S
- Antithrombin III

A deficiency of any of these constitutes a diagnosis of thrombophilia syndrome.

Thrombophilia syndrome is also diagnosed in a case of presence of abnormal antibodies called anticardiolipin and lupus anticoagulant. These antibodies are also associated with recurrent miscarriage.

What are the risks posed by deep vein thrombosis (DVT)?

The condition is painful. Untreated, thrombosis in a deep leg or thigh vein will destroy the valves in that vein. This makes the vein incompetent in transporting blood back up towards the heart. As a result, the affected person will suffer chronic pain, leg swelling and even ulceration. This is called "post-phlebitic syndrome". It can really affect the quality of life in a negative way and is a difficult condition to manage.

Having said all that, the more immediate concern is that of pulmonary embolism. This is where a dislodged clot will end up lodging in a vein of a smaller calibre in the lungs. This is a serious complication. The rough estimate is that, untreated, pulmonary embolism will kill one in eight of its victims.

Confirming the diagnosis

How can a mother-to-be suspect or recognize deep vein thrombosis (DVT)?

The affected part of the limb (usually the calf or inner thigh) will be painful and tender. The pain may be continuous or throbbing. The area may also be swollen, red and turgid.

If it is in the calf, movements of the ankle joint may cause shooting pain. If you have any of the above symptoms, even in isolation, seek prompt medical attention. Not all episodes of calf pain will be due to DVT, but it is best to leave it to the experts to make the distinction.

What sort of tests do doctors use to confirm the diagnosis?

In pregnancy, ultrasound is the first choice. However, while it is good for the thigh vein thrombosis, it is not so accurate if the suspected site is the calf. For this, a rather invasive method called venography may be used.

Even for a suspected calf vein thrombosis, the clinical impression, coupled with ultrasound results, may be judged to be enough to start treatment. If venography is used, the fetus will be shielded to minimize exposure to radiation – which is low, to begin with.

Is the risk of pulmonary embolism the same, wherever the initial clot might be?

Of the two main areas commonly affected by thrombosis in the lower limb, the upper inner thigh (femoral vein) thrombosis is potentially much more dangerous when compared to the calf thrombosis.

While it is true that calf thrombosis rarely leads to pulmonary embolism, untreated, the thrombosis in the vein could extend upwards into the thigh, thereby changing the outlook dramatically.

Treatment for thrombosis

What is the treatment for thrombosis in pregnancy?

Once the diagnosis is established, treatment will be commenced immediately. The aim is to prevent extension of the clot as well as embolism. It is also to allow the existing clot to dissolve. Heparin (or its derivatives) is used in pregnancy. The treatment is decided upon on the basis of the individual patient's circumstances. Generally, in the medium term, the mother should expect to be on heparin injections daily.

The patient will be taught to give herself the injections. The majority of patients acquire the technique easily and quickly. Alternatively, a partner or another adult may take up the task. Once all this is in place and her condition is stable, she can attend hospital as an outpatient with regular and frequent reviews.

Are there any alternatives to heparin injections?

Until a few years ago, heparin had to be administered twice or three times daily. Now, heparin derivatives are available, which are commonly known as low molecular-weight heparins. These offer a distinct advantage to the traditional heparin in that they are administered the same way but only once daily. Even though they are more expensive, many obstetric units have increasingly switched to these because of their user-friendliness. They also seem to have milder side effects. They are just as effective as traditional heparin.

There are some people who break into a cold sweat – literally! – at the mention of the word "injection". Is there no way around this?

Realistically – no. The other form of anticoagulation treatment, apart from heparin, is warfarin. Warfarin is administered orally. However, there is consensus now that warfarin is not safe to use in pregnancy. There are quite a few abnormalities that have been associated with warfarin use during pregnancy. It is also known that this may happen, at whatever stage of pregnancy the treatment is used. Abnormalities may include abnormal shape of the face, small head (microcephaly), blindness or a missing spleen.

Even though all of these are uncommon, they are serious enough to make the use of warfarin in pregnancy not worthwhile, particularly when an effective alternative is available.

Pulmonary embolism

How can pulmonary embolism be recognized?

Pulmonary embolism essentially means a blood-clot lodging in a blood vessel within the lungs. The lung section that is affected will then have its blood circulation cut off. The symptoms that the individual will experience will depend on the actual site of the blockage and the size of lung section affected.

Such symptoms may range from non-specific ones including a cough, localized chest pain, mild fever or coughing up thin blood-stained sputum.

When there is a major embolism, there could be sudden

severe crashing chest pain, shortness of breath and even passing out.

How will suspected pulmonary embolism be investigated?

When a pregnant woman or a newly delivered woman has clinical symptoms suggestive of pulmonary embolism, it is dealt with as an emergency.

If there is strong suspicion, treatment will start even before confirmatory tests are done.

This is because pulmonary embolism is a truly serious complication, which could easily and quickly lead to a fatal outcome.

Of course, if tests establish a different diagnosis, treatment can be stopped with peace of mind.

Investigations carried out include blood analysis to check gases (including oxygen and carbon dioxide), chest X-ray and ECG. All these are non-specific and the diagnosis may still remain elusive. If this is the case, then a more specialized test called a V/Q scan (also called a ventilation perfusion scan) is then performed. This is very sensitive and, even though it is not foolproof, if a pulmonary embolism is ruled out by a V/Q scan, there is almost certainly no danger to the patient.

So should everybody suspected to have a pulmonary embolism have this special (V/Q) scan performed?

Not necessarily. The attending clinicians will decide if this is the appropriate course of action. There are a lot more mundane conditions which could mimic this serious condition, including such things as muscle or ligament sprain, pressure pain from the fetal limbs in late pregnancy under the ribs and self-limiting viral respiratory infections.

But a chest X-ray involves radiation. Isn't this dangerous in pregnancy?

Yes, a chest X-ray involves radiation. So does a V/Q scan. However, precautions are taken to shield the womb and its contents. Moreover, the amount of radiation involved is considered safe. A V/Q scan involves a dose of radiation that is one-tenth of the maximum dose considered safe in pregnancy. A chest X-ray involves an even lower dose.

Treatment for pulmonary embolism

What is the treatment for pulmonary embolism?

Again, it is the anticoagulant heparin. In pulmonary embolism, this will be given in the form of continuous infusion at a much higher dose than that used in deep vein thrombosis. Special tests, will be carried out regularly to ensure that the right effective dose is being given. This may continue for a few days before switching to heparin injections. Treatment will continue for the remainder of the pregnancy and for six to eight weeks after delivery.

Is this treatment always successful?

In the majority of cases, yes. In some very serious cases, this may be insufficient and very specialized surgical intervention may be necessary as a life-saving measure. This is rare.

Is heparin safe to use in pregnancy?

Heparin does not cross the placenta and therefore, as far as the baby is concerned, it is perfectly safe. Regular tests will be carried out to ensure that an optimal dose is being given to the mother. Too much heparin can cause bleeding tendencies and, if tests show evidence of this, the dose will be adjusted downwards. Another problem associated with prolonged heparin use has been the risk of osteoporosis. In rare instances, this has been known to lead to bone fractures. The benefits of treatment far outweigh the potential risk, however.

Do the low-molecular weight heparins also pose the risk of osteoporosis?

Yes, but to a much lower extent. The preparations commonly used in the UK are known under the brand names Fragmin and Clexane.

Precautions

If a woman was treated for DVT or pulmonary embolism in one pregnancy, does she need to take any special precautions in future pregnancies?

Opinions on this differ. There is consensus that any woman with a history of pulmonary embolism in the past should start preventative heparin injections as soon she finds out she is pregnant. This advice is also relevant for those considered to be high-risk.

The high-risk group includes those with thrombophilia syndrome (see above) and those who have a history of two or more episodes of thrombosis in the past. This is regardless of whether the episodes occurred during pregnancy or not. For those who are deemed to be low-risk, the policy is less clear-cut and the attending doctor will, in most cases, decide on an individual basis.

What constitutes low-risk?

If there is only one episode of uncomplicated DVT in the mother's past history, it is considered low-risk. However, if there is an additional risk factor, such as obesity, smoking, or she has had several children, the attending doctor may advise the use of heparin as a preventative measure.

Are there any special precautions or measures that should be taken during labour and delivery?

All high-risk patients – who will already be on heparin during pregnancy – have to carry on during labour and delivery, with some minor scheduling adjustments. For low-risk patients, who may not have been on any preventative treatment, most experts agree that a short course commenced at the onset of labour and continued for a few weeks postnatally is a good idea. Again, this has to be individualized.

Post-delivery, the mother may opt to switch from injections to warfarin tablets, or she may decide to carry on with injections.

What if delivery is by caesarean section?

In this case, the advice is clear. Both low- and high-risk patients are given heparin. Operative delivery (caesarean section) is a recognized risk factor for thrombosis in its own right and anybody with a previous history has to be protected. This preventative measure may even be extended to those with no previous history of thrombosis but who have an independent risk factor, such as being overweight.

Treatment post-delivery

Why is treatment continued after delivery?

Because the risk posed by pregnancy does not disappear immediately after delivery. It tends to subside slowly and the immediate postnatal period is a risky period. The six to eight weeks of treatment is arbitrary, because it has always been difficult to know when it is entirely safe to stop altogether; the figure has more to do with tradition than science.

Does the mother have the option of warfarin after delivery?

A week after delivery, the treatment may be changed from injectable heparins to oral warfarin tablets. The concern about the risk of warfarin to the baby is, of course, no longer there.

Warfarin is also safe with breast-feeding. However, not every patient is keen to switch to warfarin. Warfarin medication necessarily entails regular and frequent blood tests to ensure that the correct dose is being taken. For heparin this is not necessary. Since heparin is self-administered, many mothers consider this to be a significant advantage, which avoids the inconvenience of frequent hospital visits. This is now reinforced by the availability of once-daily injections. Ideally, mothers are given the options in the postnatal period.

So, there is no problem with breast-feeding for both warfarin and heparin?

That is correct. The low molecular-weight heparins are also safe.

Arterial thrombosis

We have discussed thrombosis in veins. What about thrombosis in the other group of vessels, the arteries?

Arterial thrombosis is a problem that is almost exclusive to one group of patients: those with artificial heart valves. If a person has heart valve disease, the defective valves may be replaced by mechanical valves. In such a case, life-long anticoagulant medication is instituted. This is because the presence of artificial valves poses a real risk of thrombosis and embolism.

In almost all cases, the anticoagulation takes the form of warfarin tablets, which are taken daily. If an affected woman becomes pregnant, this will be changed to heparin for the duration of the pregnancy. If there is any laxity with the anticoagulation regime, arterial thrombosis is a real danger, with potentially fatal consequences.

Some physicians argue that, in cases of prosthetic heart valves, it is justified to continue using warfarin anticoagulation rather than risk switching to heparin. This is a very contentious argument and, while it has its merits, most experts hold that a switch to heparin is hardly ever problematic and can be smoothly phased in. The only difficulty may be in persuading a patient who is used to painless tablets to come round to the idea of having to put up with injections for forty weeks, give or take.

10. Thalassaemia and sickle cell disease

Introduction

These conditions are collectively called haemoglobinopathies. This is because the problem is with the oxygen-carrying component of blood called haemoglobin. The haemoglobin produced in these conditions is defective, which leads to chronic conditions characterized by anaemia and other health problems to varying degrees, depending on the severity of the defect. These are genetic conditions and therefore are of special interest where pregnancy is concerned. The parents will want to know the prospects for their child, as far as the condition is concerned. For some, at least, there is also a serious question of whether they can safely embark on a pregnancy.

Haemoglobinopathies are serious conditions, the control of which has improved a lot over the last few decades. They are complex syndromes with a number of sub-types. It is important that a prospective mother with any of these is treated during her pregnancy at a centre where there is the necessary expertise and experience.

There is ethnic preponderance for each of these conditions. Beta-thalassaemia is found mostly in people of Mediterranean origin. It follows therefore that in those areas where you don't find many immigrants from that part of the world, the doctors will inevitably lack the experience of dealing with the problems associated with this condition.

Thalassaemia

What exactly is thalassaemia?

This is a group of genetic conditions where there is a defect which leads to reduced haemoglobin in the red blood-cells. Haemoglobin is the oxygen-carrying component of the cells and therefore the direct consequence is anaemia (low haemoglobin).

Who is at risk?

Thalassaemia conditions are found among people from all parts of the world. There are areas where it is more common than others. Being a genetic condition means one either has it at birth or not. It cannot be acquired in any way later in life.

Can't it be acquired through blood transfusion?

Definitely not. Nor can it be acquired any other way. Genetic conditions are passed from parents to children. If a child is born without a particular condition – in this case thalassaemia – there is no way he or she will get it later on in life.

You have talked of "thalassaemia" as a group of conditions. How many types are there?

Actually, there are only two main types of thalassaemia, which are further subdivided into sub-groups. This is on the basis of the complexity of the genetic defect. We shall concentrate on the two main groups.

What are the two main groups of thalassaemia?

The first is called beta-thalassaemia. The highest concentration of beta-thalassaemia is the Mediterranean region. The name comes from the Greek word "thalassa", which means "sea". This is because the condition was first found among children of Greek (and Italian) immigrants.

How common is this condition?

As mentioned above, the highest concentration of carriers is in the Mediterranean and, to some extent, the Middle East. In Cyprus, for instance, the carrier rate is high, at one in seven. Compare this to the UK, where carrier rates are almost 1500 times lower at one in ten thousand.

What is the difference between thalassaemia major and minor?

To have the overt full-blown condition, one needs to inherit the two defective genes from both parents, therefore making a pair of defective genes. This will produce a clinical condition termed as "major".

This is a very serious condition requiring special treatment for the entire life of the individual. The life expectancy is also considerably reduced.

Thalassaemia minor, on the other hand, means in the particular pair of genes, there is one normal gene and one defective gene. In other words, this person will be known as a carrier of the disease.

Are people with thalassaemia minor better off health-wise?

Most definitely yes. They are much healthier, leading virtually independent lives. It is not unusual for a carrier of the defective gene (i.e. a thalassaemia minor individual) not to be aware of his or her status.

Occasionally, two individual carriers who are partners could find out for the first time about their status when the woman becomes pregnant and when tell-tale findings in routine blood tests could lead to specific diagnostic tests.

Who are more at risk of being affected, boys or girls?

Both sexes are affected equally. If the two parents are carriers, the baby will have a one in four chance of ending up with the full-blown condition: that is, thalassaemia major.

What are the chances that the baby will be completely normal (if both parents are carriers)?

Again, the chance is one in four. This leaves two in four or a 50 per cent chance of the offspring being carriers. If such a couple had four children, mathematically, they should expect one completely healthy child, two children who would be relatively healthy but carrying the beta-thalassaemia gene, and one sick child with the condition thalassaemia major. Of course, it does not work that way in real life. They could end up with four completely healthy children, four sick children or a mixture.

What are the prospects for the thalassaemia major child?

This is a difficult condition to control and treatment is life-long. In years gone by, these children were lucky to get to the age of ten. Things have improved markedly in the last two decades or so. The mainstay for the majority remains repeated blood transfusion. With this, thalassaemia major patients commonly make it to their twenties.

What is the biggest problem with frequent blood transfusion?

Infection risks in modern blood transfusion have been severely minimized but not eliminated altogether. However, the main problem in this condition is the iron overload which is inevitable with repeated transfusions. Excess iron is deposited in major vital organs – including the heart, liver and pancreas – slowly damaging them.

Eventual failure of these organs, especially the heart, leads to death.

Is there anything that can be done to curb the iron overload?

There are various forms of medication used to combat this, so far with mixed success.

Are there any other forms of treatment?

To circumvent blood transfusion, bone marrow transplants have been used, occasionally (but not always) with success. The best chance is produced by the availability of a matching donor, especially if it is a sibling. Not all siblings will match.

Is gene therapy available?

Research is still going on into the possibility of gene replacement therapy. This, if cracked, will be the fail-safe magic solution to this and many other genetic conditions. Indications are that this is still a long way off.

Can a thalassaemia major patient conceive and carry a pregnancy safely?

This is a formidable proposition. The general health of these girls means that they would have difficulty conceiving and the wise counsel for most of them would be to avoid pregnancy. This is because their already compromised vital organs (especially the heart) may fail completely under the added strain of pregnancy. There has been only a handful of reported cases of successful pregnancies in girls with thalassaemia major.

Does this mean that most thalassaemia-affected antenatal patients will only be carriers?

Yes. As mentioned earlier, thalassaemia minor is a condition compatible with good general health. However in pregnancy, there is a tendency to suffer anaemia and, if undiagnosed until then, the anaemia may trigger the definitive diagnostic tests which will confirm the diagnosis, occasionally for the first time.

Is anaemia in thalassaemia minor treated like any other form of anaemia?

To some degree, yes. While in thalassaemia major, the administration of iron supplements is absolutely contraindicated, in thalassaemia minor, iron may be given. This is because these individuals rarely need transfusions and therefore the risk of iron overload is minimal or non-existent. However, as a precaution, many experts advise a test to check the levels of iron supplements.

What about those who cannot tolerate oral iron?

Iron by injection cannot be used in thalassaemia minor. Other ways of supplementing iron – which may be dietary – have to be sought, if definitely required.

If a thalassaemia minor individual has a partner whose genes are both normal, what are the baby's prospects?

The child will never have thalassaemia major because, for this, inheritance of a defective gene from both parents is necessary. However, there is a one in four (25 per cent) chance that the child will be a carrier. This means a 75 per cent chance that the child will be normal, as far as this condition is concerned.

What is the role of folic acid?

Thalassaemia major patients require regular folic acid supplements. Sometimes it has to be given in the form of injection. It is an essential part of the long-term therapy.

Those with thalassaemia minor will need it to a much less extent. However, during pregnancy, it is strongly recommended that they take regular supplements of at least 5 mg daily. If iron stores are found to be depleted, this will be taken alongside.

Are any special measures required for labour and delivery, if the mother has thalassaemia major?

As mentioned before, this is a rare occurrence. However, common sense dictates that caesarean delivery may be a sensible option, to obviate the need for the strain that labour and delivery entail.

What about labour and delivery for a thalassaemia minor woman?

These individuals are overall quite healthy and no special measures are called for or instituted.

Is it possible to diagnose the condition before birth?

Yes. Quite early antenatal diagnosis can be made. This may be as early as twelve to thirteen weeks through the performance of placental biopsy or CVS (chorionic villi sampling). In this, a tiny portion of the developing placenta is drawn out using a needle which is inserted either through the cervix or the abdominal wall. This is done under ultrasound guidance. The DNA of the collected cells is analyzed to establish the status of the fetus.

Does this procedure (CVS) carry any risk?

It does, to a small extent; the most important is the risk of miscarriage, as a direct consequence of the procedure. This risk may be as high as 2 per cent.

Can the test give erroneous results?

In theory, yes. This can occur through contamination of the sample by maternal cells. However, specialist laboratories do have elaborate procedures to minimize this and, in practice, this kind of error is very rare indeed.

Alpha-thalassaemia

How does alpha-thalassaemia differ from beta-thalassaemia?

In several respects. However, the most important is that in alpha-thalassaemia, the problem is that of missing (rather than defective) genes. Different genes are affected (alpha, rather than beta), even though they are also to do with production of another component of haemoglobin, the oxygen-carrying substance in red cells.

Is this condition found world-wide?

Yes, but its highest concentration is in South-East Asia and, to a lesser extent, the Indian sub-continent.

Are there different sub-types of alpha-thalassaemia?

Yes, but we shall concentrate on the main types. Suffice it to mention here that alpha-thalassaemia major (where all four alpha genes are missing) is fatal. Affected babies are born very sick and survive for a few hours at most.

What is the carrier situation in alpha-thalassaemia?

There are several sub-groups, which makes this considerably more complex to describe than beta-thalassaemia.

However, the true carriers are those who have one or two missing alpha genes (there are usually four). It is called alpha-thalassaemia trait.

The carriers are clinically healthy and lead normal independent lives. Pregnancy may be the first time their compromised oxygen-carrying capacity is put under strain.

What if the individual has three missing alpha genes out of the four?

These patients tend to have chronic anaemia. This is brought about by constant destruction of the red cells in the body, the so-called haemolytic anaemia. This type of anemia is not exclusive to people with alpha-thalassaemia.

Such patients are said to have HbH disease.

Are any special measures required for pregnancy in individuals with the alpha-thalassaemia trait?

Special measures are seldom required. Their anaemia can be treated with oral iron supplements and folic acid. If severe, blood transfusion is given but not injectable iron.

Are any special measures required for pregnancy in individuals with three missing genes (HbH disease)?

As mentioned before, those patients tend to have haemolytic anaemia as a chronic problem. As such, they do not have iron deficiency, so iron is never required as a supplement. However, folic acid supplements are crucial because they have an exaggerated consumption of this in their bodies.

The minimum supplements should be 5 mg daily.

Is antenatal diagnosis possible with alpha-thalassaemia?

Yes. The fetal status can be established through DNA studies preferably following CVS or placental biopsy near the end of the first trimester (eleven to thirteen weeks). Genetic screening and counselling of parents is a prerequisite, to determine the probabilities of the fetus being affected and the extent. Then the parents need to know what they would want to do in each possible eventuality.

What are the options for the parents if the fetus is affected?

That is entirely up to them and it will depend on the degree of severity of the inherited condition.

As a general statement, both alpha-thalassaemia trait (where individuals are healthy) and HbH disease (where there is chronic anaemia but normal life expectancy) are compatible with continuing the pregnancy. When the diagnosis is that of alpha-thalassaemia major (all four genes missing or affected), the situation is more difficult.

What are the consequences of carrying a pregnancy where the diagnosis for the fetus is alpha-thalassaemia major?

The pregnancy itself is almost invariably associated with complications. The most difficult is pre-eclampsia, which can be exceptionally severe and life-threatening for the mother. If she manages to carry on, delivery is another tricky time. The fetus usually suffers from oedema (hydropsy) and vaginal delivery may be impossible. A caesarean section, possibly in the presence of severe pre-eclampsia, may in itself endanger the life of the mother. Add to all these, the fact the baby will survive for minutes, at most hours.

This is one prenatal diagnosis that should lead to termination of pregnancy. The final decision, of course, rests with the parents.

Will the child of an alpha-thalassaemia trait mother inherit the defective gene?

Not necessarily. Since she contributes two of the four alpha genes (the father contributing the other two), and since she has two or three normal genes herself, she may very well contribute the normal ones; if the father is not affected, this particular child will be unaffected. As can be seen, there is an element of lottery on whether the child is affected or not. The chances of what happens depends on how many defective genes she is carrying as well as whether or not the father is also a carrier.

The pre-pregnancy or pre-test counselling is meant partly to deal with this issue in detail for each particular couple.

Are any special measures required for delivery?

Pregnancies for carriers of alpha-thalassaemia are largely routine affairs, even if the baby inherits the defect. The only exception is when the fetus ends up with alpha-thalassaemia major (as discussed above). As such, no special measures are called for during pregnancy, other than folic acid and sometimes iron oral supplements. Likewise, delivery does not call for any special measures.

Sickle cell disease

What is sickle cell disease?

This is a condition where the haemoglobin is defective. Haemoglobin is the oxygen-carrying component of the red blood-cells. It is a defect of part of that haemoglobin which renders the cells susceptible to destruction in the body, in certain conditions.

How did this condition acquire its name?

The cells carrying this defective haemoglobin tend to acquire a characteristic "sickle" shape in certain unfavourable conditions, hence the name "sickle" cell.

What are the conditions that lead to this distortion in the shape of the cells?

This is not a simple straightforward affair. However, any condition which reduces oxygen in the bloodstream (such as pneumonia and malaria), high altitude (so mountaineering is not a suitable hobby) and such conditions as dehydration – even body cooling – could lead to a "sickling" crisis.

Why is "sickling" of the cells described as a crisis?

Any person with the condition will tell you that such episodes are very aptly described as crises.

When "sickling" happens, the cells cannot move freely within the bloodstream in the smallest blood vessels, and affected areas are denied oxygen as a result. This could be in bones, joints, kidneys or other organs. This causes severe pain for the sufferer, which can barely be controlled by even the strongest painkillers.

Are any particular measures recommended to prevent the crises from occurring?

It is impossible to completely eliminate the risk of a sickling crisis. This is because some episodes are precipitated by ill-defined causes.

However, it is possible to minimize this risk by a meticulous observation of general measures which prevent the conditions which favour a crisis.

The sufferer has to ensure that she is not short of oxygen (e.g. unduly stressful physical exercises), dehydrated or exposed to very low temperatures for prolonged periods.

Infection is probably the leading trigger of sickling crises. This is worsened by the fact that dehydration often accompanies infections. Early detection and aggressive treatment of infections is therefore one of the principal treatment measures.

There is also a place for preventative steps in the form of antibiotics.

Apart from the crises, what other problems are associated with sickle cell disease?

People with sickle cell disease are chronically anaemic. Their haemoglobin levels hardly ever rise above 9.5 g/dl. Compare this to the normal levels of 12.5–15.0 g/dl for the average woman.

The chronic anaemia is largely due to the recurrent destruction of the blood-cells in the body. The cells are vulnerable from carrying the defective haemoglobin. SCD is also known as "sickle cell anaemia" simply because anaemia is virtually a permanent feature.

What about those individuals who are carriers only?

To be affected by sickle cell disease, an individual has to inherit the defective gene from both parents. If only one defective gene is inherited from either parent, the child will be a carrier but will not have the disease. This is known as "sickle cell trait". These individuals are usually healthy and do not suffer the clinical manifestations of sickle cell disease. However, in very extreme conditions, a sickle cell trait individual may suffer a sickling crisis, usually relatively mild. This is rare.

Are there any special problems suffered by women with sickle cell disease (SCD) in pregnancy?

Pregnancy puts a considerable strain on the body systems of sickle cell disease sufferers. The chronic anaemia and impaired oxygen supply mean these women suffer a higher rate of such complications as miscarriage, preterm labour and even stillbirth.

Do people with sickle cell trait have the same rate of increased risk in pregnancy?

No. The carriers or sickle cell trait individuals usually have normal pregnancies and the risks of the potential pregnancy complications above are comparable to those of the average population.

Are there special precautions required by a sickle cell disease sufferer before she conceives?

Yes. If a SCD sufferer is planning to become pregnant, she should see her doctor, who will need to sort out a few things.

One will be to offer counselling regarding the potential problems and outcome. There will also be genetic counselling. Since a SCD sufferer will inevitably pass on a defective gene to the child, it is important that the status of the partner is established, in order to calculate the chances of the child being affected and to what degree.

For instance, if the father is neither a sufferer nor a carrier (i.e. he has normal haemoglobin), the child will inherit a defective gene from the mother and a normal gene from the father. This means the child will be sickle cell trait or a carrier. This and all the other possible permutations have to be discussed and fully understood.

The other important aspect to be dealt with is the mother's general health pre-pregnancy. One of the organs that sickle cell disease tends to affect is the kidneys. It is imperative therefore that kidney function is assessed, to ensure that they can take the extra strain placed on them by pregnancy.

Finally, it is important that the mother's overall health status is optimized, so she can start her pregnancy from a relatively healthy position.

What special measures do these women require during pregnancy?

Nothing can substitute meticulous antenatal care. Apart from the general measures that every pregnant woman benefits from, SCD sufferers will need regular screening of their renal (kidney) function, and checks for possible urinary tract infection and development of such complications as pre-eclampsia and liver function.

The single most important measure will be to track her haemoglobin level and many affected women will require blood transfusion, sometimes several times, during pregnancy.

Why is blood transfusion likely to be necessary for SCD sufferers?

These women are chronically anaemic and pregnancy will inevitably worsen this. Anaemia puts a strain on vital organs, including the heart, and weakens the individual. This has to be prevented as much as possible.

Moreover, by giving sufferers "normal" blood, the proportion of defective blood is reduced. This reduces the chances of sickling crises. Sickling could be potentially catastrophic in pregnancy as these episodes are directly responsible for many – if not most – of the fetal losses in sufferers.

If blood transfusion is that beneficial, why is it not given as a matter of course to every pregnant SCD sufferer?

One wishes solutions were that simple and straightforward!

Even though modern blood transfusion is extremely safe, problems remain. The potential for these problems increases with the number of transfusions.

The transmission of viral infections via blood transfusion has been virtually eliminated, but there is always a risk, however tiny this might be. That is why the universal wisdom of not to transfuse unless necessary still holds true.

There is also the virtually unpreventable risk of developing what are known as atypical antibodies as a result of repeated transfusions. These antibodies could affect the fetus to the extent of triggering preterm delivery and exchange transfusions at birth.

This means that transfusions should be offered and given only when a meticulous assessment shows that it is necessary.

Are there any circumstances where blood transfusion is considered necessary as a matter of course?

Yes. If a general anaesthetic is required, let's say for a caesarean section, then blood transfusion will be given, usually beforehand unless the urgency for the operation means this is impractical. In such a case, alternative forms of anaesthesia (such as a spinal) may be considered and adopted.

What preparations will be necessary for labour and delivery?

For SCD sufferers, it is imperative that any conditions which could precipitate a crisis are avoided. Dehydration can be prevented by ensuring adequate fluid intake, usually by the intravenous route. Screening for possible urinary tract infection is normally done regularly, especially towards the end of pregnancy. It will need to be done at the onset of labour as well.

Labour itself will be managed actively to ensure that there is no maternal distress, exhaustion or prolonged labour. Blood will always be available, in case transfusion becomes necessary.

What about those women with sickle cell trait in labour?

While no special measures are normally required for these women during pregnancy, the story is different for labour and delivery. Virtually all experts agree that these women should be managed actively along the lines of SCD sufferers (see above). Experience has shown that complications and occasionally unexpected (rare) fatalities have occurred in women with sickle cell trait. Investigations in such cases tend to show that severe dehydration and/or hypoxia (oxygen deficiency) are the precipitating factors. Labour and delivery should therefore be regarded as extreme conditions which could push sufferers beyond the barrier that normally makes them not susceptible to "sickling".

What about monitoring of the fetus during labour?

Continuous electronic fetal heart monitoring will take place for sickle cell disease sufferers.

Will there be any special measures in the period immediately after delivery?

Yes, for both SCD and sickle cell trait women, during the post-delivery period (especially the first twenty-four to forty-eight hours), the measures taken during labour will be maintained. These should include prevention of dehydration and hypoxia.

Simple measures which ensure adequate fluid intake and rest for the mother are normally sufficient. If an infection was being treated, this should be completed.

Who is at risk?

Sickle cell disease, like the other so-called haemoglobinopathies, is a genetic disease. The defective genes are inherited from parents.

If one parent passes on the relevant defective gene, the child will be a carrier with what is known as sickle cell trait. If the defective gene is inherited from both parents, the child ends up with a complete pair of the defective genes and will have the full-blown condition known as sickle cell disease (SCD).

Is there any ethnic propensity for this condition?

Different ethnic groups are known to be more prone to different genetic conditions by virtue of their evolutionary genetic inheritance. Just like cystic fibrosis is prevalent among northern Europeans and beta-Thalassaemia among people of Mediterranean extraction, sickle cell disease is prevalent among people of black African origin.

The condition is also found among people from Saudi Arabia, India and the Mediterranean areas. It is, however, less prevalent among these peoples. Inter-ethnic marriages mean that the possibility of finding any of these conditions in a member of another ethnic group is improbable but is far from impossible.

11. Thyroid disease in pregnancy

Introduction

There are two broad categories of thyroid disease.

These are hyperthyroidism, where more thyroid hormone is produced than the body requires, and hypothyroidism, where less thyroid hormone is produced. Both conditions have a significant impact on the ability to conceive, the successful carrying of pregnancy and on the fetus itself.

Hyperthyroidism is not one simple condition. It may be caused by a variety of diseases, all leading to a common consequence: the production of excess hormone by the thyroid gland. The outward and physiological effects will, therefore, be more or less the same. This condition is quite common and affects roughly two out of every thousand pregnant women. Most of these will have a condition known as Graves' disease, which is explained in this chapter. There are several other less common causes of hyperthyroidism, also explained below.

Ideally, the condition should be recognized before conception; this is not always the case, as the symptoms may be so mild that they do not cause undue concern. Sometimes, the diagnosis is made during investigations for fertility difficulties, and often the condition is discovered for the first time during pregnancy.

Treatment for hyperthyroidism needs to be maintained during pregnancy to optimize the successful outcome of the pregnancy. Some forms of medication are completely safe in pregnancy, while others are not. All this is clearly discussed in this chapter.

Some forms of hyperthyroidism may affect the newborn and the details on this are found in this chapter. However, these effects are usually transient and relatively easy to treat.

Hypothyroidism or deficiency of the thyroid hormone is also important with regard to fertility and successful pregnancy.

Investigations for infertility or reduced fertility will, in most instances, include thyroid function tests, as there is firm evidence that hypothyroidism can make conception difficult. Moreover, untreated hypothyroidism sometimes causes various minor and occasionally serious problems in pregnancy. We have explained all these in this chapter.

Treatment of hypothyroidism in the pre-conception and pregnancy period is by simple replacement of the hormone. It is safe, inexpensive and very effective.

Thyroid disease and fertility

Can thyroid disease interfere with fertility?

Yes. A woman suffering from hypothyroidism or low thyroid hormone may have difficulty conceiving.

Some women with hypothyroidism contact their doctor about infertility and the condition is discovered in the process of investigating the cause of infertility.

Hypothyroidism

Why would low thyroid hormone cause infertility?

It causes failure to ovulate. This may be through an interference with the normal hormonal environment in the body.

Can low thyroid hormone (hypothyroidism) cause problems in pregnancy?

For women who conceive in spite of the thyroid hormone deficiency, a number of problems may be encountered:

- There is an increased tendency to miscarry. Ironically they may also have prolonged pregnancy, requiring intervention in the form of labour induction.
- There is increased susceptibility to pregnancy complications such as anaemia, placental abruption, pre-eclampsia and postpartum haemorrhage.
- The baby may be of low birth weight and generally in this group of women, the loss of babies during the birth is slightly higher than average.

Is there any treatment for a pregnant woman who has hypothyroidism?

Yes; the treatment is simple, safe and effective. Thyroxine – which is the thyroid hormone – is administered orally daily, at a dose determined after a specific blood test.

Can a woman taking thyroxine breast-feed?

Yes. It is completely safe.

Can a woman suffering from hypothyroidism recognize the condition?

Unfortunately, it is rather difficult because the symptoms are quite non-specific. For the majority, the condition is stumbled upon in the course of investigation other – seemingly unrelated – problems such as infertility, menstrual irregularities or weight problems.

Symptoms may include a general sense of lethargy that is difficult to shake off, feeling cold (even in quite warm weather), weight gain, heavy periods which tend to be irregular or lack of periods altogether.

Thyrotoxicosis or hyperthyroidism

What about the effect of increased thyroid hormone in pregnancy?

This condition, also called thyrotoxicosis or simply hyper-thyroidism, can affect pregnancy in a number of ways. These may include:

- miscarriage
- death of the fetus in the womb
- premature delivery
- growth restriction
- fetal hyperthyroidism.

What is Graves' disease?

This is a variant of hyperthyroidism. It is actually the most common cause of hyperthyroidism in pregnancy. It is associated with antibodies which cause or stimulate the production of excessive thyroid hormone. The antibodies can cross over to the fetus to cause the same effect there.

What would make a woman suspect that she has hyperthyroidism?

Again, it is difficult, as the symptoms are non-specific. They may include weight loss (or inability to gain weight), increased appetite, palpitations, sleep disturbances, tremors of the hands and sweaty palms.

Most cases of hyperthyroidism are discovered before the affected woman has conceived and therefore most of the affected women are already being treated when they become pregnant.

How common is this condition?

It is estimated to affect about one in every 500 pregnancies.

Is there any treatment for this condition in pregnancy?

Yes; there are two main types of medication that can be used in pregnancy. Both are considered safe but one – propythrouracil (PTU) – is preferred in North America and the other is used more in most of Europe. This is carbimazole. They are both very effective.

Does this mean these drugs do not cross the placenta to the baby?

They both cross the placenta. This is why just the optimal dose needs to be used to control the disease. Excessive doses have the potential of suppressing the developing thyroid gland of the fetus. Evidence shows that in optimal doses, these two drugs are quite safe for the baby.

I have heard of people with hyperthyroidism being treated with radioactive iodine. Can this be used during pregnancy?

No. This can permanently destroy the fetal thyroid gland.

What about surgery to treat the condition?

Yes, this is an option. If medical treatment fails to control the hyperthyroidism, then partial resection of the thyroid gland may be undertaken. This is normally only considered after twenty weeks of gestation. It is unusual to resort to this treatment method during pregnancy.

Is the baby in the clear once the maternal condition is controlled?

In cases where the hyperthyroidism was due to Graves' disease, there is still a risk that the baby will be affected, regardless of the level of control in the mother. At least one in ten such babies are born with Graves' disease because of passage of the antibodies from mother to baby across the placenta.

The drugs suppress the production of the hormone but do not eliminate the rogue antibodies. The condition in the baby is transient.

Does pregnancy itself have any effect at all on the disease?

Yes. Graves' disease will tend to go into partial remission during pregnancy. None the less, treatment will still be required in almost all cases, even though for those already on treatment, the dose may be reduced. Delivery will be followed by exacerbation of the condition.

Can a woman taking prapylthiouracil (PTU) breast-feed?

Yes. Even though a very small amount of the drug is found in breast-milk, it is not considered to be in sufficient quantities to cause unwanted effects.

Can a woman taking carbimazole breast-feed?

Yes. The advice is actually similar as for PTU above. The lowest effective dose should be used and the baby's growth progress monitored.

What is a "thyroid storm"?

This is a rare complication of hyperthyroidism. It may be triggered by infection, labour or surgery (such as caesarean section). It may also complicate surgery undertaken to treat the disease itself.

It is a result of a release of massive quantities of the thyroid hormone into the bloodstream. It is characterized by a very high temperature, high heart rate (and palpitations), dehydration and extreme agitation.

Is thyroid storm dangerous?

Yes, and intensive and sustained efforts to control the symptoms and suppress the thyroid hormone are required. When appropriately managed, the condition is brought under control in a relatively short time.

Can hyperthyroidism cause excessive vomiting?

In a small proportion of women who suffer excessive nausea and vomiting in early pregnancy, hyperthyroidism is found to be the associated factor. Control of the hyperthyroidism is usually followed by subsiding of the nausea and vomiting. Most mothers presenting with excessive nausea and vomiting in early pregnancy have normal thyroid function.

Can hyperthyroidism or hypothyroidism occur for the first time after delivery?

Yes. There is a unique condition called postpartum thyroiditis. This is characterized by transient hyperthyroidism with all the hallmarks of raised thyroid hormone. In a few days, this turns to hypothyroidism. That may take several months to clear up, as it does in over 90 per cent of affected patients. In a small minority, it remains permanently as hypothyroidism, requiring thyroid hormone supplements for life.

Does postpartum thyroiditis recur in subsequent pregnancies?

It might, but this is not always the case.

12. Epilepsy in pregnancy

Introduction

Epilepsy is a relatively common condition among young people. However, large strides have been made in controlling epileptic seizures using medication. This has meant that the majority of epileptics lead virtually independent lives with little risk of convulsions.

Pregnancy presents a unique challenge in the life of an epileptic. This is not only because of anxiety about what effect pregnancy might have on the condition (which is unpredictable), but also because of such factors as the effect of the pregnancy on the dose of medication.

There is also the fear of convulsions and its potential consequences on the pregnancy, the effect of the anticonvulsant medication on the fetus and many more.

All these questions and many others have been tackled in this chapter. Not all the answers are known and it will be pretentious for any physician to suggest otherwise. However, as in most chronic conditions that individuals learn to live with, the optimal result – both in terms of a problem-free pregnancy and a good outcome – lies in the meticulous control of the condition. The buck, as the old adage goes, ultimately stops with the individual. The decision to take medication as recommended always lies with the patient.

As we shall see while answering specific questions, there is no such thing as a "safe" anticonvulsant. The potential for adverse effect on the baby does, however, differ from one group of anticonvulsants to another; such consequences are uncommon, even in collective terms. Moreover, changing from one anticonvulsant to another that may be deemed relatively safer is usually quite limited in real life. This is because there may be anxiety about abandoning a drug with proven effectiveness for another, which may not be as good in that particular individual. Moreover, a switch needs to be made before conception, to be effective in skirting the potential adverse effects on the fetus. Many pregnancies among epileptics are "discovered" at a five to six week stage, too late for any such measure. All these subjects are dealt with in detail in this chapter.

The effects of epilepsy on pregnancy and the fetus

As an epileptic on medication, how should I expect pregnancy to affect my condition?

It is impossible for anybody to predict. Roughly 50 per cent of patients see no change in the seizure frequency. Of the remainder, some will experience more seizures and some fewer.

Can the fact that I have epilepsy cause complications to the pregnancy?

The aim of managing epilepsy in pregnancy will be to prevent seizures, as these could lead to injury to you and may cause a late miscarriage or premature delivery, with consequent loss of your baby.

Apart from that, there is known to be a slight increase in the risk of bleeding in pregnancy. Bleeding, when it occurs, is usually light and painless. It very rarely threatens the well-being of the pregnancy. Epilepsy does not make you more prone to develop other pregnancy-related problems, such as pre-eclampsia.

What about the baby?

Yes, there is an increased risk (compared to the general population) of major malformations, especially those of the skull, mouth or heart. Most of these can be detected by ultrasound scanning, optimally at around eighteen to twenty weeks of gestation. Nine out of ten of babies born to epileptic mothers are free of any malformations.

Can the risk of malformations be reduced or eliminated by stopping anticonvulsant medication?

No. The increase in the risk of malformations is inherently there by having epilepsy. This background risk remains the same, whether you are on anticonvulsants or not. It is probably more important to concentrate on the positive aspect that your baby has a 90 per cent chance of being completely normal.

Does medication add to the risk of malformation?

The answer to this is, broadly, yes. However, there is a wide variety of anticonvulsant medication and new ones are coming on the market all the time.

Of the traditional anticonvulsants, carbamazepine (tegretol) is considered to be the safest, in relative terms. It is, however, not completely free of side-effects to the fetus, and may occasionally cause defects, mostly minor. Phenytoin may cause some defects of the skull bones, digits and occasionally may have long-term consequences including mental retardation, with learning difficulties. It should be emphasized here that all these are quite uncommon.

Should anticonvulsant medication be stopped if I am planning to conceive?

The issue of continuing with medication during pregnancy is rather complex.

For the majority of women with epilepsy, continuing with medication is not only desirable but imperative. In carefully selected cases, where there have been no seizures for at least two years, an attempt to stop anticonvulsants in the pre-conception period could be made. If she remains free of seizures, she could be treated by observation alone. Unfortunately, 30 per cent of all patients who try this strategy have a recurrence of seizures and have to be put back on medication.

It is considered unwise to adopt this strategy if you are already pregnant. In this case, medication should be continued.

What about types of anticonvulsants?

A few patients may be maintained on valproic acid and trimethadione. These are not commonly used. If a patient is on one of these, it may be changed to a safer variety such as carbamazepine. Both trimethadione and valproic acid have been associated with a variety of birth-defects and valproic acid is notorious for causing spina bifida and other defects of the spinal column.

The decision to change medication is not always automatic or straightforward since you may have tried the apparently safer alternatives in the past with disappointing results. Alternatively, you may have a history of seizures that are very difficult to control and your doctor may judge it unsafe to take the gamble.

Does an epileptic mother need to take any other precautions during the course of the pregnancy?

Anticonvulsant medication makes the epileptic mother vulnerable to developing a folic acid deficiency. Folic acid will be recommended as a supplement, preferably throughout the course of pregnancy.

Hereditary effects of epilepsy

If the father of the baby is an epileptic, does that still carry an increased risk of malformations for the fetus?

Yes. The risk of fetal malformations as a result of parental epilepsy is roughly the same if one or the other parent is epileptic.

However, if the father is the affected parent, the baby will not be at risk of those malformations associated with anticonvulsant medication.

What are the chances of the baby developing epilepsy himself or herself, later on in life?

Approximately 10 per cent. Again, this is regardless of which parent is affected. It is important, though, to remember that 90 per cent of all children born to an epileptic parent will not be affected by this condition.

Medication changes in pregnancy, labour and postnatally

Are any changes required in the dosage of the anticonvulsant medication during pregnancy?

In theory, you may require an increase in the dose of your medication. In practice, most physicians have found this to be unnecessary and therefore tend to stick to the same pre-pregnancy regime.

Your doctor may, however, want to check the drug levels in your blood from time to time. If this is found to be well below the acceptable therapeutic range, the case for increasing the dose may be compelling, even in the absence of seizures. After all, the aim is to prevent these from occurring.

Are any special measures required in labour?

No. Labour does not increase the risk of seizures and no special measures are called for.

Are any special measures required after delivery?

For the mother, no, but you will be strongly advised to have vitamin K given to the baby, which counters the increased bleeding tendency that these babies are especially prone to. The case for vitamin K is certainly stronger for these babies, even though vitamin K is recommended for and administered to practically all newborns.

What place does pre-conception counselling have?

The various issues touched upon here make it clear that pre-conception counselling is ideal. It is essential that the issue of fetal anomalies associated with this condition and its treatment is fully discussed and understood. It is also important to explore possibilities of either stopping or changing medication in the period leading to pregnancy, i.e. before starting to try for a baby. For those on sodium valproate (valproic acid), if it is not possible to change, pre-conception use of folic acid will be strongly advised, as it will minimize the risk of spina bifida (associated with this type of medication).

13. Diabetes in pregnancy

Introduction

Diabetes – a condition where the pancreas does not produce enough insulin, which is needed for the body to absorb sugar (glucose) into cells and process it – is one of those chronic conditions that has significant potential of wreaking havoc during a pregnancy.

Many diabetic women who become pregnant will be on insulin. Through the course of the pregnancy, the needs of the body for insulin will continually change and dosage adjustments are inevitable. This means that monitoring of the condition will need to be closer and almost always involves not only the obstetrician but a specialist physician (for diabetes) as well as the GP, midwife and probably a diabetic liaison nurse: a classic multi-disciplinary approach.

This is not meant to cause anxiety to the mother but to provide a close and coordinated service to ensure the best possible outcome.

There is no doubt that if a pregnant diabetic woman has poor blood-sugar control, the chances of a poor outcome are high. Not only that, but there is the possibility of very serious diabetic complications which could be life-threatening to the mother herself.

There is a group of women who become diabetic for the first time in pregnancy and whose diabetes ends with their pregnancy. This condition is aptly called "gestational diabetes". This will also require special measures, which will differ from person to person. All this is explained in detail in response to specific questions in this chapter.

Diabetes is one of those conditions which can be quite effectively controlled, to the point where pregnancy seems uncomplicated.

This, however, entails a very interventionist approach, which many women may find unacceptable. The onus is on the health-care professionals, from the midwife and GP through to the hospital-based professionals, to ensure the mother understands why a particular management plan is required and why each specific measure needs to be taken.

Gestational diabetes

Can diabetes occur for the first time in pregnancy?
Yes. A number of women are found to be diabetic for the first time in their lives while pregnant. Pregnancy has been described as a "diabetogenic condition". This simply means it can trigger the development of diabetes.

Is gestational diabetes (diabetes occurring in pregnancy) different from classical diabetes?
In a few ways, yes. It is, however, important to concentrate on the aspects where it is similar to classical diabetes. In either type, when the condition is not controlled, it can have serious consequences for both the mother and the baby.

So, how does it differ?
It differs in the sense that the gestational type of diabetes is easier to control and usually clears up soon after delivery.

Is there any association between gestational diabetes and the classical diabetes?
In some cases there is. It is recognized that some women who have the symptoms of gestational diabetes actually have mild diabetes prior to conception and pregnancy helps to unmask the condition. Naturally, with these women, the condition does not completely clear up after delivery.

Are any long-term consequences to be expected?
As mentioned above, some patients have latent diabetes and delivery may just take them back to the quiescent state with no symptoms and no need for treatment. These may constitute anything between 10 and 20 per cent of all gestational diabetes patients. For these, diabetes develops in the medium or long-term. Conversely, for over 80 per cent of

mothers with gestational diabetes, the condition clears up entirely shortly after delivery.

Who is at risk of developing gestational diabetes?

Mothers who:

- have symptoms of increased water intake (feeling abnormally thirsty), urinary frequency and feeling hungry and peckish more often than normal
- are overweight or obese
- have close relatives with diabetes
- have a history of delivering large babies in the past
- gain an excessive amount of weight during pregnancy
- have a previous history of gestational diabetes
- are aged thirty or over.

What do you mean by previous gestational diabetes?

There is a risk of recurrence of gestational diabetes of one in two; that is, up to 50 per cent of affected mothers will experience a recurrence in a subsequent pregnancy.

Can a prospective mother reduce the risk of getting gestational diabetes?

A woman can reduce this risk by acting upon some factors, such as being overweight. Controlling or reducing the body weight to a level around the ideal for her body height will significantly reduce the risk of gestational diabetes.

Is there anything a mother can do to check whether she might have latent diabetes?

Yes. If a woman has suffered from gestational diabetes in a previous pregnancy and she is planning another baby, she can arrange for her doctor to perform a blood screening test for diabetes before she conceives. This will tell her whether she has latent diabetes or not. For a woman who does not have latent diabetes, this test will always be negative.

Is there another test, such as a urine test, to screen for diabetes?

Afraid not. The only definitive screening and diagnostic test is a blood test. A urine test is very unreliable as a screening tool and is most certainly not diagnostic.

How is the diagnostic test conducted?

You will hear the term Glucose Tolerance Test or, more often, GTT. It simply involves the person fasting for several hours overnight and taking a measured sugary drink in the morning. A series of blood samples are taken, normally every thirty minutes for the next two hours. Levels of sugar in each sample are analyzed.

What does the GTT tell the doctor?

It will tell the doctor whether the mother's body is processing sugars (and other carbohydrates) efficiently. If this is the case, it will mean she is not diabetic.

It could, on the other hand, show that the control of blood-sugars is not optimal – which will be termed "impaired glucose tolerance".

It could show that blood-sugar level control has been completely lost. This will mean she has gestational diabetes.

What are the implications of impaired glucose tolerance?

Well, she does not have diabetes, so things are not too bad. The standard control of this is purely dietary. Her doctors and midwife will give her advice on the kind of changes she needs to make in her diet. In most cases, a dietician is involved, to give personalized specialist dietary advice. Regular blood-sugar tests will be done for the remainder of the pregnancy.

Can the baby be affected by impaired glucose tolerance?

When this diagnosis is made, the mother is bound to have a closer follow-up of her pregnancy. Sometimes impaired glucose tolerance progresses into gestational diabetes, which may call for changes in the management strategy. If impaired glucose tolerance is well controlled, there is no evidence of any adverse effects to the growing fetus in the womb.

What if she has gestational diabetes?

A careful assessment of her condition is made. The decision will then be taken whether to stick to dietary control of her condition or to start her on insulin. If her obstetrician opts for the former, she will be asked to have frequent timed blood-sugar tests. It is of absolute importance that she sticks to the monitoring regime. If the dietary management alone does not seem to give good control, then insulin needs to be used. The aim is to achieve blood-sugar levels that stay within the normal range.

Is there a role for exercise?
Yes. Strenuous exercise is out, as it can cause a dangerous fall in the blood-sugar level. On the other hand, a complete lack of exercise does make blood-sugar control that little bit more difficult. The midwife and doctors will advise the mother on the recommended type and extent of exercise. It is never necessary to go to the gym, however.

How is insulin administered?
The mother will be taught how to self-administer insulin injections. Most people find this quite easy to learn. The injection causes very little pain and is relatively superficial.

Some diabetics use tablets for their condition. Can't these be used for gestational diabetes?
No. Tablets used in the classical form of diabetes cannot be used in pregnancy. Patients who are on these tablets will be switched to insulin injection during the course of their pregnancy. This is because the tablets are less reliable in pregnancy and could harm the fetus.

Does the diagnosis of impaired glucose tolerance influence the timing of delivery?
No. If this condition has not progressed into gestational diabetes, it should not influence the timing of delivery, because it cannot harm the mother or the baby. If any intervention is recommended, this will be done on the basis of other complicating factors and not because of impaired glucose tolerance.

Does gestational diabetes influence the timing of delivery?
Debate still rages about this. There is no doubt that for patients where the gestational diabetes was controlled by diet alone, there is little justification to intervene, unless there are other complicating factors. For those who needed insulin,

debate is whether they should be allowed to go beyond forty weeks of gestation. Historically, because of increased unexplained stillbirth among diabetic expectant mothers after thirty-eight weeks, delivery used to be planned around this stage. The argument now is that the control of diabetes in pregnancy and the ability to monitor the fetal well-being has advanced so much that this is no longer necessary.

Not everybody agrees with this contention. Certainly, some cases of unexplained stillbirth near term, in the presence of seemingly good diabetic control, still occur but these are very few and far between. The body of opinion seems to be moving towards managing these pregnancies like any other, provided the blood-sugar control is impeccable. Most obstetricians will hesitate at the idea of allowing the pregnancy to go beyond forty-one weeks.

Ultimately, the condition of the fetus, the obstetrician's opinion and, most importantly, the mother's own wishes will determine the timing of delivery.

What is likely to be the method of delivery?

Again, this depends on all the other factors in pregnancy. If there is no contraindication to vaginal delivery, this will be the natural choice. Gestational diabetes itself should not directly influence the mode of delivery. However, if the fetus is estimated to weigh significantly above average (over 4.5 kg or 10 lbs), the mother may be advised to have a caesarean section unless, of course, she has had a baby of similar or higher weight in the past vaginally, and without problems.

Should labour be expected to be different?

In many ways, no. However she will have a drip (intravenous infusion) throughout. This is necessary to ensure that her blood-sugar is well controlled throughout labour. Her blood-sugar level will be checked at least every hour. She may have an insulin infusion as well, if this is found to be necessary.

Why is this very close blood-sugar control suddenly necessary in labour?

If good control is not achieved in labour, control of the baby's blood-sugar could be difficult. In fact, the baby's blood-sugar may drop quite steeply shortly after he or she is born, putting him or her at risk of brain damage.

What happens to the mother after delivery?

Her insulin requirements drop sharply immediately after delivery and therefore she will still have her blood-sugar monitored closely, especially in the first twenty-four hours, to determine how much (if any) insulin she requires.

In the medium term (i.e. one day after delivery), virtually all gestational diabetics have their insulin stopped.

In the long term, a small group may continue to have diabetes, which will need some form of management. This group consists of those who had latent diabetes and pregnancy helped to unmask it.

Could a woman who has had gestational diabetes do anything after delivery to check whether she had or has latent diabetes?

Yes, she could ask her doctor for the diagnostic test (GTT) to be performed, at least two months after delivery. A negative result means latent diabetes is very unlikely.

Is there increased risk of fetal malformations among those with gestational diabetes?

No.

Classical diabetes

I am an insulin-dependent diabetic and I am planning to conceive. Is there anything special I need to know?

Yes. Good diabetic control before conception is of utmost importance for your own and your baby's ultimate well-being. If you have decided to try for a baby, your doctor can arrange a simple blood test to determine how good your blood-sugar control has been.

If this is found to be unsatisfactory, it is best to put your plans on hold until the diabetes control has been optimized. Alteration in the insulin regime will be made until the blood-sugar level control is good and stable. This may take several weeks to achieve, but is well worth it. There is no doubt that poor diabetes control at the time of conception is by far the leading cause of major fetal malformation among diabetic mothers. The rate of such malformations (about 3 per cent) is similar among diabetics where pre-conceptual control has been good and among non-diabetics. In the case of poor pre-conceptual control, however, the rate of such malformation increases up to six times.

If I am insulin-dependent and I discovered that I was pregnant, even though this was unplanned, can I do anything in the early stages of the pregnancy to eliminate the increased risk of fetal malformations?

As stated before, if your blood-sugar control has been good, the risk of such malformation is not increased. On the other hand, if this has been unsatisfactory (you can have this verified by a simple blood test), it is in most cases too late to influence occurrence of malformations. There is strong evidence that most malformations are already in place by eight weeks of gestation. Any intervention in correcting blood-sugar control has to be in place by five weeks of gestation, otherwise it is too late.

How and when will a mother know if her baby is affected?

The only reliable test to detect possible major malformation is an ultrasound scan ideally performed at about eighteen to twenty weeks of gestation. Detection is possible a few weeks earlier, but a negative result may not be as reliable. Most major malformations will be detected.

As an insulin-dependent diabetic, what changes should I expect when I become pregnant?

In the beginning (i.e. the first ten to twelve weeks), the tendency is for insulin requirements to decrease. This is because blood glucose is being transported from the mother's bloodstream to the fetus. This means she ends up with less blood glucose and is prone to low blood glucose (hypo-glycaemia). Gradually, she develops insulin resistance and this means her insulin requirements will start going up again.

In summary, at the beginning, the tendency is to require less insulin and, about one third of the way through, the trend is towards more insulin. What all this means is, she should expect a few adjustments in the insulin regime during her pregnancy.

What are the consequences of poor blood-sugar control?

The mother could become very seriously ill if her blood-sugar is allowed to drift wildly. Both very low and very high blood-sugar can be dangerous, even life-threatening. As for the fetus, poor diabetic control is estimated to be responsible for close to half of all babies lost either in the form of stillbirth or infant death soon after delivery.

What sort of blood glucose levels should a mother aim for?

The affected mother will need to check her blood glucose anything between two and five times a day throughout the course of the pregnancy.

She should be aiming for a level of between four and seven. The glucose level should be nearer four before her breakfast and nearer seven two hours after her main meal. In reality, this is difficult to achieve and a drift by a factor of one from this range is generally considered acceptable, provided it is not persistent.

If a mother has eye complications as result of diabetes, will pregnancy make these worse?

The most common diabetic eye complication is retinopathy. If she already has this, the symptoms may get worse. This is, however, strictly temporary and her eyes will go back to the pre-pregnancy status soon after the end of the pregnancy. All diabetic expectant mothers should have their eyes examined during pregnancy, to keep track of existing retinopathy and to detect any retinopathy which may develop for the first time during pregnancy.

What if her kidneys have been affected by diabetes?

It depends on the extent of renal (kidney) disease. If the only detectable problem is loss of protein in the urine, then pregnancy should not have any significant effect. It would not make the renal disease worse and there will be only a slight increase in fetal growth restriction. She is, however, at a slightly increased risk of developing pre-eclampsia.

If, on the other hand, her renal disease has already caused hypertension, then the risk of developing pre-eclampsia is quite significantly increased. This, in turn, may lead to significant fetal growth restriction and/or prematurity. More than a third of such patients have premature delivery.

What should a diabetic mother expect if the baby is delivered prematurely?

In any situation, it depends on the degree of prematurity. As a rule, babies of diabetic mothers tend to fare less well at every stage of the pregnancy. Good diabetic control quite significantly reduces the difference, but it does not eliminate it altogether. The doctors will strive to minimize the possibility of a premature delivery as much as they can, but this is not always possible. In the presence of complications, the mother's own well-being is paramount and early delivery may become inevitable as a life-saving measure.

What are the main problems afflicting premature babies?

The biggest problem is usually lung function.

Babies of diabetic mothers are particularly prone to poor lung function. Normally, when a premature delivery is anticipated, a short course of steroid injections over twenty-four to forty-eight hours is administered. The steroids stimulate the fetal lungs to produce a chemical which helps to facilitate good lung function.

For diabetic patients, however, this is not a straightforward affair. Firstly, steroids disrupt diabetic control as they increase insulin resistance, which will make the mother prone to high blood-sugar. Secondly, the fetus of a diabetic mother does not respond as well to steroids. Most obstetricians agree, however, that if prematurity is a distinct possibility, steroids should be given and close and intensive blood-sugar surveillance maintained.

When should a diabetic mother expect to deliver?

In the absence of complications and with good blood-sugar control, she is likely to be allowed to go into labour at term. If she does not go into labour by her due date (at forty weeks), whether she is allowed to go beyond this stage will ultimately depend on her wishes and her obstetrician's opinion. Because such pregnancies are intensively monitored, most mothers do not want to wait beyond their due date, and it is probably unfair and unwise for the obstetrician to try to persuade her otherwise. As for how safe going post-date is, the honest answer is that nobody knows.

What if the blood-sugar control has not been optimal during the pregnancy?

If it appears that the mother's blood glucose control has been poor, an obstetrician is faced with a difficult decision. Leaving delivery too late clearly courts the risk of stillbirth. Early delivery could result in prematurity complications that could be difficult to manage. The compromise may be to admit the mother into hospital and try to bring the blood-sugar under control.

If this is achieved, then she may remain in hospital and be delivered after thirty-eight weeks of gestation. If control is not secured even in hospital, then a close surveillance of the fetal condition is maintained (in hospital) and delivery may be at any time, if and when the fetal condition appears unsatisfactory. Otherwise, if all appears to be going well while in hospital, she may deliver at thirty-eight weeks.

If the baby is delivered at thirty-eight weeks, is he or she still prone to lung maturity problems?

Unfortunately, yes, especially if diabetic control has not been good. This is, however, uncommon at this gestation and, when present, can be controlled satisfactorily in most maternity units.

What is the likely method of delivery?

Diabetes in itself is not an indication for caesarean section. If this is recommended it will be for the usual obstetric reasons, such as fetal distress or abnormal lie of the fetus.

What about the size of the baby?

Diabetic mothers are prone to have big babies, which obviously increases the probability of a caesarean delivery. This problem is minimized by good diabetes control.

What happens during labour?

There are different regimes in different centres but all are based on the principle of continuous infusion of both dextrose (glucose) and insulin. The mother's blood-sugar is checked every hour and adjustments in the rate of the infusions made accordingly. This is aimed at maintaining her blood-sugar within a strict (normal) range, to minimize complications to the baby after delivery.

What are the possible immediate complications, post-delivery?

If blood-sugar control has been poor during labour, the baby may soon develop severe hypoglycaemia (low blood-sugar) as well as an imbalance of some essential minerals such as calcium and magnesium. This may be in addition to respiratory difficulties to which these babies are prone. The baby's condition may deteriorate quite rapidly, requiring intensive care.

Is it true that the baby will be prone to develop jaundice?

Yes, but this is hardly ever serious. This develops a few days after delivery and is usually quite mild. The level of the pigment (bilirubin) causing the jaundice will be checked in the baby's blood. If this is found to be significantly raised, treatment by being put under a special light (phototherapy) may be administered. This is rarely necessary.

What happens to the mother after delivery?

Her insulin requirement goes down, immediately after delivery. In some cases, it may be necessary to stop insulin temporarily (for twenty-four to forty-eight hours) before resuming at a dose used before conception. In any case, her blood-sugar will be monitored closely in the first twenty-four hours to determine her individual requirements.

The final word?

Good blood-sugar control is key to controlling the condition before conception, in pregnancy, and during labour and delivery. If this is achieved, the mother's expectations and outcome should be similar to anybody else's.

14. Blood pressure and pregnancy

Introduction

Hypertension or high blood pressure is one of the more serious complications that can affect a pregnancy.

A small percentage of pregnant women who have raised blood pressure will have it as a pre-existing condition and may be on medication even before conception. This is chronic hypertension, also known as "essential hypertension".

There is a small group of women who may have pre-existing hypertension because of a known underlying disease, usually of the kidneys. In such women, the hypertension is, strictly speaking, not a pregnancy complication. Rather, it is a concomitant condition that will need to be monitored and controlled during the course of the pregnancy. This is because pre-existing hypertension has a potential for worsening or being complicated by turning into pre-eclampsia.

This brings us to the main hypertensive condition to affect pregnancy: pre-eclampsia. The majority of women who develop pre-eclampsia have no identifiable underlying cause.

Pre-eclampsia is also known as "pregnancy induced hypertension" (PIH) and also by the older term "pre-eclamptic toxaemia" (PET). In North America, it has also been known as "EPH gestosis". All these terms mean exactly the same thing.

This condition is significant because, if poorly managed, it may lead to loss of the baby. More serious still, both the mother's and the baby's lives could be in danger. Pre-eclampsia cannot be cured while the woman is still pregnant. All the measures that are taken are meant to control the condition, to allow the fetus to grow to a viable stage. This is why preterm delivery and caesarean section are common and predictable consequences of this condition. On the other hand, if the condition is well controlled, as is sometimes the case, the pregnancy will be allowed to go to term and, with a bit of luck, there will be a spontaneous labour and normal delivery. However, no woman with this condition should convince herself that this is what is aimed for. It should be seen as a bonus if it is achieved.

In this chapter, we set out to answer specific questions about pre-eclampsia and other hypertensive conditions in pregnancy.

Blood pressure in pregnancy

What happens to the blood pressure in pregnancy?

The normal tendency is for the blood pressure to fall slightly during pregnancy. It may reach a nadir about halfway through, at around eighteen to twenty weeks of gestation. It tends to stay there and then may rise back towards the pre-pregnancy levels towards the end of the pregnancy. This is the experience of the majority of pregnant women.

Can the blood pressure fall to a dangerous level?

This is extremely unusual and this possibility can safely be ignored. Occasionally, women may experience light-headedness and feeling faint during pregnancy. This tends to occur on prolonged standing, walking in the sun or rising rapidly from a sitting position. Rarely, actual blackouts have been reported.

What should a woman do if she experiences any of the above?

The sensible thing is to avoid the precipitating factors although it is an unnecessary overkill for the mother to put restrictive limits to her activities, just because she has had the odd feeling of faintness in pregnancy. As a rule, the fall in blood pressure is temporary and lasts a few seconds before the self-regulatory mechanism kicks in to correct it. It should never be an overriding worry.

What about raised blood pressure (hypertension)?

This is a problem.

There is no point in any doctor or midwife trying to say "not to worry" when a mother is noted to have raised blood pressure in pregnancy. The action that is taken is the important issue for the expectant mother to concentrate upon. As raised blood pressure (hypertension) is a vast subject, we shall try to explain it in as concise a way as possible.

How many types of hypertension (in pregnancy) are there?

There are two broad groups. These are:
- pre-existing hypertension
- pregnancy-induced hypertension

Pre-existing hypertension can also be termed "chronic hypertension" or, when the cause is unknown (as is mostly the case), "essential hypertension". If you happen to suffer from hypertension, you will encounter these terms many times.

Pregnancy-induced hypertension is more popularly known as pre-eclampsia and was also once known as "toxaemia of pregnancy", "pre-eclamptic toxaemia" (PET) and, across the Atlantic, "EPH gestosis". These terms may crop up occasionally but they are largely historical now.

Hypertension and pre-eclampsia

What causes pre-existing (chronic) hypertension?

Chronic hypertension is uncommon in the young and starts to become a significant feature in the late thirties and early forties. For the majority of people known to have chronic hypertension, the cause is unknown. That is why this is known as essential hypertension. For the remainder, the hypertension may be associated with such diseases as diabetes, kidney disease or SLE. Obesity is an associated factor.

What causes pre-eclampsia?

As mentioned before, pre-eclampsia is a purely pregnancy-related condition. It does not occur otherwise.

We, do, however, have to be careful here. The classification of hypertensive conditions in pregnancy is not mutually exclusive. Women with pre-existing hypertension are certainly more at risk of developing pre-eclampsia. That is, their uncomplicated hypertension may evolve into pre-eclampsia. Otherwise, the cause of pre-eclampsia remains unknown.

What is the difference between hypertension and pre-eclampsia?

One is part of the other.

Hypertension is simply higher than normal blood pressure. In pregnancy, this is generally taken to be a blood pressure of 140/90 or above. This is a convenient cut-off and not always significant. Its importance differs among individuals.

Pre-eclampsia is a syndrome which includes hypertension and loss of protein in the urine. Almost invariably (but not necessarily) there is oedema.

Is chronic hypertension a risk factor in pregnancy?

Yes, though not to the same extent as pre-eclampsia.

Firstly, there is a tendency among hypertensive expectant mothers to have abnormal blood vessel development in the uterus and placenta. This may mean that the fetus does not get sufficient nutrients and oxygen and the intrauterine growth may be restricted to some degree. This, however, is uncommon in the presence of well-controlled hypertension and in the absence of pre-eclampsia.

Secondly, chronic hypertension could evolve into pre-eclampsia, where the normal antihypertensive medication is ineffective and which may lead to premature delivery.

Thirdly, hypertension is associated with an increased risk of placental abruption, which is the premature separation of the afterbirth, with grave consequences to the fetus and even the mother. This subject is discussed in greater detail in Chapter 19, "Bleeding in Pregnancy".

Should a woman continue to use antihypertensive medication in pregnancy if she suffers from chronic hypertension?

Generally, yes. She should talk to her doctor when trying to conceive, and the doctor will advise her.

The reason is, while continuing to use medication is desirable, there are some types of antihypertensive drugs which have been associated with adverse effects on the growing fetus in the womb or whose safety in relation to the fetus cannot be guaranteed.

In such a situation, the accepted advice is to switch to the type of medication known to be safe in pregnancy. This should ideally be done before conception. When medication has been taken in the critical first ten to twelve weeks of pregnancy, for whatever reason, it is debatable whether advising to change at this stage is worthwhile. The exception will be those types of drugs which affect fetal development. Her doctor, together with her obstetrician, should be able to explain and discuss this with her, depending on what she is taking. There are many classes of antihypertensive drugs and no blanket rule can apply to all or even to most of them.

What should an expectant mother do if she is found to have pre-eclampsia?

The only effective treatment of pre-eclampsia is delivery.

It is therefore important to be clear that, whatever other measures the doctor may institute, the aim is to try to control the condition and not to eliminate it.

Pre-eclampsia can have quite devastating effects on both fetus and mother and the doctor will try to prevent those complications. The doctor will therefore try to ensure that the condition does not worsen; that the fetus continues to grow at an acceptable rate; and that neither the mother's life nor that of the fetus is put at risk.

So what are they likely to do?

She will almost invariably be advised to rest.

Because one of the hallmarks of pre-eclampsia is reduced blood-flow to the uterus, the placenta and ultimately the fetus, rest is meant to make the best of a bad situation. It means that blood which would normally be diverted to the active muscles when the mother engages in physical activities is, with rest, allowed to go to the uterus.

Rest is the mainstay of pre-eclampsia control.

Medication: She may be put on medication to try to control the blood pressure. The sole aim of using antihypertensive medication is to protect the mother from dangerously raised blood pressure, which may cause such things as stroke. It is therefore, purely a complication prevention measure and not a treatment for pre-eclampsia. It does not prevent the core progression of the disease.

Monitoring: The blood pressure will be monitored closely. How closely will depend on how high it is, as well as how abnormal the other parameters are.

What are the other parameters?

Pre-eclampsia can only be diagnosed if the raised blood pressure is accompanied by loss of protein in the urine. This is brought about by the effects of the disease on the kidneys. The mother will, therefore, have her urine checked very frequently for the level of protein loss. This is one of the principal means of determining the progression of the condition. If she is hospitalized, she may have her total urine collected for twenty-four hours, for a quantitative analysis of the protein loss. This is considered superior as a way of analyzing and determining the extent of the protein loss and, by implication, the severity of the condition.

Will she be hospitalized?

She might be. If the obstetrician looking after her feels it unsafe to monitor the condition at home, she may be advised to stay in hospital for a closer, continuous observation of her condition. This will:

- include monitoring symptoms
- monitoring blood pressure
- protein in the urine
- urine output (reduction in amount is not a good sign)
- a battery of blood tests.

If the condition is judged to be only mild, she will be monitored at home, probably with visits from the community midwife; the frequency of the visits could range from daily to twice weekly or so, depending on her obstetrician's assessment and opinion. Rest will, however, be part of any plan of management.

Should the mother read anything into oedema (or swelling) of limbs?

Not much. Eighty per cent of pregnant women have some degree of swelling of limbs – mostly the feet, ankles and fingers (rings are tight!). Some will have gross oedema without any hint of raised blood pressure.

The oedema is largely a function of the normal physiological changes happening during pregnancy.

However, patients with pre-eclampsia have an increased tendency to develop pronounced oedema which may also be more generalized, affecting such unusual areas as the face.

The bottom line, however, is that the presence of oedema does not diagnose pre-eclampsia, and, more significantly, its absence does not rule out the condition or lessen its severity.

What will ultimately be done?

The aim is to ensure delivery of a healthy baby without putting the mother at risk.

If the condition is getting worse in spite of all the measures, immediate delivery is the only option. This is to prevent eclampsia, which could potentially seriously harm both the mother and the baby. It could even kill them.

If the mother is very far from term, the method of delivery is likely to be a caesarean section, as induction of labour is unlikely to be successful – at least, not quickly enough. If she is nearer to term, let's say thirty-five weeks of gestation or more, induction of labour is a viable alternative. The mother's condition will be closely monitored all the time and, if it is seen to be worsening, the induction process may be halted and delivery achieved by caesarean section.

The decision on how to proceed will depend on a combination of factors including the severity of the condition, whether the mother can be induced, fetal condition (which may be compromised), and the mother's own wishes.

Each individual case is unique and there are no fixed rules.

Overall, what are the potential complications of pre-eclampsia?

Apart from affecting the growing fetus, the disease affects various organs in the mother's body.

- The fetus might be retarded in growth and therefore will be very small with all the attendant potential problems.
- There is a high rate of prematurity which is associated with higher rates of morbidity and mortality.
- Premature separation of the afterbirth (placental abruption) may occur. The rate of fetal loss, as a consequence, is very high.
- The mother may suffer vital organ failure, such as liver or kidneys.
- Increased bleeding complications as a result of the inability of blood to clot. This is one of the less common but potentially very serious complications of severe pre-eclampsia.

- Stroke may result from severe pre-eclampsia.
- Eclampsia.

What is eclampsia?

Pre-eclampsia gets its name from the fact that, it is the condition which precedes eclampsia. Historically, eclampsia was an issue because, with less than perfect antenatal care, this was sadly, a common culmination of this syndrome. Nowadays, it is not uncommon for a doctor to go through training and practice to retirement without seeing a case of eclampsia.

Basically, eclampsia is generalized convulsions or seizures with loss of consciousness, indistinguishable from an epileptic seizure. It is the ultimate complication of pre-eclampsia. All measures instituted in pre-eclampsia are geared towards preventing this from happening.

Will delivery prevent eclampsia?

Not always. Delivery is certainly the beginning of the end of pre-eclampsia. There is, however, a critical period of about forty-eight to seventy-two hours following delivery in severe pre-eclampsia, where eclampsia might still happen. That is why intensive monitoring of the condition continues unabated in this period. Eclamptic fits have been reported to occur up to seven days after delivery, but this is so rare that it can be safely discounted.

Occasionally, antihypertensive medication may need to be continued for several weeks after delivery to control the blood pressure. The risk of eclampsia, however, recedes rapidly after delivery and virtually disappears after the first four days. Other potential complications of raised blood pressure, such as stroke, remain – hence the need to ensure well-controlled blood pressure.

Will the pre-eclampsia recur in the next pregnancy?

The odds are that it will not. If this was the mother's first pregnancy, she has a one in four (25 per cent) chance of having the condition in her subsequent pregnancy. If she was affected in her second or later pregnancy, the risk is higher, up to one in two, i.e. 50 per cent.

In a small group of patients, pre-eclampsia recurs in every pregnancy. These women are considered to have an underlying latent essential hypertension.

What are the affected mother's chances of developing chronic hypertension later on in life?

For the majority of women who suffer from pre-eclampsia in one pregnancy (usually the first), the risk is similar to that of the general population, i.e. it is not increased. The story is different for those who experience recurrent pre-eclampsia in each pregnancy. Here, as mentioned before, the risk of chronic hypertension later on in life is significantly above average.

Recurrent pre-eclampsia is therefore regarded as a sign of latent hypertension.

Can one do anything to prevent pre-eclampsia?

No. Medical science as it stands now does not offer any measures to prevent pre-eclampsia from developing.

Are there any factors that increase the risk of pre-eclampsia developing in pregnancy?

Yes, but most will be out of the mother's control.
These include:
- pre-existing hypertension
- multiple pregnancy
- chronic renal disease
- molar pregnancy (*see* Chapter 17, "Cancer and pregnancy")
- diabetes.

There is no evidence that good diabetes control reduces the risk of pre-eclampsia.

What about drug use and pre-eclampsia?

Drug abuse, especially with cocaine has been associated with hypertension and increased risk of placental abruption and fetal loss. It has not been associated with pre-eclampsia.

On the other hand, those who abuse heroin are not advised to withdraw during pregnancy. Instead, a switch to a better-controlled agent in the form of methadone is advised. This is because heroin withdrawal can cause a significant rise in blood pressure. Neither use nor withdrawal is associated with pre-eclampsia.

Can pre-eclampsia cause fetal malformations or abnormalities?

No.

How safe is the oral contraceptive pill after suffering from pre-eclampsia?

Very safe. Once the blood pressure has settled, which may be within two or three weeks of delivery (but occasionally longer) and in the absence of contraindications to its use, the pill can be safely taken.

Note: In the last chapter of this book, there is a section on the most asked questions as compiled by some of the leading pregnancy and childbirth organizations. One of the contributors is APEC, the Association for Pre-eclampsia. There are some very interesting questions addressed there that readers of this chapter are likely to find useful.

15. Problems of amniotic fluid

Introduction

The "waters" or amniotic fluid is a crucial integral part of the pregnancy "unit". There is a womb or uterus carrying the pregnancy, there is the fetus (baby), there is the placenta (afterbirth) and there is amniotic fluid, also known as "liquor". These are the four major components of the pregnancy unit.

In the majority of pregnancies, the amniotic fluid volume is normal. The volume changes according to the stage of the pregnancy. It tends to increase steadily throughout most of the course of the pregnancy, slowing down in the final ten weeks of pregnancy, peaking at about thirty-six weeks before plateauing, and then by thirty-eight weeks starting to go down again. This means that, at each stage of the pregnancy, there is a range of volumes that is considered normal. Any measurements that fall outside of this range are considered abnormal and may be a cause for concern.

Ultrasound scanning is the commonly available means of measuring the volume and tracking the trend of how the volume is changing. It is not perfect but is the best available tool for the job.

The term "oligohydramnios" means below normal fluid volume, while "polyhydramnios", an equal mouthful, means above normal fluid volume. In this chapter, we have set out to explain the possible causes of these, how they are investigated, how the progress of pregnancy is monitored and the possible effects of each.

It is important to emphasize from the outset that in many – if not most – cases, the cause for the fluid volume abnormality is never found and that nothing untoward happens to the baby. None the less, identified cases of abnormal fluid volume need to be investigated because, in those cases where the cause is identifiable, specific action may be imperative to ensure a successful pregnancy.

Amniotic fluid

Where does the fluid around the baby come from?

This fluid is known as amniotic fluid. It is also called liquor.

As the pregnancy grows beyond the twelve-weeks mark, fetal urination becomes the main source of amniotic fluid. The main means of the removal of the fluid is by the fetus swallowing it. This means that there is a continuous circulation of the fluid.

What is the normal volume of fluid?

At each stage of pregnancy, there is a range that is considered normal for that gestation.

When the estimation (usually by ultrasound scan) falls below the lower border of the range, the volume is considered subnormal. Likewise, if it is seen to be above the normal range, the doctor may arrange for some tests to establish the possible cause.

Any experienced midwife or doctor can detect increased amniotic fluid volume on examination alone. Reduced volume can also be suspected through feeling the abdomen, but is not as obvious.

As a rough guide, volumes are about 30 ml at ten weeks, 300 ml at twenty weeks, 600 ml at 30 weeks and about a litre at thirty-eight weeks. Beyond this point, the volume gradually falls and will be about 700 ml at forty weeks and lower still if the pregnancy continues to forty-one or forty-two weeks. It is important to emphasize that these figures are averages and that, at each mentioned stage, there is a range of volumes that will be considered perfectly normal.

Reduced fluid volume

Is reduced amniotic fluid volume a matter for concern?

Yes. Even though, in a good number of cases, no cause for the reduction of the volume is ever established, reduced fluid volume may signal such problems as fetal abnormality, suboptimal placental function, unrecognized rupture of membranes or even wrong dates. Reduced amniotic fluid volume always calls for closer monitoring of the pregnancy.

What sort of fetal abnormalities would one worry about in the presence of reduced fluid volume?

The main concern is kidney or other urinary tract abnormalities.

If the baby has one of the few serious kidney abnormalities that makes them unable to produce urine, then there will be very little – almost undetectable – amniotic fluid. This is usually apparent very early, probably around twenty weeks of gestation. An ultrasound scan will go a long way in establishing the diagnosis but this is not always possible.

If there is a condition that obstructs the flow of the urine, again there will be reduced fluid volume.

As a rule, the defects have to be bilateral (affecting both kidneys) to produce this effect.

Is there anything that can be done in the presence of such abnormalities?

It depends on the diagnosis or potential diagnosis. Some kidney abnormalities are incompatible with life outside the womb. Most obstructive conditions can be relieved before delivery, if this is found to be necessary. This is usually a stopgap measure.

The attending obstetrician will explain in detail what the suspected or confirmed diagnosis is and the proposed course of action.

What about sub-optimal placental function?

If the placenta, for whatever reason, is not functioning efficiently, this may be reflected in reduced amniotic fluid volume. There will also be restricted growth of the fetus.

If these features are apparent, the progress of the pregnancy will be monitored closely and there is a high possibility of induction of labour even before reaching term. Each case is obviously assessed on its own merit, and there is no hard and fast rule.

Can genetic or chromosomal abnormalities cause reduction of fluid volume?

Yes. Some chromosomal abnormalities are characterized by a chronically reduced fluid volume, almost always accompanied by fetal growth restriction. Because many of these abnormalities occur with other physical abnormalities, the diagnosis may be suspected before delivery. If this is the case, fluid could be taken from around the baby (by a procedure called amniocentesis) for analysis, to establish the diagnosis.

Does reduced fluid volume have any adverse effect on the growing fetus?

Yes. The most feared effect is poor lung development. Normal lung development depends on the presence of sufficient amounts of fluid. If the reduced volume starts very early and does not improve, lung development could be very poor and this is an extremely difficult problem to overcome. The severity of this problem also depends on the degree of reduction in the fluid volume.

What are the other complications of low fluid volume?

The baby may be born with limb deformities, which are normally correctable. It is usually the feet that are affected (known as talipes or "club foot"). There is also an increased risk of fetal distress and delivery by caesarean section. As mentioned before, premature delivery – either spontaneous or induced – may be unavoidable.

What about rupture of the membranes ?

Yes, this is also a cause of reduced amniotic fluid volume. In virtually all cases, this is immediately apparent. A complication unique to this is the risk of infection affecting the pregnancy. This increases the risk of losing the baby quite significantly. Labour tends to occur soon after rupture of the membranes: that is, within days. It is, however, not unknown for the pregnancy to continue for several weeks after rupture of the membranes.

Can the membranes reseal after a rupture has occurred?

There is no conclusive evidence that this ever happens.

Can anything be done to prevent infection following a rupture of the membranes?

The main preventative measure is a hands-off approach – literally. This is supplemented with close surveillance, in order to detect infection at an early stage before it establishes itself. Taking antibiotics to prevent infections has not been shown to have any significant effect.

Are there any maternal complications from reduced amniotic fluid?

Not directly. There is the potential complication arising from the primary cause of fluid reduction, for instance, infection in ruptured membranes. There is also the increased risk of caesarean delivery as a result of fetal distress, to which these babies are prone.

Is the cause of reduced amniotic fluid always identifiable?

Not always. It is estimated that even with exhaustive investigations, 10 per cent of cases of reduced amniotic fluid volume remain unexplained.

Is this state of affairs (reduced fluid) known by any special name?

Yes. In medi-speak it is called "oligohydramnios". A situation where the amniotic fluid volume is increased above the normal range is called "polyhydramnios". If they sound like a mouthful, it is because they are! They are worth mentioning though, so if you heard them being bandied about, you would know what was meant.

Can fluid be added artificially in the presence of reduced amniotic fluid volume?

This procedure, called "amnio-infusion", is still in its infancy and its place in mainstream obstetric practice is yet to be established. In this, sterile fluid is injected into the gestational sac. Results in various pilot studies have been variable, some showing moderate benefit and others showing none at all. It certainly needs further evaluation.

Increased fluid volume

What are the probable causes of an increase in the amniotic fluid volume?

There are many known causes of abnormally high amniotic fluid volume. The most common ones include:

- diabetes
- impaired fetal swallowing, because of obstruction in the gut or some kind of paralysis
- increased urine output, which may result from twin-to-twin transfusion or a rare condition known as diabetes insipidus (twin-to-twin transfusion is discussed in Chapter 25, "Twins and multiple pregnancy")
- fetal heart failure – for instance, resulting from severe anaemia or a viral infection affecting the fetal heart.

So diabetes causes increase in fluid volume?

Yes, even though this is not in every case. Any woman who has an unexplained increase in fluid volume – usually in the last ten to twelve weeks of pregnancy – will have a simple blood test to rule out diabetes. If this condition occurs earlier in pregnancy, it is unlikely to be due to diabetes.

What could cause impaired fetal swallowing?

As mentioned before, fetal swallowing is the principle means of removing amniotic fluid from circulation. (The fluid is continually produced and removed, hence the term "circulation".) If swallowing is impaired, there will be an imbalance, as the fluid is being produced but not removed.

Some babies have a developmental anomaly of gut obstruction. This means that although they can swallow, the fluid does not get anywhere. In other babies, the problem is neurological. If the baby has the severe brain anomaly called anencephaly – which in reality means there is no brain tissue – it will be unable to swallow. This condition is almost always recognizable early in pregnancy on the ultrasound scan and will almost certainly be picked up at the eighteen to twenty weeks routine anatomy scan.

There are other conditions that affect the muscles where the fetus is unable to effectively perform any activity requiring the use of muscles, including the act of swallowing: such as an infection caused by a virus called Coxsackie B, which causes temporary paralysis (and clears up in a couple of weeks). In the meantime, the mother will not feel any fetal movements at all.

What could cause the heart of the unborn baby to fail?

The heart is made up of muscle and, to function properly, it requires oxygen. If the amount of oxygen supplied to the heart muscle is insufficient, the heart will gradually fail. This can happen if the fetus is severely anaemic. Such severe anaemia may be caused by a condition destroying the baby's blood-cells – this may happen in a mother with a Rhesus negative blood group if she becomes sensitized: that is, if the fetus is Rhesus positive, when blood-cells from the fetus find their way into the mother's circulation for the first time, they will trigger the production of antibodies against them. If it happens again, this will trigger a bigger production of the antibodies, which attack and destroy Rhesus positive cells. This is the main reason why any Rhesus negative mother should be protected against possible sensitization.

The baby's heart may also fail as a result of infection by some viruses which home in to the heart muscles. This is a rare occurrence. There are various other causes of fetal heart failure which your doctor may wish to discuss with you. They are, however, uncommon.

What makes the fetus produce excessive amounts of urine?

If the fetus has inherited a condition known as diabetes insipidus, then the problem may appear as an increase in fluid volume. Individuals who have this condition have an impairment in the regulatory mechanism in urine production. They end up producing excessive amounts of urine; in the case of the fetus, this overwhelms the fluid removal mechanism.

A relatively commoner cause of excessive urine production by the fetus is in cases of identical twins who develop a complication of twin-to-twin transfusion. This means that one twin's blood is transfused into the other's circulation. The recipient twin tries to cope by increasing its urine production. This condition may cause a rapidly increasing abdominal girth, which may cause extreme discomfort to the mother. It is a dangerous condition that might end up with the loss of one or both twins. (This is discussed further in Chapter 25, "Twins and multiple pregnancy").

What makes a pregnant woman suspect that she has developed increased fluid volume?

It is difficult. Most cases of increased amniotic fluid volume develop insidiously. A midwife or a doctor may be the first person to draw attention to the fact that the fluid may be increased, during a routine examination. Occasionally, the uterine distension produced by the excess fluid may cause abdominal discomfort. This creeps in by stealth. The only exception to this presentation is in twin-to-twin transfusion. Here, the development of excess fluid is rapid and therefore the discomfort appears quickly and can be quite marked and distressing to the mother.

How does excess fluid affect the outcome of the pregnancy?

It depends on the cause of the excess. There is no doubt that, taken overall as a group, excess fluid (polyhydramnios) has a less favourable outcome compared to where fluid volume is normal. However, this is a heterogeneous group covering a wide spectrum.

At one end there is the group with severe abnormalities such as anencephaly (absent brain tissue). This condition is incompatible with life outside the womb. At the other end, there is excess fluid where the cause cannot be found. Almost all of these have a good outcome. In the middle, there are various causes whose result will depend on their cause and how severe it is. It is worth mentioning here that the result of excess fluid associated with gestational diabetes depends on how well-controlled the diabetes is. Poorly controlled diabetes in pregnancy leads to an uncertain – even poor – result.

Does the mother with excess fluid suffer from any adverse effects?

If the abdominal distension is excessive, then there could be considerable discomfort and backache. She may not be able to find a comfortable sleeping position. In extreme cases, she may even get breathless. These are exceptional circumstances.

The risk of a caesarean delivery is higher in this group of women, regardless of the cause of increased fluid volume. This is because the fact that there is excess fluid makes her prone to complications such as placental abruption, abnormal lie of the fetus and premature labour, all of which may make caesarean section unavoidable.

Treating the problems

Are there any effective treatment methods for excess fluid?

Again, treatment will depend on the cause. The mainstay of any treatment regime is to ensure the relief of symptoms for the mother and to prolong pregnancy to prevent prematurity, whenever possible.

Rest is generally advised and avoidance of physical overexertion may be useful in preventing preterm labour.

In conditions like anencephaly, where the baby has no hope of survival outside the womb, termination of pregnancy is advised unless the mother has moral or other objections to this.

Indomethacin is one drug that may be used both to control the amount of amniotic fluid (through reduction of the fetal urine output) and to prolong the pregnancy (through suppression of the uterine activity). It is not always successful and sometimes causes fetal complications of its own; its use is limited to below thirty-five weeks of gestation. In some conditions, such as twin-to-twin transfusion, its use is probably unwise.

What is the most effective method of relieving the symptoms?

In very excessive fluid accumulation, the one effective method of relieving the symptoms is to repeatedly drain the fluid. This is called "amnio-reduction". A certain amount of fluid is removed each time using a long needle through the abdominal wall, under ultrasound guidance. The relief from symptoms usually lasts a short time, certainly not more than a day or two. The procedure has to be repeated several times.

Are there any risks arising from the procedure of amnio-reduction?

Yes. It could lead to rupture of the membranes, which will almost certainly lead to labour within days, if not hours.

The procedure could also provoke a more serious condition in the form of placental abruption which, in most cases, calls for immediate delivery by caesarean section. This could be at an extremely premature stage and the baby may not survive.

The other major risk is that of introducing infection, which may also lead to the baby not surviving.

All these are serious potential complications but are uncommon. Your obstetrician will discuss the situation with you to allow you to decide, on balance, how to proceed. Decisions are never easy in such circumstances.

16. Trauma in pregnancy

Introduction

Sadly, trauma is a fact of life for the pregnant women as much as for others. This may be in the form of a physical assault, a motor traffic accident, a domestic accident or an accident at work.

When a pregnant woman is injured, especially if it is somewhere around the abdomen or pelvis, the ensuing anxiety becomes two-pronged. "Am I all right and is my baby all right?" This concern is readily understandable and explainable. The natural maternal instinct is for the preservation of her child. However, it is also true that nature makes pregnancies fairly safe from considerable trauma, even when this is directly inflicted on the abdomen or pelvis. Miscarriage or premature labour are not common consequences, even of major trauma. However, there may be other less serious consequences of trauma that may call for specific actions. This chapter sets out to explain these and other related questions.

Causes

Is trauma a major issue in pregnancy?

Look at it in this context. Among women of childbearing age (16–45 years), trauma is a leading cause of hospitalization and occupies one of the three top spots in causes of death among people of this age group throughout the Western world. Pregnant women are included in these statistics.

What are the causes of trauma in pregnancy?

Violent assaults – usually from another member of the family – and road traffic accidents are the leading causes of trauma in pregnancy. There are also accidental injuries, sustained at home or in the workplace. Falls are particularly common.

How often does trauma to the pregnant woman lead to fetal loss or premature labour?

This is a difficult, if not impossible, question to answer.

The outcome depends on several independent factors, including the area of injury, the severity of the injury, the gestational age and, not least, the psychological fallout, especially if it was a case of assault.

Area and severity of trauma

What is the importance of the area of injury?

For obvious reasons, the farther the injury is from the abdomen, the better the prospects for the pregnancy. If the injury is completely away from the pregnant uterus, then the prognosis for the pregnancy is good. A direct penetrating trauma to the uterus reduces the prospects for the fetus quite substantially. It is not always so well spelt-out, however. A remote injury could be so severe that part of the treatment could involve the sacrifice of the pregnancy. This is rare.

What about the severity of the injury?

An injury sustained on the pregnant abdomen could lead to fetal demise simply because of its severity. This may be in the form of direct trauma to the fetus itself, or perforation of the womb, with resultant severe internal bleeding.

It could also lacerate the placenta (afterbirth). All these make the fetal prognosis quite poor.

It is said that, in cases of direct abdominal trauma, the baby may protect the mother: how is this?

This is tragic but true role-reversal. In advanced pregnancy, trauma sustained directly on the abdomen, when very severe, may kill the baby but leave the mother in a less serious condition. This is simply because the pregnant uterus offers an effective physical shield against injury to the vital organs in the abdomen.

Even though there have been hundreds of recorded gunshot wounds to the abdomen of pregnant women throughout the twentieth century, the last recorded maternal death from such an injury was in 1912! There are several more advantages to being pregnant than you ever imagined. . .

Why is gestational age of importance?

Direct trauma to the abdomen below twelve weeks of gestation is unlikely to affect the pregnancy, because the uterus is still entirely in the pelvic cavity up to that stage.

Trauma sustained in the early second trimester up to about twenty-four weeks may lead to miscarriage; or if it is twenty-four weeks or beyond, it can cause preterm labour, if it is severe enough. The eventual consequence is pregnancy loss because most severely premature babies are lost, even if born alive.

Penetrating trauma sustained in the latter phase of pregnancy (third trimester) has a 40–70 per cent chance of leading to fetal loss. Indirect trauma leading to preterm labour has a less adverse outcome.

Psychological "fallout" from trauma has been mentioned as a factor in the likely outcome. What does this mean?

Researchers have repeatedly observed that there is no consistent relationship between the severity of the injury and fetal outcome in trauma during pregnancy. This is particularly observed when trauma was a result of inter-personal violence usually involving a husband or boyfriend.

It has been observed that in some cases where the maternal injury severity score was 0 (i.e. virtually no physical injury), the woman went on to lose the pregnancy. It is believed that the weight of mental and psychological distress resulting from the assault leads to this outcome. This is why it is important to ensure that all victims of assault are given not only the medical treatment for the physical injury (if there), but psychological support as well.

Results of trauma

If trauma sustained in pregnancy leads to heavy blood loss, does this put the pregnancy at a particularly increased risk?

Yes. When there is severe haemorrhage as a result of an injury to any part of the body, the body does not classify the pregnant uterus as a vital organ. If you are going into shock, blood will be diverted from your uterus to organs such as your heart, lungs and brain. If you think about it, this is logical. What is the point of ensuring fetal survival, if the mother is going to be killed in the process?

Prolonged shock from severe haemorrhage will almost inevitably lead to fetal loss.

What is the best position for a bleeding pregnant woman who has sustained trauma?

Place her on her left side and avoid putting her in a supine (lying on her back) position. This will allow adequate blood to continue flowing to the fetus. It will also prevent increased bleeding from injured lower limbs, a feature associated with a supine position.

Is caesarean section on the cards for a woman presenting with an injury?

Very much so, but this will depend on a few factors. As a rule, caesarean section will only be considered where fetal viability outside the womb is a realistic prospect.

Caesarean section will be considered in cases of:
- fetal distress that cannot be relieved otherwise
- penetrating injury to the uterus, putting maternal or fetal life at risk
- some forms of spinal injury
- a need for extensive treatment to the mother in the abdominal area where the pregnant uterus is in the way.

Is fetal death an indication for caesarean section?

No. The exception, which is quite uncommon, is where this measure is deemed an essential part of treatment for the injured mother.

If abdominal surgery was performed late in pregnancy but the uterus was left untouched, will this mean an inevitable caesarean delivery?

Not at all. The mother may be anxious that her abdominal scar is still too fresh and therefore not strong enough to withstand the rigours of labour. This is not so and even a two-week-old scar will withstand labour.

If injuries sustained in pregnancy include pelvic fracture, will this necessarily mean a caesarean delivery?

No. Any decision on the method of delivery will depend on the extent and type of fracture, and the duration since it occurred, as well as the usual obstetric considerations.

If the fracture is still unstable, then vaginal delivery is out of the question.

If healing has resulted in no deformity and the fracture occurred at least eight weeks before, then a vaginal delivery is possible.

Is there any risk of ending up with a hysterectomy?

Following severe trauma, it may be impossible to do the necessary life-saving surgical procedure without removing the uterus. In such a situation, the doctor has no choice but to perform a hysterectomy. Also, sometimes attempts to control bleeding from an injured uterus repeatedly fail, putting the woman's life in peril, and a hysterectomy may be the only solution.

It has to be emphasized that such situations and outcomes are rare.

If severe trauma results in maternal death, what are the prospects for the baby?

Pretty dire. Circumstances in most cases dictate that the baby too is lost.

In theory, following cardiac arrest, if the baby is delivered within five minutes, it will be in reasonably good condition. It can still be successfully resuscitated if delivery is within fifteen minutes. Beyond this, survival is unlikely. All this depends on whether the fetus itself sustained a direct injury and whether it was at a viable gestational age.

17. Cancer and pregnancy

Introduction

Cancer. The dreaded word.

Pregnant women are inevitably in their youth or occasionally in their early middle age. This means that they are at risk of those cancers that affect people in this age range. Cancer of the cervix, ovary, breast, blood (leukaemia), skin (melanoma) and lymphatic system (lymphoma) come to mind. While it is true that most of these are commoner in late middle age and beyond, they are also seen in the younger reproductive age groups. This is why roughly one in a thousand pregnant women will be found to have cancer.

This obviously raises very serious questions. Is it treatable? Is the treatment compatible with continuing pregnancy? Will it affect the baby? Should a termination be performed and is this an acceptable proposition? And many more.

Cancers are a very diverse group and no short overall summaries are possible. For some, such as cervical cancer, treatment is required almost promptly or at the very least within a few short weeks of diagnosis to maximize the chances of a favourable outcome. Nor is treatment compatible with continuing pregnancy or even future pregnancy. These facts are discussed in detail here.

Other forms of cancer treatment – such as that of the breast or thyroid – may be compatible with continuing pregnancy, depending on the stage of the disease and the pregnancy itself. Again, all these facts are tackled here. There are never any cut and dried answers with cancer, let alone where pregnancy adds another dimension to the equation.

Cancer and the fetus

Does pregnancy increase the possibility of developing cancer?

No. A woman's risk of developing any of the various forms of cancer remains the same when pregnant.

If a woman develops cancer during pregnancy, will the fetus be affected?

Not directly. The action that is likely to be taken to treat the condition is more likely to have an adverse effect on the fetus than the actual cancer. It depends on the type of cancer, the form of treatment adopted and the stage of pregnancy.

Can the cancer spread to the fetus?

This is exceedingly rare. Only a handful of cases have ever been reported in the world. The working assumption is always that this is not going to happen.

How will cancer diagnosed in pregnancy be treated?

Again, this depends on the type of cancer, the stage of the disease and occasionally the patient's wishes, as we shall see below. If the treatment of choice is radiotherapy, especially in the first half of pregnancy, the fetus is very unlikely to survive: even less so if the cancer is in the pelvic cavity or abdomen.

If chemotherapy is the chosen treatment, this is usually safe for the fetus, provided that the pregnancy has gone past the crucial first twelve weeks during which the fetus's body organs are formed. Chemotherapy used in the last twenty-five weeks of pregnancy cannot cause developmental fetal abnormalities.

If surgery is the treatment of choice, the fetus is usually safe, provided the operation is not on the womb itself.

Does pregnancy make cancer grow faster or more aggressively?

Only one type of cancer – malignant melanoma – has ever been reported to show features of increased aggressiveness during pregnancy. Malignant melanoma is a relatively rare form of skin cancer. It can also arise in the eye. Other forms of cancer behave the same, regardless of pregnancy.

Breast cancer

Is breast cancer more difficult to diagnose in pregnancy?

Unfortunately, yes. Because of the natural changes to the breast consistent with pregnancy, abnormal breast lumps are that little bit more difficult to identify. As a result, diagnosis tends to be late, which consequently substantially reduces the chance of the mother's survival.

Should a woman diagnosed with breast cancer in pregnancy have the pregnancy terminated?

Termination of pregnancy does not influence the course of the disease one way or the other.

If radiotherapy is the chosen form of treatment, then the mother will miscarry anyway.

If treatment is surgery only or surgery and chemotherapy, there is no point in terminating the pregnancy.

The various aspects of the disease will be assessed in each particular patient before she is advised on the options. In advanced disease, where cure is unrealistic, the woman may choose a form of treatment which ensures palliation, as well as continuation of pregnancy.

What advice will be given to a woman with breast cancer regarding breast-feeding?

There is no evidence that breast-feeding will have any adverse effect either on the mother or baby. This is regardless of whether she is on chemotherapy or not.

Should a woman successfully treated for breast cancer be advised against future pregnancy?

Absolutely not. There is no documented evidence to suggest that future pregnancy may trigger recurrence.

Should a woman suspecting a malignant breast lump during pregnancy have a mammogram? Is it safe for the fetus and is it effective in diagnosis?

A mammogram is less reliable in pregnancy because of the changes to the breast. It does, however, have a place – albeit limited – in trying to diagnose breast cancer, even in pregnancy.

As far as the safety of the fetus is concerned, experts agree that the amount of radiation is negligible and the fetus is perfectly safe. The definitive diagnosis, however, depends on needle aspiration of any suspicious lumps for the cells to be analyzed in the laboratory.

It is said that breast-feeding may protect the mother against future development of breast cancer. Is this true?

Yes. Studies have shown that having children confers some protection against future development of breast cancer. This benefit is further increased among those who breast-feed. Women who breast-feed their children have a significantly lower incidence of breast cancer compared to those who never had children or those who did not breast-feed.

How common is breast cancer in pregnancy?

In the Western world, roughly one in every 3000 pregnant women will have breast cancer. The figure is thought to be much lower in developing countries, presumably partly because of the higher prevalence of breast-feeding.

Cancer of the cervix

Is cervical cancer more likely to occur in pregnancy?

No. The behaviour of this type of cancer is the same in pregnancy as in a non-pregnant state. It is one of the commoner malignancies seen during pregnancy, simply because it is a fairly common type of cancer in women of childbearing age.

So what are the symptoms of cervical cancer in pregnancy?

The same as in a non-pregnant state, i.e. abnormal vaginal bleeding, abnormal vaginal discharge and vaginal bleeding following sexual intercourse.

There is usually no pain unless the disease is advanced.

What will be done to diagnose the cancer?

If a woman has symptoms suggestive of cancer of the cervix, colposcopic examination of the cervix will be carried out immediately. This is an examination of the cervix, using a special microscope and applying a special chemical to it. Both the instrument and the chemicals used are perfectly safe in pregnancy. Normally a biopsy (tissue sample) will be taken for histological analysis (i.e. a microscopic examination of the tissue sample), which is the only way the diagnosis can be confirmed or refuted. Further treatment will depend on the results.

If cervical cancer is diagnosed, can the pregnancy still be saved?

If cervical cancer is confirmed, termination of the pregnancy is virtually inevitable. This is because both forms of treatment used in this type of cancer are incompatible with continuing pregnancy. Treatment will either be in the form of surgery (where a hysterectomy will need to be done) or radiotherapy, or occasionally both.

If cervical cancer is discovered in pregnancy and the pregnancy is advanced, is vaginal delivery an option?

Yes. The doctors will need to make a careful assessment of the cancer lesion on the cervix. Because vaginal delivery involves the progressive dilatation (opening) of the cervix in labour, it is important to ensure there is little or no risk of heavy bleeding from the cancer lesion. Vaginal delivery will not worsen the disease in any way. However, most experts will advise caesarean delivery, because surgery for treating the cancer can be carried out at the same time. This will be in the form of a hysterectomy after delivering the baby.

Is there any form of treatment of cervical cancer that still allows for future pregnancy?

No. Cervical cancer is either treated by hysterectomy – where the cervix and the rest of the womb is removed – or radiotherapy, which permanently eliminates the ability of the womb to carry a pregnancy.

What are the criteria for choosing surgery or radiotherapy as the form of treatment?

The extent of the disease. In the early stages, both radio-therapy and surgery are equally effective. In the advanced stages, radiotherapy is the best treatment.

Will a woman treated for cervical cancer go into induced menopause?

Not necessarily. Most experts try to preserve ovarian function in a young woman treated for ovarian cancer, so as to avoid premature menopause. This is not always feasible, in which case hormone replacement therapy (HRT) will be necessary. HRT has no adverse effect on the behaviour of the disease.

If cervical cancer is discovered at a stage of pregnancy where the fetus is unlikely to survive, is it safe to wait for a "few weeks" to allow the survival of the baby before beginning treatment?

This is an extremely difficult question. Obviously, if it is early pregnancy (i.e. below twenty weeks), many experts will find it extremely difficult to consider waiting. In cases over twenty weeks of gestation, where waiting will be confined to two to four weeks, the idea could be given serious thought, if this is what the mother wants. It is impossible to know what is a safe interval between diagnosis and successful treatment of the cancer, as the disease behaves differently in different individuals. Most experts would prefer to start treatment within days of confirming diagnosis, to maximize the chances of a successful treatment.

Ovarian cancer

Should a woman worry if she is found to have an ovarian cyst during her pregnancy?

In most cases, no. Ovarian cysts are rather common in pregnancy, especially in the first half. The overwhelming majority of these cysts are innocent, the so-called "functional cysts".

If an ovarian cyst is found while performing an ultrasound scan of the pelvis in pregnancy, the features are analyzed to see if it looks suspicious. It is usually checked with a follow-up ultrasound. If it appears to be increasing in size or changing in character, an operation will be performed to remove the cyst, usually around sixteen to twenty weeks of gestation. This poses little risk to the pregnancy, is technically not difficult to perform and avoids undue delay in confirming diagnosis. Small cysts of less than 8 cm diameter do not merit any intervention, provided they are not growing.

Are there any other potential complications of an ovarian cyst in pregnancy?

Yes. About one in six large ovarian cysts in pregnancy undergo torsion or twisting, which causes quite severe pain. This normally occurs in the first half of pregnancy and is rarer in advanced pregnancy. Torsion can occur a few days after delivery.

If ovarian cancer is diagnosed during pregnancy, what are the options?

It depends on the type of ovarian cancer, the stage of the disease and the patient's wishes. Most types of ovarian cancer can be treated adequately with surgery where the ovary and tube are removed and the pregnancy is left to continue. This is provided that the disease is caught at an early stage. If it is more advanced, more extensive surgery may be required while still preserving the pregnancy. The surgery will be followed by chemotherapy which, beyond the first twelve to fifteen weeks of pregnancy, is considered safe for the fetus. Surgery can, of course, provoke a miscarriage.

Are there forms of ovarian cancer that require treatment with radiotherapy?

Yes. There is a form of ovarian cancer – relatively common in the younger woman – which responds quite well to radiotherapy. It is called a "dysgerminoma". The best treatment for the disease in the early stages is still surgery but, if it is more advanced, radiotherapy may be necessary for a complete cure. If the diagnosis is made in early pregnancy, the radiotherapy part of treatment may be deferred until the fetus is viable. This approach requires very careful analysis of all the factors and, of course, the mother's wishes.

How common is ovarian cancer in pregnancy?

Rare. The estimated figure is one in 20,000. An average district hospital with 2,500 deliveries per year will encounter a case of ovarian cancer in pregnancy once every eight to ten years.

Malignant melanoma

What is malignant melanoma?

This is a type of cancer, usually of the skin but occasionally arising from the eye; it tends to arise from pigmented "birthmarks" but can appear anywhere on the skin surface.

Why is malignant melanoma especially important in pregnancy?

Firstly, it is relatively common in pregnancy, affecting up to one in every four hundred pregnant women; secondly, it is probably the one malignancy that is definitely known to be adversely affected by pregnancy, being more aggressive at this time; and thirdly, it is one of the very rare forms of cancer which could metastasize (extend to) the placenta and/or the fetus. On a positive note, regression of the cancer can occur following the end of the pregnancy.

Should a pigmented birthmark be considered for surgical removal before trying to conceive?

It is fair to say that most birthmarks will remain innocent and without any changes throughout life. It is, however, prudent to ask a doctor to look at a birthmark, not only before conception but early in life, to see if it may have potential for malignant transformation. Any changes to such lesions, however innocuous they may seem, require immediate medical attention. Such changes may be an increase in size, a change in shape or colour, or development of irritation. There is no time to waste because malignant melanoma can be incredibly aggressive.

What will be the treatment if malignant melanoma is diagnosed in pregnancy?

As in the non-pregnant state, surgery is the mainstay. There is usually no need to terminate the pregnancy. If the disease is discovered at a late stage and surgery is unable to remove the disease entirely, chemotherapy is supplemented. This is not very effective. Radiotherapy is hardly ever useful.

Hodgkin's disease

Why is Hodgkin's disease important in relation to pregnancy?

Only because this is a type of cancer relatively common in young people. The peak incidence of this disease is in the early to mid-thirties. Pregnancy itself has no effect on the disease.

How can one suspect development of Hodgkin's disease?

Enlargement of lymph glands (lymph nodes), especially in the neck area, is the most common presentation. Other symptoms may include fatigue, weight loss and night sweats. Such symptoms should be immediately reported to the doctor. If an enlarged lymph node is found, a biopsy will be taken for analysis. This should establish the diagnosis. The whole process takes only a few days.

Once the diagnosis of Hodgkin's disease is made, what then?

In relative terms, this is a type of cancer with a good prognosis because it responds to treatment. However, most treatment forms are incompatible with pregnancy.

The form of treatment adopted will depend on the stage at which the diagnosis is made. The obstetrician, together with the oncologist (cancer specialist), will explain everything exhaustively for the expectant mother to make an informed choice.

In summary, in the early stages, the disease is best treated with radiotherapy. Termination of pregnancy is necessary, in most cases. However, if the disease is confined to the upper part of the body, a form of shielding of the uterus and its contents is possible. The advanced disease is treated by combined chemotherapy. Unfortunately, the types of drugs used for this disease are incompatible with pregnancy and therefore termination is mandatory. Some patients insist on waiting until the fetus has reached a viable stage before terminating the pregnancy. This is a risky strategy, as the intervening days or weeks could make the difference between successful treatment and missing the boat. The patient is made aware of all these facts.

If a woman is treated with radiotherapy, that is surely the end of her fertile days?

No. The ovaries will be shielded effectively against radiation and fertility after treatment is not usually affected.

What is the effect on fertility after chemotherapy?

There might be reduced fertility following chemotherapy. Hormonal manipulation, sometimes employing the oral contraceptive pill, may help to counteract the adverse effects on the ovary. Combination treatment, where both radiotherapy and chemotherapy have been used, tends to have a more adverse effect on fertility. Even among those who successfully conceive, the rates of both miscarriage and fetal malformation are increased.

What is the advice regarding future pregnancy after successful treatment of Hodgkin's disease?

It is considered wise to wait for at least two years before trying to conceive again. This is because if there is a recurrence in this period, it would inevitably require very aggressive treatment, which will be incompatible with pregnancy.

Molar pregnancy

What is trophoblastic disease?

This is a group of conditions that occur almost exclusively in pregnancy. They range from the benign but potentially malignant hydatidform mole (molar pregnancy) to the frankly malignant choriocarcinoma.

So what exactly is hydatidform mole (molar pregnancy)?

This is a condition where, following conception, the baby does not grow. Instead, tissue consisting only of vesicles (a sac filled with clear fluid) develop. The "pregnant" woman will have normal pregnancy symptoms and body changes. In fact, in some cases, symptoms such as nausea and vomiting may be quite pronounced and may be the first warning of something amiss. It is important to emphasize from the outset that molar pregnancy is not a malignant condition. It appears in this chapter for reasons explained below.

What are the symptoms of molar pregnancy?

There may be exaggerated pregnancy symptoms. This is by
no means always the case. More commonly, the woman will
have light vaginal bleeding or a brownish discharge. More
than half of such patients are found to have a uterus which
feels bigger than the apparent gestation of the pregnancy. A
significant proportion, however, will have the uterus feeling
smaller than the gestation. The diagnosis will be confirmed
by an ultrasound scan which shows a characteristic image.
Very occasionally the patient will pass some vesicles.

What follows the diagnosis of molar pregnancy?

The uterus will be emptied of its contents, usually by suction
curettage under a general anaesthetic.

Occasionally, severe bleeding complicates the procedure
and blood transfusion may be necessary.

What kind of follow-up is required after treatment for molar pregnancy?

Molar pregnancy is a benign condition but with a malignant
potential. The potential remains for several months after the
evacuation of the uterus. Follow-up is recommended for
about one or two years, during which you should not try to
conceive. Most experts consider one year to be adequate.

Follow-up normally involves the patient giving urine
samples at timed intervals, which may be weekly at first, then
fortnightly, monthly and so on. Pregnancy hormone levels in
the urine are quantified. These are expected to fall steeply to
virtually undetectable levels within weeks of the evacuation.
Needless to say, pregnancy, during this follow-up period will
complicate the picture.

What happens if the hormone levels do not fall as expected during the follow-up?

It may mean that the patient has what is known as
"persistent mole", an invasive mole or, more seriously, a
malignant transformation into what is known as choriocarcinoma. Tests will be carried out to verify which is which.
Treatment in the form of chemotherapy will almost certainly
be embarked on. Success with treatment is excellent, even
with choriocarcinoma, provided it is started in time. This is
the essence of close follow-up.

What proportion of molar pregnancies will transform into the malignant form (choriocarcinoma)?

Probably less than 5 per cent. The risk of transformation depends on several factors and is higher among those who have a previous history of molar pregnancy and older mothers (i.e. those above thirty-nine years of age). It is, however, important to say that all affected mothers need the close follow-up.

Are there any known predisposing factors to molar pregnancy?

No. Curiously, this condition is most common in the Far East where, in some countries such as Taiwan, molar pregnancies constitute about 1 per cent of all pregnancies. Compare this with less than 0.05 per cent in western Europe (or one in 2000), which means it is more than twenty times commoner in some countries of the Far East compared to western Europe.

Does this mean it is likely to be environmental or genetic?

No. If it was environmental, you would expect Caucasians in the Far East to have increased incidence, to match the natives of those countries. This has not happened. On the other hand, in countries such as the USA with a large immigrant community from the Far East, the incidence of molar pregnancy appears to be the same as that of other ethnic groups and is nowhere near that seen in their ancestral lands. The important predisposing factors therefore remain elusive.

Does the use of chemotherapy after molar pregnancy mean that it has turned into cancer?

Not at all. About one in five patients with molar pregnancy will need chemotherapy. In fact, for the majority of these, it will be because of what is known as a persistent mole. This is a warning sign that malignant transformation may follow. Chemotherapy is therefore a pre-emptive strike. Less than a quarter of those receiving chemotherapy do so because of a malignant transformation.

What kind of cancer is choriocarcinoma?

This is an aggressive tumour, which is associated with pregnancy in the overwhelming majority of those affected.

The preceding pregnancy could be molar, normal, ectopic or even a miscarriage. The majority (over 50 per cent) of choriocarcinoma follow a molar pregnancy, about a quarter follow normal pregnancy, and a smaller proportion follow miscarriage or ectopic pregnancies.

Choriocarcinoma is fortunately very sensitive to chemotherapy and the cure rate approaches 100 per cent, especially when it is caught in the early stages.

Does choriocarcinoma follow immediately after the pregnancy?

In most cases, it is discovered within days or weeks. Unfortunately, in some cases, it may occur several months – even years – after the initial pregnancy, which may make suspicion and therefore diagnosis quite difficult.

What are the symptoms of choriocarcinoma?

This depends on its timing (following the initial pregnancy) and site. Symptoms may include irregular vaginal bleeding, absence of periods, pelvic pain, chest discomfort and/or a cough, with or without blood-stained sputum. The important thing is for the doctor to suspect it and carry out the necessary diagnostic tests.

Do chest symptoms mean the spread of disease outside the womb?

Yes. Choriocarcinoma can spread to the lungs, liver, spleen, kidneys, brain and other organs. It remains treatable, even at this stage. Spread to the brain makes complete cure a little more difficult, but not impossible.

Following a molar pregnancy, what are the chances of a recurrence in a subsequent pregnancy?

About 1 per cent. However, the probability rises quite exponentially, following two molar pregnancies. This in itself is a rare occurrence.

What is the recommended contraception during the period of follow-up before the all-clear?

The combined oral contraceptive pill is the best method. If this cannot be used, for any particular reason, then barrier methods could be employed. The intrauterine device (coil), though effective, is not recommended in this situation.

Leukaemia

What is leukaemia?

This is simply known as cancer of the blood. In actual fact, it is a cancerous proliferation of the cells in the bone marrow, which gives rise to the different types of blood-cells in circulation. The cancerous cells in the marrow spill over into the circulation. In acute leukaemia (the aggressive form of the disease which can become very serious in a matter of days and, without treatment, can kill the patient in two or three months, as opposed to chronic leukaemia, which is slowly progressive and may go on for years, even without treatment), there will be a severe deficiency of red blood-cells, white blood-cells and platelets. Untreated, death ensues within about three months.

How common is leukaemia in pregnancy?

Acute leukaemia is a disease of the younger age groups. In fact, of cancer-related deaths in the reproductive age group (sixteen to forty years), acute leukaemia is the second most common! In absolute terms, however, it remains rare. The incidence is about one in 75,000 pregnancies. An average district hospital will encounter one pregnant woman with leukaemia once every twenty years or so.

Does pregnancy make leukaemia more likely to occur?

No.

Does pregnancy have an adverse effect on the course of the disease?

In an oblique way, yes. Pregnancy itself will not affect the course of the disease. However, it may actually cause a delay in diagnosis, which could be critical. At the outset, the symptoms of acute leukaemia include non-specific clinical features such as fatigue and breathlessness. These are not uncommon in pregnancy.

A routine blood test at an early stage may reveal anaemia as the only abnormality. Again, this is not uncommon in pregnancy and all the symptoms may be put down to this. The unsuspecting doctor may then send the expectant mother away with a prescription of iron supplements and dietary advice. This can be catastrophic, because a delay of a few days in diagnosis could actually mean the difference between life and death for both the mother and the baby.

Once diagnosed, how is acute leukaemia treated?

There are different types of acute leukaemia and treatment will partly depend on this. Generally speaking, treatment is by combination chemotherapy and the response on the whole is good. This is in the short and medium term. There is usually a period of maintenance therapy, once the condition has gone into remission. Relapse is not uncommon and tends to occur within two to five years.

Can the fetus survive chemotherapy or must there be a termination?

The fetus is not unduly harmed by chemotherapy, unless the diagnosis was made and treatment commenced in very early pregnancy. As a matter of fact, chemotherapy ensures the survival of the fetus through the survival of the mother, who stands no chance without it. Termination of pregnancy does not offer any advantage to the treatment.

What if acute leukaemia is diagnosed before conception?

In such a case, the woman will be advised not to embark on pregnancy and effective contraception should be taken. It is inadvisable to conceive whilst on chemotherapy, since this will expose the embryo to these noxious agents at its most sensitive and vulnerable stage.

Will a woman who has been treated for acute leukaemia retain her ability to have children?

A majority of affected women retain their fertility. Nor will a future pregnancy carry any special risk because of her history.

If acute leukaemia is diagnosed in the first trimester of pregnancy (the first twelve to thirteen weeks), should termination be contemplated then?

In acute leukaemia, there is no time to lose. Once the diagnosis is made, treatment has to commence promptly. If the pregnancy is in its early part, when the embryo is quite vulnerable, there is an increased risk of miscarriage as a result of chemotherapy. There is also a risk of fetal abnormalities as a direct result of this. This risk is estimated to be in the region of 10 per cent. In reality, there is no dilemma posed. Chemotherapy has to be given and one hopes for the best for the fetus. The alternative to this is to withhold treatment, where the outcome is not in doubt: both mother and baby will be lost. Termination of pregnancy simply doesn't feature in the scheme of things.

If a child was exposed to chemotherapy in the womb as a result of leukaemia treatment for the mother, what are his or her long-term prospects?

Leukaemia in pregnancy is a rare condition and whatever we know about children is necessarily based on this very small sample. As such, we have to be cautious in our pronouncements. Insofar as we know, there are no long-term adverse effects on the child as a result of exposure to these drugs in the womb. More information may emerge in the future, which might alter this perception

Can acute leukaemia be transmitted from the mother to the fetus in the womb?

This is so exceedingly rare that it should, to all intents and purposes, be ignored. In the last hundred years, only two cases of maternal to fetus transmission of leukaemia have been reported world-wide.

We have discussed acute leukaemias, what about chronic leukaemias?

There are relatively few cases of chronic leukaemia associated with pregnancy in the medical literature. One type of chronic leukaemia is mainly found in the elderly, so it is exceedingly rare to be associated with pregnancy. This is the chronic lymphocytic leukaemia (CLL).

Overall, chronic leukaemias are much less aggressive and can run a very long course, often with long spells without need for treatment. When chemotherapy is required, if the woman is not pregnant yet but planning to conceive, thorough counselling is mandatory to explore the options. These should include effective contraception during the time of treatment. Chemotherapy immediately before conception or in the early trimester is considered a risk factor (for the fetus) that is best removed by avoiding pregnancy in the meantime. If the woman is already pregnant and chemotherapy begins later on in pregnancy, the only anticipated problems for the fetus are preterm delivery and low birthweight. These are the same problems encountered with chemotherapy use in acute leukaemias.

18. Spina bifida and related abnormalities

Introduction

Spina bifida is one of the many (and probably most widely recognized) anomalies that can affect a developing fetus. Ultrasound has revolutionized the realm of prenatal diagnosis and today – in the developed world, at least – it is unusual for an unrecognized spina bifida baby to be born.

There are other less common but arguably more serious anomalies which affect what is known as the craniospinal column. This is basically made up of the cranium (skull) and the spine. Abnormalities of the skull will range from the most serious anencephaly (where the skull is missing – a condition which is incompatible with life) through hydrocephaly (increased size of head) to microcephaly (small head).

This is a wide field in the sense that there are several "in between" anomalies, and a variety of underlying causes – which may be genetic, or even as a result of infections or alcohol abuse during pregnancy. There is also the fact that many of these conditions may be associated with other abnormalities elsewhere, such as the heart or the gut. It will therefore be presumptuous to say we have given answers to all pertinent questions on this. We have, however, tried to give clear answers to most of the obvious questions on this subject.

Whether a parent will choose to have a termination as a result of a diagnosis of a particular condition is a complex question. While there has been candid imparting of facts about which condition is compatible with life (and which is not), there is a realization on our part that this is not the only important question in this situation. Ultimately, the mother is the one who is going to have to live with the after-effects of her decision, whichever this might be. She is therefore the one best placed to know what she can be at peace with.

One simple but profound "discovery" of the last twenty years is the fact that taking folic acid at no more than 5 mg daily before conception and during the early weeks of pregnancy dramatically reduces the chances of the baby being affected by spina bifida. It is a simple, inexpensive and safe preventative measure. However, as we have emphasized below, the fetal spine is already formed by six weeks of gestation. This stresses the importance of timing in this condition. Any measures instituted after the mother has missed even one period are unlikely to have any effect on this.

And, in the course of setting the record straight, the issue of hydrocephaly needs to be mentioned. This is widely but erroneously known as "water on the brain". In this condition the water is around rather than on the brain. The only abnormality is therefore the increase in the quantity of the fluid, a state of affairs that might stifle brain development.

Spina bifida

What is spina bifida?

This is the most common of a group of abnormalities collectively known as "neural tube defects" (NTDs). The spine is made up of several small bones called vertebrae, which are stuck neatly together. Each vertebra is closed, leaving a hole in the centre. The holes of the spinal vertebrae form a hollow "tube", into which the spinal cord runs. The spinal cord is therefore completely covered all round.

When there is a defect on one or more of the vertebrae, part of the spinal cord will not be covered. This defect is what is known as spina bifida. It is usually on the lower part of the spine.

Are there different types of spina bifida?

There are two major groups. The more serious type – which is immediately obvious – is where only a thin membrane covers the spinal cord from the elements. The less common and less serious "occult" spina bifida is where, even though there is a defect on the bony spine, the skin over the defect is intact.

This may be missed antenatally and could conceivably go unrecognized for years. Only one in ten cases of spina bifida are of this hidden type.

What are the related abnormalities?

These are known as "cephaloceles". Cephaloceles generally mean bone defects on the skull.

Because the skull closure is supposed to take place quite early in pregnancy (before six weeks of gestation), when there is failure of this occurrence, the growing brain may protrude through the defect. In about 10 per cent of spina bifida cases, there is also a cephalocele.

How is spina bifida (or the related neural tube defects) detected?

The screening tests performed early in the second trimester are crucial in this. One of the chemicals looked for in the blood test variably known as the "triple test" or the "double test" is called alpha-fetoprotein or AFP.

AFP is a chemical produced by the fetal liver. It eventually reaches the maternal circulation by diffusion across the placenta.

When there is an open neural tube defect, the amount of AFP that reaches the maternal bloodstream is quite markedly increased. By checking levels of AFP in maternal blood, one can therefore suspect whether there is a significant possibility of a neural tube defect such as spina bifida being present.

What if the neural tube defect is of the closed type?

In such a case, the AFP levels will be normal. This test is therefore not useful in detecting this kind of defect.

Is AFP raised only in cases of neural tube defects?

No. This is why high levels alone are not diagnostic, only suggestive. Such a result only raises the possibility of the presence of such a defect. Other causes of high levels of AFP include:

- abdominal wall defects
- placental tumours
- fetal bowel obstruction
- fetal skin disorders
- fetal growth restriction.

Raised AFP appears to always be a sign of something serious.

Not at all. There are innocent causes such as multiple pregnancy and wrong gestational age. If the pregnancy is more advanced than the mother thinks, levels will be (erroneously) interpreted to be higher than normal.

Not infrequently, the cause of the raised AFP cannot be identified, in spite of an exhaustive search, and the baby is born healthy.

What follows a suspicious blood test result (raised AFP)?

The blood test is ideally done at around sixteen to seventeen weeks of gestation. Once the results have been obtained, a detailed anatomy ultrasound scan will be performed. This will, first of all, establish the gestational age with fairly good accuracy. The margin of error at this stage of pregnancy is one week either way, at most.

The next step will be a systematic search for any possible abnormality. The cranium (skull), spine and the rest of the body will be systematically and minutely examined. A case of spina bifida or a cephalocele is usually fairly easily identified.

How big is the possibility of missing a spina bifida on the scan?

Pretty remote. It is very unusual to miss a neural tube defect. However, like any other technical undertaking, the detection success rate will depend on such factors as the quality of the equipment used (in this case, the ultrasound machine), the expertise and experience of the operator, and the ease with which the procedure is carried out. Marked obesity on the part of the mother can make a detailed ultrasound examination a very difficult undertaking.

Since the chemical AFP used to screen for neural tube defects is not raised in "closed" defects, how sensitive is ultrasound in detecting these?

Very sensitive. The possibility of missing a defect on ultrasound is very low and even then it will occur where the defect is very small and the equipment resolution poor.

Are there any known risk factors which make a mother prone to have a baby with a neural tube defect such as spina bifida?

Yes. A family history of neural tube defect is regarded as a risk factor. In fact, if one or the other parent is affected, the risk is increased ten-fold, compared to the general population rate. The increase in the risk is similar if one of the siblings is so affected.

Even with an affected second degree relative (such as an aunt or uncle), there is some increase in the risk, though modest.

Are there any other known risk factors, apart from family history?

Yes. Diabetics on insulin have an increased risk of about four-fold.

Epileptic mothers taking valproic acid (Epilim) medication at conception and in the immediate period after are also at increased risk.

What is the general population prevalence of neural tube defects?

It actually differs from country to country and from area to area in the same country. In established multi-racial societies like the United States, it has been observed that the rate is twice as high among Caucasians compared to the black community.

In the UK, some parts of Scotland were noted in the late 1970s to have rates which were two or three times higher than the rates in other parts of the country.

As for gender: girls, for some obscure reasons, are more affected than boys.

The overall prevalence is estimated to be one or two per thousand.

What can be done once a diagnosis of spina bifida is confirmed?

This is a difficult and very complex issue. The prognosis of a child affected by spina bifida is difficult to predict accurately and will be influenced by several other factors.

One important factor is to search for the presence of other associated abnormalities such as a cephalocele. Presence of this makes the baby's prospects pretty bleak. It is also important to try and look for abnormalities in other organs such as the heart, lungs and bowel. Presence of such anomalies alongside a spina bifida defect may actually signify a possible underlying genetic or chromosomal disorder. If facilities allow, the specific disorder may be screened for. Such disorders, if confirmed, mean the outlook is bad.

In a case of an isolated spina bifida defect, with no evidence of any other abnormality, the prognosis is significantly better. The management of any such case will involve, among others, the obstetrician, radiologist, clinical geneticist, paediatrician and a paediatric neurologist. This kind of intensive consultation can overwhelm the parents and is always handled carefully, to keep the parents in control.

A detailed discussion with the parents is required to explain the medium and long-term prospects. All questions will be exhaustively answered before the parents make any major decisions. Parents invariably make all the major decisions and are encouraged to take their time in reaching any decisions, which is never easy.

If the spina bifida is isolated and there does not appear to be any underlying genetic disorder, what are the likely long-term prospects for the affected child?

Again, one has to be cautious when pronouncing the long-term prognosis. However the outlook is much better for such a child. For open spina bifida, paralysis of the lower limbs is virtually invariable. Complications such as the development of hydrocephaly may develop but surgical techniques have improved significantly and shunts are used to relieve this with modest success. (Shunts are devices used to shift fluid from the brain channels to the blood circulation.)

Many spina bifida children have now grown into adults who have made a success of their lives. It is important when citing this not to trivialize the considerable problems and obstacles that such a child is bound to face.

What is the situation regarding closed (occult) spina bifida?

As mentioned before, these defects are covered with intact skin. The prognosis is almost always good and these children tend to have no neurological deficit. They are therefore capable of leading full independent lives.

What is the general trend in cases of spina bifida diagnosis?

Overall, most parents opt for termination of pregnancy in cases of "open" spina bifida. Whether this trend will evolve in the opposite direction over time remains to be seen.

What if the diagnosis is that of a cephalocele rather than spina bifida?

As mentioned before, with a cephalocele, the bony defect is on the skull rather than the spine. Again, if what is protruding through the defect is only a fluid-filled bag of membranes, the prognosis is good and the defect can be repaired after delivery.

However, in many cases, the brain itself is protruding through the defect and the head remains abnormally small, so-called "microcephaly". In other cases, there is hydrocephaly with poor brain development. In such cases, there is usually serious neurological deficit and the prognosis for the baby is poor. If there is an associated genetic or chromosomal disorder, then the outlook may verge on the hopeless. Again, the various relevant experts will give their opinion and advice before a decision is made on how to proceed.

If pregnancy has not been terminated and/or the diagnosis is made late in pregnancy, what will be the method of delivery?

Since, in most cases, the situation is unsalvageable, an endeavour is made to achieve a vaginal delivery. If, however, the prognosis for the baby is judged to be promising and where delivery through the vaginal route risks causing trauma, a caesarean section may be opted for.

What are the chances of a cephalocele recurring?

It is rather high, at one in twenty. There is, in other words, a 5 per cent chance of the child in a subsequent pregnancy being similarly affected. Looking at it positively: the child in a subsequent pregnancy has a 95 per cent chance of not being affected.

Anencephaly

What is an anencephaly?

This is a much more serious condition in which there is virtually no brain and most of the skull vault is missing.

What are the prospects for such a baby?

Invariably fatal. Without intervention, a full-term anencephalic baby dies shortly after birth.

Can anencephaly occur together with spina bifida?

Yes. Such a concurrence is not uncommon.

How is anencephaly diagnosed?

If an ultrasound scan is performed after about twelve weeks of gestation, the anomaly is fairly obvious. At eighteen to twenty weeks, when most routine scans are performed, it is almost impossible to miss an anencephaly. It provides a definitive diagnosis.

Alternatively, like in "open" spina bifida, the initial suspicion may arise following a "triple" or a "double" test. Levels of the chemical AFP are markedly elevated with anencephaly, as they are with "open" spina bifida. In fact, these two conditions are the most common causes of raised AFP.

How common is anencephaly?

It is as common as spina bifida and in some areas it has been observed to be more common. The incidence ranges anywhere between one and six per 1000 deliveries.

For some unclear reason, there is a racial difference as well. Anencephaly is less common among the black community and people from south-east Asia, compared to Caucasians.

Like spina bifida, anencephaly affects girls more than boys.

Is anencephaly associated with underlying genetic disorders?

Occasionally, yes. In such cases, even the recurrence rate may be quite high: up to one in four (25 per cent).

Once anencephaly has been diagnosed, what then?

Anencephaly is invariably fatal. In fact, many such babies are stillborn and those born alive survive for minutes or, at most, hours. With such prospects, the doctor will advise the only sensible avenue – which is pregnancy termination.

The mother – for moral, religious or other reasons – may decline and decide to continue with the pregnancy. In such a case, she is given the required antenatal care and support. Most mothers opt for termination.

What are the likely problems if she opts to continue with such a pregnancy?

There are no specific or unique problems associated with an anencephalic pregnancy. However, this pregnancy is more prone to such complications as polyhydramnios. This simply means excessive amounts of amniotic fluid. This can be very uncomfortable and physically distressing. Another potential complication is fetal demise and subsequent stillbirth.

Are there any potential labour problems?

There is a slight increase in the incidence of pregnancy continuing beyond term in such cases. There is also an increased tendency for the fetus to be lying abnormally. This may render labour and vaginal delivery difficult, if not impossible. Apart from these, labour should be expected to be normal.

If an anencephalic baby is born alive, will attempts be made to keep him or her so?

This is neither desirable nor justifiable. It will be cruel to both the mother and the baby to embark on such a pointless endeavour. An anencephalic baby should always be allowed to die peacefully.

Hydrocephalus

What is hydrocephalus?

This condition, also known as "hydrocephaly", is an abnormal enlargement of the head that is caused by abnormal increase in the amount of cerebro-spinal fluid. Hydrocephalus is not a neural tube defect. However, it is frequently associated with these.

What is "cerebro-spinal fluid"?

There are channels within the brain which contain a circulating fluid. This is called cerebro-spinal fluid, by virtue of its location. The short form is CSF. This fluid is continually produced by some parts of the brain and it circulates continuously. If there is an obstruction to the flow of this fluid during fetal life or in early infancy, the fluid builds up. This will squeeze the brain, effectively impeding its growth and causing enlargement of the head, hence hydrocephalus.

Is this occurrence always associated with a neural tube defect such as spina bifida?

Not at all. In the UK, about three per 10,000 babies are born with hydrocephalus not associated with any neural tube defect.

Are there any known causes of congenital hydrocephalus?

There are several known causes. Hydrocephalus may result from a structural abnormality during brain formation, where the fluid channels do not have a free passage.

Another known cause is infection affecting the fetal brain. This may lead to scarring and blockage of the fluid channels.

Obstruction of the fluid channels may also result from bleeding inside the brain or from growth of a tumour.

The list above gives causes of obstruction of the fluid channels. Is this the only mechanism through which hydrocephalus develops?

Channel obstruction is the most common but not the only cause of hydrocephalus. Occasionally, the cause is a defect in the membrane that is responsible for absorption of the fluid. In this case, the fluid continues to be produced but is not removed. The inevitable consequence is fluid build-up and hence hydrocephalus.

There are many cases of hydrocephalus that remain unexplained.

How is hydrocephalus diagnosed?

By using ultrasound. Mild forms of hydrocephalus may be difficult to ascertain and may require several scans over a number of weeks to confirm the diagnosis. When hydrocephalus is advanced, the diagnosis is relatively easier and may not need a repeat scan to confirm.

What happens after the diagnosis of hydrocephalus is confirmed?

A detailed ultrasound examination of the fetus will be made to check whether there are any other associated or concurrent abnormalities. These could be in other organs such as the heart and lungs. A sample of amniotic fluid from around the baby will be taken for analysis. This is to check whether there is any underlying chromosomal disorder.

Once the status has been established, the relevant experts will carefully evaluate the situation to try and determine the possible prognosis. This will then be discussed with the prospective parents, who will be helped to decide on how best to proceed.

What is the likelihood that a hydrocephalic baby has an underlying chromosomal disorder?

About one in ten. That is why this is an important test as it will influence advice given regarding future pregnancies as well.

What are the possibilities and likely scenarios?

If hydrocephalus is isolated with no serious underlying chromosomal aberration, the prognosis is not so bad.

The progression of this condition will be closely monitored and delivery will be planned, depending on how fast the size of the head is increasing. In most cases, delivery is undertaken when fetal lung maturity is reasonably adequate. This could be between thirty and thirty-four weeks of gestation. Occasionally, the pregnancy is allowed to continue further if the progression of the condition is assessed to be very slow.

Delivery is usually, but not always, by caesarean section.

Is there any possibility of hydrocephalus resolving spontaneously?

This has been known to happen but is evidently very rare.

What if progression of the condition is rapid and the fetus is still too immature to survive outside the womb?

There are various methods of trying to relieve pressure on the fetal brain. The most popular is insertion of a shunt, which allows the trapped fluid to flow into the amniotic cavity. It also prevents subsequent build-up.

A decision to perform this procedure is not taken lightly since up to 10 per cent of fetuses are lost as a direct result of the procedure.

It may be unwise to consider a shunt for a fetus that has got other major organ abnormalities and whose prognosis is poor anyway.

What are the prospects of babies diagnosed to have hydrocephalus?

Variable. It has to be emphasized that a respectable percentage of these children grow up to be normal both physically and in intellectual attainment. Others have mild learning difficulties but some will be profoundly retarded. This last group forms roughly 20 per cent of the total.

Early shunting is known to improve the prospects of intellectual outcome.

Is it true that hydrocephalus can occur after birth?

Yes. The same kind of injuries that lead to hydrocephalus in the womb can occur in early infancy and cause this condition to develop.

Meningitis, or a more widespread infection termed "meningo-encephalitis", if occurring in the early months of life, can cause sufficient scarring in the fluid channels in the brain to cause obstruction. Hydrocephalus will follow.

Bleeding inside the brain substance may also lead to the same consequence. Premature infants are particularly prone to this.

Is there any way that this can be prevented?

Meningitis needs to be recognized and treated early and aggressively if such devastating consequences are to be avoided.

For preterm infants, it is strongly believed that administration of vitamin K soon after birth significantly reduces the risk of spontaneous bleeding inside the brain (as well as in other organs).

How does vitamin K work?

It helps to accelerate maturation of the clotting system in the body. Since this system is immature and not very efficient in the newborn (and more so, in the premature infant), the risk of accidental bleeding in vital organs – including the brain and lungs – is substantial. In fact, vitamin K is recommended to be given to all babies at birth, regardless of the gestation.

Where does folic acid come in?

Folic acid is now known for certain to reduce the occurrence of neural tube defects such as spina bifida and the others. For it to be effective, supplements need to be taken in the period before conception and through the weeks of the first trimester of pregnancy. There is no doubt that dietary deficiency of folic acid (or deficiency caused by any other factors) increases the risk of neural tube defects. Epileptic women taking valproic acid (sodium valproate) are particularly advised to use folic acid in the period leading to conception, since use of this drug is associated with a high rate of neural tube defects.

Is hydrocephalus a neural tube defect as well?

No. Folic acid therefore has no role to play in this condition.

19. Bleeding in pregnancy

Introduction

There are few more anxiety-provoking incidents in pregnancy than vaginal bleeding. In early pregnancy, this invokes panic of an impending miscarriage. In spite of the understandable fright, in the majority of cases, the bleeding will pass off unexplained and without any lasting effect on the pregnancy. The figures speak for themselves. In an average pregnant woman where a pregnancy has already been clinically recognized, there is only a 10 per cent chance of a miscarriage before the halfway (twenty weeks) mark. The possibility of late miscarriage or preterm labour is even less – in fact much less – than this.

There is a minority group of women who are more prone to miscarriage than others and where bleeding in early pregnancy will be a comparatively more ominous sign. We explain these facts in detail in this chapter.

Bleeding in early pregnancy may also be an early warning of something wrong with the pregnancy from the outset. Conditions such as ectopic pregnancy, missed abortion and molar pregnancy may have bleeding as the first symptom. It all boils down to one conclusion: each and every case of early pregnancy vaginal bleeding should be investigated. An ultrasound scan, which is a perfectly safe test, will in most cases establish the status of the pregnancy. In many cases, however, it does not settle the question of why there is bleeding.

Bleeding in the later part of the pregnancy is slightly different. It does not necessarily warn of impending labour or delivery. In most cases, the cause remains unknown and it may be a recurrent phenomenon throughout the remainder of the pregnancy. In some cases, it may be a sign of a serious underlying condition, such as placenta praevia or placental abruption. These conditions and their management are fully explained here.

Bleeding at any stage of pregnancy is a cause for concern and should never be ignored. However, it is also true that, in most cases, it will pass without further problems.

Bleeding in early pregnancy

How common is vaginal bleeding in pregnancy?

Very common. It is arguably the most common problem doctors have to deal with among pregnant women.

Is vaginal bleeding in early pregnancy significant?

Yes. No bleeding at any stage of pregnancy should be ignored. For the majority, it is of no consequence, but this fact has to be verified. About one in five pregnant women experience vaginal bleeding in the first twelve to fourteen weeks of pregnancy.

What could cause bleeding at such an early stage of pregnancy?

The causes are many and we can only mention the most common. These are threatened miscarriage, ectopic pregnancy, intrauterine fetal demise and cervical problems.

What proportion of women with early pregnancy vaginal bleeding go on to miscarry?

The first thing that should be done if a pregnant woman has mild or moderate vaginal bleeding is for the doctor to examine her and then perform an ultrasound scan. This will establish where the pregnancy is located (in or outside the womb) and, if it is inside the womb, whether it is viable.

For those where the fetal heartbeat is identified, about 10 per cent will still go on to miscarry. For the remaining 90 per cent, the bleeding stops sooner or later and the pregnancy carries on normally.

How soon can an ultrasound detect the fetal heartbeat?

At five weeks of gestation (calculated from the last menstrual period) the fetal heartbeat is just visible. A clear heartbeat should be seen at six weeks of gestation, if the doctor is using a vaginal probe. If an abdominal probe is used, it may be difficult to detect a heartbeat at five weeks and even at six weeks if the mother is of big build or overweight.

How safe is an ultrasound scan, especially at this stage of the pregnancy?

These machines use sound waves and there is no radiation at all. They have been used extensively over many years now and no adverse effect has been demonstrated. They are considered to be safe.

Does a pregnancy implanting outside the womb (ectopic pregnancy) cause vaginal bleeding?

Yes. This may be one of the warning signs usually (but not necessarily) accompanied by abdominal pain. The symptoms of ectopic pregnancy may occur in all sorts of fashions and bleeding may well be absent.

If the diagnosis turns out to be threatened miscarriage, can anything be done to pre-empt miscarriage?

No. It has to be emphasized that about 90 per cent of threatened miscarriages resolve themselves. There are no measures which the pregnant mother or the doctor can take to influence the outcome.

Surely bed-rest is beneficial if miscarriage in threatening?

No. The standard advice is to try to avoid physical and mental stress. This may actually be achieved by trying to carry on as normally as possible. There is no evidence at all that bed-rest actually improves chances of avoiding a miscarriage. It may be important to focus on the positive – which is the fact that the possibility of a successful resolution is, on the balance of probabilities, really quite high.

How is fetal demise diagnosed?

Sometimes the fetus dies at an early stage of the pregnancy but actual miscarriage does not take place. This is termed "missed abortion". The warning may come in the form of disappearance of the pregnancy symptoms and/or a light blood-stained or dark-brown vaginal discharge. Sometimes there is light vaginal bleeding which tends to be painless. An ultrasound will confirm presence of an intrauterine pregnancy and absence of fetal heartbeat.

How is fetal demise (missed abortion) managed by doctors?

There are options. If there is some doubt to the diagnosis, advice is given to do nothing and have a repeat scan in about a week's time. This will remove any doubts one way or the other.

If the diagnosis is not in doubt, the mother may opt for the conservative approach, where she waits for spontaneous miscarriage to take place; medication may be given to expedite the process of miscarriage. The final alternative is to have the contents of the uterus evacuated surgically, normally under a general anaesthetic. This is a minor procedure which normally takes less than fifteen minutes to perform. The woman is usually fit to go home two or three hours later.

What if an ultrasound scan shows that miscarriage has already taken place?

Then the question the doctor has to answer is whether the miscarriage is complete or whether there are still some products of conception retained in the uterine cavity (known as incomplete abortion). If it is complete, then nothing further need be done. If it is incomplete, then the woman may be given the options of either allowing the miscarriage to complete naturally (provided that the bleeding has settled and appears insignificant) or be taken to theatre to evacuate the remnants.

Is anything else required?

Yes. If the woman's blood group is Rhesus negative, she needs an injection of anti-D. This is administered to all Rhesus negative women who bleed in pregnancy, regardless of the stage of pregnancy and also regardless of whether the pregnancy is still viable or not. It is meant to protect her from developing antibodies in her blood which could have an adverse effect on future pregnancies.

Rhesus positive women require no such injection.

Can this anti-D treatment be administered any other way?

No. It is only in the form of injection.

Bleeding in late pregnancy

What about bleeding in late pregnancy?

If we refer to pregnancy beyond twenty-four weeks of gestation as late pregnancy, then bleeding after this stage is much less common but still a significant problem.

We know that in the first trimester (the first twelve to thirteen weeks), up to 20 per cent of pregnant women will experience vaginal bleeding. After twenty-four weeks, the figure is less than 5 per cent.

What could possibly cause bleeding in late pregnancy?

The causes are many and varied. The important statistic is that in up to 50 per cent of cases, the cause of the bleeding is never established. Among those that are identifiable, the important causes are placenta praevia, placental abruption and cervical pathology.

Placenta praevia

What is placenta praevia?

This basically means that the placenta is low-lying.

Normally, the placenta (afterbirth) is implanted well away from the neck of the womb. In some cases, however, the placenta is very close to and even overlying the opening of the neck of the womb (cervix). This makes it prone to bleed in the course of the pregnancy.

How serious is placenta praevia?

It really depends on the degree of how close it is to the cervical opening. When it is actually covering the cervical opening, it is very serious indeed and most obstetricians will admit such a patient to hospital at a certain stage of the pregnancy, to stay in for the remainder of the pregnancy.

This is even in the absence of any bleeding. The main

reason is because bleeding in major placenta praevia can be so abrupt and heavy as to endanger the lives of both mother and fetus within minutes.

Are all patients with placenta praevia delivered by caesarean section?

The majority are. Only the ones with minor placenta praevia (and all else being well) are actually allowed to have vaginal delivery. The attending obstetrician should be able to explain why he or she is advising a particular method of delivery.

What about the timing of the delivery in cases of placenta praevia?

In the absence of bleeding, efforts will be made to allow the pregnancy to get as close to term as possible. Of course, if it is major placenta praevia, the final weeks – which may be as many as six to ten – will be spent in hospital. The aim is to prevent unnecessary prematurity, whenever possible. If the mother starts bleeding and if bleeding is heavy or recurrent, then there will be no option but to deliver the baby.

Some mothers with placenta praevia have no symptoms until they suffer from heavy vaginal bleeding and delivery has to be made immediately. Delivery before thirty-seven weeks of gestation will have to be carried out in almost 40 per cent of such mothers.

Does this mean prematurity is a serious problem in cases of placenta praevia?

Yes. In fact, it is the leading cause of losing a baby, in this condition: the loss of babies born before twenty-eight weeks of gestation is very high. Even those who survive suffer from significant illness because of prematurity.

Are there any other problems associated with the diagnosis of placenta praevia?

Yes. Growth restriction of the fetus in the womb is commoner among women with placenta praevia, affecting almost one in six of them – a much higher incidence than in most pregnant women.

The risk of serious malformations of the fetus are also almost doubled.

For the mother herself, there is the dramatically increased risk of caesarean delivery, serious blood loss (even after delivery), and increased susceptibility to infection in the post-delivery period.

Should a woman panic if she is told that she has a low-lying placenta at her eighteen to twenty weeks ultrasound scan?

No. About 18 per cent of all pregnant women (almost one in five) have a low-lying placenta at that stage of the pregnancy.

At term, only about 2 per cent (one in fifty) have placenta praevia. For the majority, changes in the course of the pregnancy result in the placenta being in a normal location. However, if a woman said to have a low-lying placenta at twenty weeks bleeds vaginally at any point, she should see her doctor promptly. She might turn out to be one of the few with whom the placental location remains low.

There is normally no indication to arrange a routine repeat scan, as this will be done whenever there is a clinical indication.

Are there any known causes of placenta praevia?

No causes are known but there are certainly predisposing factors. These include:

- multiple pregnancy (twins or more)
- multiple previous deliveries,
- older mothers (above age thirty-five)
- previous caesarean section
- smoking during pregnancy.

Does placenta praevia recur?

Yes, but not that commonly. It recurs in about 5 per cent of affected women.

Placental abruption

What is placental abruption?

This is the separation or detachment of the placenta from its implantation site during pregnancy. The placenta is supposed to remain attached to its base until the baby has been delivered. If detachment occurs any time before, that is placental abruption or "abruptio placenta", as the condition is classically known.

It sounds like a serious pregnancy complication

Yes, it is. Of course, the outcome depends on when it occurs during the pregnancy and the extent of the detachment.

What are the symptoms of placental abruption?

Normally, abdominal pain and vaginal bleeding. It can, however, occur with no revealed bleeding at all and only with abdominal pain which varies in intensity.

Is placental abruption dangerous?

Yes. When the bleeding is heavy – which is not uncommon in this condition – the pregnant woman will go into shock quite quickly. The bleeding can also cause other complications. Even after delivery, bleeding may still be a difficult problem to contain. Placental abruption causes maternal deaths and between 1984 and 1987, four women died in England and Wales as a consequence of placental abruption.

The baby fares badly, too. Figures published in various developed countries show that anything between 14 and 65 per cent of these babies are lost as a direct consequence. Half of these are stillborn, the remainder dying shortly after birth.

Are there any other problems?

Yes. Babies in pregnancies affected by this condition tend to be growth-restricted. In fact, four out of five such babies will have some degree of growth restriction at birth.

The birth itself is also usually premature.

These babies are also more prone to have major malformations – almost twice the average expected rate.

By the nature of the condition, even a baby born alive may have quite severe anaemia, requiring emergency transfusion soon after birth.

Are there any predisposing factors to placental abruption?

Yes. Hypertension is the most significant risk factor; this is regardless of whether this is pre-existing or it developed during pregnancy. Other risk factors are:

- trauma, especially if it is directly to the abdomen
- cigarette smoking
- drug abuse, particularly cocaine
- older mothers (over thirty-five years).

In a significant proportion of affected mothers, no risk factor can be identified.

Does placental abruption recur?

Yes, there is a tendency for this to happen. If you have had one abruption, the risk of this recurring in a subsequent pregnancy is one in twenty, that is about 5 per cent. If it occurs in two consecutive pregnancies, the risk jumps to one in four, i.e. about 25 per cent. Pregnancies following an abruption are regarded as high risk and are managed as such.

Can an ultrasound scan diagnose abruption?

The diagnosis of this condition is largely clinical: that is, it depends on the symptoms a woman has and the doctor's findings on examination. A scan has a very small role to play in diagnosis and will miss well over 90 per cent of abruption cases. It is, however, useful in verifying the condition of the fetus when the diagnosis is made or suspected.

A special blood test may confirm the diagnosis by identifying the presence of fetal cells in the mother's circulation.

What is the method of delivery?

This depends on several factors. If there is significant abruption and the fetus is alive, the only option is an emergency caesarean delivery. Several factors do influence the method and timing of delivery:

- Gestational age: if the fetus is severely premature and there is no realistic chance of survival outside the womb, a caesarean section is probably unwise, unless the extent of bleeding makes it unavoidable.
- If the bleeding is not continuous but assessment shows that vaginal delivery is unlikely to be achieved in a reasonable space of time, then a caesarean section becomes inevitable.
- If the woman is already in labour and the fetal condition is stable, then vaginal delivery may be aimed for.
- If the baby is dead and the patient is stable, the strategy is usually a vaginal delivery. If she is not already in labour, this is usually induced.

Cervical bleeding

How common is bleeding from the cervix during pregnancy?

Fairly common, in relative terms. Minor – usually painless – vaginal bleeding is experienced by many women during pregnancy. Examination may reveal that the bleeding is coming from the cervix. This is usually a result of what is popularly known as cervical erosion, a common occurrence during pregnancy and among those taking the pill.

It is important to emphasize the fact that erosion is an erroneous term because there is no actual erosion. The main point is that the changes make the cervix prone to easy bleeding. Bleeding from the cervix may be provoked by sexual intercourse or douching. It may also occur unprovoked.

The cervix may also bleed as a result of inflammation, a condition known as "cervicitis". Bleeding is typically light and self-limiting. It may be recurrent.

What is a show?

Labour is normally preceded by a "show". This is usually a mucous plug which is occasionally blood-stained; the blood accompanying the show could be substantial, to the extent of causing anxiety. The early contraction pains and/or backache may reinforce the anxiety that something is wrong. In any case, any bleeding in pregnancy should be verified by an expert.

20. Smoking and alcohol use in pregnancy

Introduction

In the UK, two depressing statistics are: one, that about 28 per cent of the population are smokers and two, that young girls are overtaking boys on the uptake of smoking. All this means that smoking is a major issue in pregnancy and childbirth.

These are general facts in the public arena: that smoking is likely to cause fetal growth restriction in the womb (with all the spin-off consequences of this), that the baby of a smoking mother (or father) is more prone to cot death and that the child is several times more likely to suffer from glue-ear. There are other less well-known facts such as the increase in the likelihood of preterm labour and fetal death in the womb.

However independently minded a prospective mother might be, she will in most cases concede that pregnancy does import an added responsibility on her. This is the well-being of another person. As such, pregnancy quite often turns out to be the time when the mother faces up to her lifestyle and examines whether she should continue smoking or not. Many women find this to be that elusive impetus they needed to quit smoking.

And alcohol . . .

The effects of alcohol on pregnancy are quite different from those of smoking. There is no doubt that alcohol in moderation is safe in pregnancy. However, heavy and sustained drinking in pregnancy has a potential for serious adverse effects, which may include a profoundly disabled child. The issue of alcohol use and abuse is a broad one and is not confined to the narrow question of whether the baby will be affected or not. There are other relevant facts: that an alcohol-dependent mother is more prone to physical trauma and life-threatening infections such as Hepatitis B, HIV etc. There are also other ramifications – all laid bare in this chapter.

Cigarette-smoking and alcohol abuse can never be good for the pregnancy: that much is made clear here. What is probably more important is the fact that there is no room for indifference, either.

Smoking

What are the likely effects of smoking during pregnancy?

There is no doubt that smoking is bad for your pregnancy. Among the likely adverse effects of this habit are spontaneous miscarriage, low birth-weight, bleeding conditions in pregnancy (APH), and increase in the perinatal mortality (the death of the baby just before or soon after birth).

Why is smoking in pregnancy harmful?

When you smoke, you are sending nicotine, carbon monoxide and cyanide into your circulation. These act to reduce oxygen supply to the growing baby. The higher the amount of nicotine in the cigarette brand you smoke and the higher the number of cigarettes smoked daily, the higher the risk of adverse effects. No rate of smoking is considered completely safe.

Why would smoking increase the risk of bleeding complication in pregnancy?

It is a direct effect of the reduced oxygenation of the afterbirth. The two major causes of bleeding in pregnancy – which are placental abruption and placenta praevia – are both more common among smokers. Both these complications can lead to fetal loss, with placental abruption being riskier.

Why is low birth-weight so bad?

This is a direct result of the fetus being subjected to chronic oxygen starvation. It increases the risk of death or illness at birth. A small fetus copes less well with the stresses and strains of labour and this increases the risk of emergency caesarean section.

Why is baby loss higher among mothers who smoke?

Death of the baby at or just before birth is twice as high among mothers who smoke in pregnancy compared to those who do not. These babies are lost as a result of an increase in complications such as severe bleeding in a pregnancy, preterm delivery and preterm rupture of membranes, all of which could be a direct consequence of smoking.

Surely spontaneous miscarriage cannot be blamed on smoking?

Rates of spontaneous miscarriage are over 25 per cent higher among smokers and, in England and Wales alone, over 4000 miscarriages are directly blamed on maternal smoking every year. It is thought that in the older mother (over 35 years of age), smoking may increase the risk of chromosomal anomalies, which in turn increases the risk of miscarriage further still.

Is the mother who smokes out of the woods, once she has delivered safely?

Unfortunately not. Cot death has been partly blamed on parental smoking. The risk of this happening to the baby of a mother who smokes is calculated to be increased two to five times compared to those in non-smoking households. In fact, a quarter of all cot deaths are directly attributable to maternal smoking, especially if death occurs in the first ten weeks of life.

Are there any long-term effects of smoking?

Children born to smokers on average suffer more from poor physical and intellectual growth. In fact, the latter is quite marked and study after study has shown that educational attainment is significantly lower for those children whose mothers smoked during pregnancy and after birth. On the physical front, though less marked, they achieve lower weight and height.

Is it beneficial to stop smoking during pregnancy?

Yes. The damage from smoking is cumulative. When you stop smoking, you halve the damage. Obviously, the earlier you stop, the bigger the benefit to your baby.

Moreover, since smoking has all sorts of health problems for pregnant women as well, pregnancy is a good time to quit smoking permanently. Certainly, the incentive is bigger. In the UK, about 30 per cent of smoking mothers manage to stop smoking during pregnancy. Over half of these stay off cigarettes permanently.

Are there any other problems for the child?

Yes. If you are a smoker, your child is at increased risk of suffering from asthma and "glue ear", a leading cause of deafness in children. Moreover, if you are planning to breast-feed, you may find it quite problematic because smoking interferes with milk production.

Will stopping smoking during pregnancy have any adverse effect on the baby?

Absolutely none. It may be very difficult to achieve and sustain on your part but, once achieved, all you have done to yourself and your baby is good.

Alcohol

Does alcohol consumption during pregnancy have any adverse effects?

Yes. The extent of the negative effect on the baby depends on the amount consumed during the course of the pregnancy.

Does this mean there is a degree of drinking that is considered safe?

Yes. An average consumption of fifteen units of alcohol per week has not been shown to have any adverse effect. This message has to be given with a note of caution. Since biological phenomena hardly ever obey strict rules, it is probably wiser to stick below this level. Any person who averages fifteen units per week is certainly not dependent and cutting down should be quite easy.

What are the adverse effects of alcohol?

A moderately heavy drinker – at an average consumption of eighteen to twenty units per week – runs the risk of ending up with a low birth-weight baby. Smaller babies are more likely to suffer illness in the immediate post-delivery period.

A heavy drinker imbibing more than twenty units of alcohol per week runs a far more serious risk. This is in the form of what is known as "fetal alcohol syndrome". This syndrome is characterized by fetal growth restriction (worse than that seen in moderate drinking), neurological abnormalities, developmental delay, intellectual impairment and facial deformities.

How common is fetal alcohol syndrome?

Statistics differ from country to country. In the UK, no national figures are available but in France, thirty-three babies are born with this very serious condition out of every 10,000 live births. The figure is seventeen per 10,000 in Sweden. There is no strict consistency in the susceptibility to the condition and other factors such as smoking, drug abuse and nutritional deficiencies may play a part. It is, however, true that with alcohol intake in excess of eight units per day (fifty-six units per week), the risk is very high indeed.

Do all such heavy drinkers end up with babies with fetal alcohol syndrome?

No. In fact, only about one in three such mothers deliver babies with the condition. This reinforces the assumption that the condition is due to a number of factors, though heavy alcohol intake is crucial.

What is a unit of alcohol?

It is equivalent to 10 grams of alcohol. This is found in:
- one glass of wine
- half a pint of beer, lager or cider
- one measure of a "short", if you are drinking spirits.

Is fetal alcohol syndrome immediately recognizable at birth?

Not always, especially if the history of alcohol abuse is not known to the health professionals looking after the mother and the facial deformities are not immediately obvious. In such a case, the warning may come late with the manifestations of neurological abnormalities. This may be in the form of infant irritability and hyperactivity, later still.

Intellectual impairment will be manifest in due course.

Is fetal alcohol syndrome that serious?

There is no doubt about it. In the USA, it is the leading documented cause of mental retardation.

That is the baby; what about the mother?

Excessive alcohol consumption has all the dangers to the mother in pregnancy as in the non-pregnant state. It may affect her health (weakening it), and may have adverse effects on the liver, pancreas and the brain. Some of these may be serious and life-threatening.

Should a pregnant mother be weaned off alcohol, if she is using it in excess?

Yes. However, since this may be difficult – to the extent of using medication to control withdrawal symptoms – admission into hospital is necessary. The acute detoxification period may last for anything between three and seven days. The period immediately after should be used to identify and start correcting nutritional deficiencies. Vitamin supplements are required, in most cases.

Does "Antabuse" have a role to play in weaning a pregnant mother off alcohol?

No. This is a drug whose real name is disulfiram. It is not used in pregnancy as its safety to the fetus cannot be guaranteed.

If I am an excessive drinker and have become dependent, can I just stop without medical help?

This is not advised. Withdrawal symptoms can be devastating and may endanger life and limb. Epilepsy-like grand mal seizures may occur within a day of stopping the alcohol. If you are alcohol-dependent, withdrawal should be done in hospital or in a dedicated detoxification centre.

What happens after delivery?

If the mother has made a successful withdrawal during her pregnancy, then the achievement should be reinforced in the postnatal period. Counselling, support and self-help measures will be instituted and maintained, to help her stop drifting back into dependency.

Should a woman taking excess alcohol consider breast-feeding?

This is controversial. Alcohol is secreted freely in breast-milk and the breast-fed baby gets as much alcohol as the mother. By virtue of this fact alone, it may be wise to consider not to breast-feed. An additional disincentive is the fact that alcohol has an inhibitory effect on milk production, which could lead to the baby not getting enough and therefore being irritable, which in turn leads the mother to more alcohol abuse, her crutch in any sort of crisis – a classic vicious circle.

21. Drug abuse in pregnancy

Introduction

Drug abuse is a scourge that is now a fact of life and has to be confronted as such. While it has, mercifully, remained a "minority sport", some communities in the UK and elsewhere have been quite significantly hit.

Pregnancy adds a new dimension to the whole issue of drug abuse. There are various groups of drugs that have different effects on pregnancy, some more serious than others. It is important to stress that no abused drug is considered safe in pregnancy. The management of a situation where a woman conceives while dependent on a substance will depend on the type of substance and the degree of addiction.

For some – such as cocaine, which has several different effects on the central nervous system – the only logical management option is withdrawal. Let's not kid ourselves: this may not be easy. In fact, it could be extremely difficult, needing the admission of the mother into a specialist detoxification unit. For other drugs, such as heroin, various options may be available, as detailed in this chapter.

Various other substances have also been dealt with here.

Substance abuse goes much further than the narrow perspective of what is likely to happen to the fetus in the womb. The wider issues are discussed here.

Heroin

How does heroin abuse affect pregnancy?

The spectrum of adverse effects to the fetus range from premature delivery, through growth restriction to stillbirth. Nor does the problem stop at delivery, as such babies suffer serious withdrawal symptoms, needing treatment which may last several days, even weeks. More than half of heroin addict babies are born prematurely; a substantial proportion of these do not make it.

What is the alternative to heroin?

If you are already addicted to heroin and you find yourself pregnant, the advice is to switch to methadone, which is a related drug. Methadone is administered at scheduled intervals (as opposed to haphazard heroin use) which helps to keep blood levels of the drug relatively stable. This helps minimize withdrawal, which is the scourge of heroin addiction for both mother and baby.

If I am already on methadone, should I wean myself off when pregnant?

Preferably not. If you do this, you are likely to unleash withdrawal in the fetus, which could be disastrous. Continue taking methadone as per schedule and, with expert help, careful attempts to reduce the amounts taken could be started, if this is desired. Attempts to quit altogether, though noble, should only be made after delivery.

If I use methadone in pregnancy, will my baby not suffer from withdrawal when he or she is born?

This is inevitable. The degree of withdrawal symptoms will depend on the dose of methadone you were maintained on: i.e. the higher the dose, the more severe the withdrawal symptoms. About one in five babies of such mothers have withdrawal symptoms mild enough not to require any treatment; for the rest, some kind of treatment will be required.

Does withdrawal occur immediately after the baby is born?

Unfortunately not. Methadone withdrawal in the baby will occur several days – sometimes more than a week – after delivery. This means it may all happen after the mother has been discharged from hospital. It is therefore important that the mother should know the withdrawal symptoms, to enable her to seek medical attention quickly and in time.

What are the methadone withdrawal symptoms in babies?

These include:
- severe irritability
- restlessness,
- a high-pitched cry
- refusing to feed,
- rapid and laboured breathing
- general distress.

These are similar to heroin withdrawal symptoms, except that with heroin, the symptoms appear within a day or two after delivery.

Can I breast-feed if I am on heroin or methadone?

Small amounts of both these drugs cross into the milk. If you cannot stop the drug habit, you should consider bottle-feeding.

Cocaine

If I am abusing cocaine in pregnancy, what are the likely adverse effects to the fetus?

The fetus of a cocaine-abusing mother is in peril throughout the course of the pregnancy. The miscarriage rate among cocaine abusers is more than double that of non-abusers. For those fetuses who survive to the second half of the pregnancy, a substantial proportion will be found to be growth-restricted and many are born prematurely. At least one in twenty will be stillborn, a far higher rate than in non-users. The rate of placental abruption (premature separation of the afterbirth) is also high and most of the affected babies die.

In fact, this complication is life-threatening to the mother as well. Any mother using cocaine in pregnancy should remember these five complications, since she is a prime candidate: miscarriage, growth restriction, prematurity, stillbirth and placental abruption.

It is a pretty dire picture; what is one to do?

The only way to avoid these problems is to stop abusing the drug. This may be difficult but there is really no alternative.

If I manage to scrape through and deliver a healthy baby, am I in the clear?

No. First of all, your baby may have various forms of major malformation as a direct consequence of being exposed to the drug in the womb.

Secondly, the baby will suffer severe withdrawal symptoms requiring hospitalization.

Thirdly, and more ominous, is that the baby is at great risk of cot death. The rate of this among cocaine-abusing mothers is increased more than thirty-fold compared to the general population.

Should I breast-feed if I am still using cocaine?

Don't even consider it. Cocaine appears in breast-milk in significant quantities and its effects on the baby could be catastrophic.

Is a baby born to a cocaine-abusing mother at risk of anything other than the mentioned cot death?

The baby may have abnormalities of the visual system. Haemorrhages of the retina in the eyes are rather common and the effects could be long-lasting.

There is evidence also that children exposed to cocaine in the uterus are more likely to suffer from attention-deficit disorders when compared to the general population.

Cannabis

What about use of cannabis (marijuana)?

There are, without doubt, a number of people who would baulk at the term "abuse" in reference to cannabis use. We will not attempt here to argue the merits of this debate one way or the other. But, when it comes to pregnancy, cannabis use is undoubtedly a bad idea. Many of the adverse effects of cigarette smoking can be encountered with cannabis use. Of course, research on this has repeatedly been frustrated by the fact that many – if not most – of those who use cannabis are cigarette smokers as well.

What is known for sure is that cannabis use independently causes intrauterine growth restriction with all the potential problems associated with this. It also causes fetal malformations occasionally, with babies born with dysmorphic features. The baby may display behavioural and sleep abnormalities, especially in the first few weeks. There may be delay in cognitive development as well.

When a woman using cannabis becomes pregnant, she should be encouraged to give up. This is safe to do during pregnancy. Most, if not all, hospitals have got rehabilitation units where individuals with a problem of substance abuse are helped by professionals to give up. Such a woman should be referred to such a unit.

22. Taking medicines during pregnancy

Introduction

It is a fact of life that many – probably most – pregnant women are prescribed medicine for brief or even prolonged periods during their pregnancy. It is also true that since the 1960s and 70s, medication use during pregnancy has significantly declined.

Prescription drugs used mostly include the common supplements, such as iron and folic acid. Also used commonly are drugs to combat "morning sickness" (anti-emetics), painkillers and laxatives to combat the common complaint of constipation.

Antibiotics are also frequently prescribed, especially for urinary tract infections, a relatively common problem in pregnancy. There are several other groups of drugs used during pregnancy.

Common to all these is the question: are they safe? After the tragedy of thalidomide, this is no longer an idle muse.

As a general, rather sweeping, statement: the majority of drugs prescribed during pregnancy are perfectly safe for the majority of women. A significant proportion of pregnant women throughout the world use iron. It is safe. However, it may not be safe for women with conditions such as sickle cell disease or thalassaemia, common among people of African and Mediterranean descent respectively. These facts need to be established. Penicillin is a widely used antibiotic that is quite safe at any stage of the pregnancy, but some people are allergic to them – so this fact needs to be established as well.

Some antibiotics are unsafe only at a certain stage of pregnancy, so the doctor needs to be sure of the gestation when prescribing them.

All these and many other issues pertaining to the subject of medication during pregnancy are discussed in this chapter.

Drugs and their effects

How common is the use of prescription and non-prescription drugs during pregnancy?

Fairly common. In the UK, three to four out of every ten pregnant women take some kind of medicine at least once during their pregnancies. This does not include iron or folic acid. In the USA, the figure is considerably higher.

What sort of medicines do women take commonly during pregnancy?

Mostly are the simple painkillers, paracetamol being the leader. Also commonly taken are antibiotics and drugs to relieve heartburn (antacids).

Non-prescription medicines are taken far less nowadays, compared to twenty or thirty years ago.

The main concern of many, if not all, pregnant women, is the transfer of the drug across the placenta to the fetus. What is the general rule?

It is important to know that most drugs are transferred across the placenta to the fetus. The main issues are the rate of transfer, which differs from drug to drug, and the effect the drug is likely to have on the fetus. These will be discussed in due course.

What proportion of birth defects can be blamed on medicine taken during pregnancy?

The figure is not known for sure. However, in the Western world, where approximate figures are available, it is estimated that about one in forty (2.5 per cent) of babies born with defects end up that way because of medicines takes by the mother during pregnancy.

This is about one in 1500 of all newborns, since babies with birth defects account for 2–3 per cent of all newborns.

Is there a particular period in pregnancy which can be described as especially sensitive?

Yes. The embryonic phase of pregnancy, which stretches up to the eighth week, is particularly sensitive to any foreign chemicals. This is the time when organs are being formed. Any damage occurring at this stage is irreversible. A word of caution: not all types of medication will cause damage to the fetus, even if taken in this sensitive period, and some medications taken outside this period could still inflict harm.

Antibiotics

What are the antibiotics considered to be safe at any stage of pregnancy?

Penicillin is known by several different names and is known to be safe. Common penicillin drugs include amoxycillin, cloxacillin and methicillin. There are many other types.

Another group of antibiotics which are not known to cause any harm to the fetus are the cephalosporins. These too are known in a variety of names. Those commonly used include cephradine, cefuroxime, cefotaxime, cephalexin, cefaclor, and cefadroxil.

What about tetracyclines?

These are known to be harmful in the second half of pregnancy, where they can be incorporated in the developing bones and the forming teeth. With the latter, the discoloration caused is permanent.

Even though the confirmed harm appears to be confined to the second half of pregnancy, the standard advice is to avoid them throughout pregnancy. The advice also applies to the period after delivery, if the mother is breast-feeding.

What about trimethoprim?

This drug, which is commonly prescribed for urinary tract infection, is frowned upon by most doctors when it comes to use in pregnancy. There is a theoretical risk, yet to be confirmed, that the baby may be harmed. Most doctors would prefer to use alternatives.

What about septrin (Co-trimoxazole)?

Septrin is a well known antibacterial drug. Its actual name is Co-trimoxazole. It is actually a combination of two drugs, one of which is trimethoprim. Because of the concern mentioned above for trimethoprim, the advice for septrin is the same: avoid it, if possible.

Sedatives and antidepressants

What is advice regarding commonly used sedatives such as Diazepam?

There is no known harm in one-off use of drugs such as Diazepam. However, long-term use during pregnancy has been associated with defects such as cleft lip and palate, particularly so if taken in the critical first eight weeks.

Late pregnancy use, just before delivery, is associated with depression of respiration and very low muscle-tone of the newborn. In fact, this may be so bad that the baby may not cry and may be unable to feed for up to twenty-four hours after birth. This will require special care and can be extremely worrying to the parents.

What is the effect of commonly used antidepressant medication?

The most commonly used drugs for depression are the tricyclic antidepressants. The commonly known drugs are imipramine (Tofranyl), amitriptyline (Lentizol) and dothiepin (Prothiaden).

These are not known to cause any birth defects.

Another group of drugs which have been around only for a few years are the SSRIs. The name stands for Serotonin Selective Re-uptake Inhibitors. The most famous SSRI antidepressant is prozac. Its generic name is fluoxetine.

There are other, less famous SSRIs, including seroxat (Paroxetine) and faverin (Fluvoxamine). All these have no known detrimental effect on the fetus. The advice, however, is to avoid them unless necessary. This is because doctors do not have enough experience of these drugs to be sure.

What about drugs used in psychotic conditions?

The most common anti-psychotic drugs are the group known as phenothiazines. These include chlorpromazine (Largactil), haloperidol (Serenace), fluphenazine (Modecate), and thioridazine (Melleril). There is no known evidence of birth defects as a result of using these drugs.

Another commonly used anti-psychotic drug is lithium. This is to be avoided in pregnancy at all costs. Lithium is known to cause major heart defects and more than 10 per cent of babies born to mothers using the drugs in pregnancy will be affected.

Nausea and vomiting

Morning sickness is the bane of early pregnancy. What of the drugs commonly used to remedy this?

Nausea and/or vomiting is quite common, especially in the initial ten to fourteen weeks of pregnancy. Many women manage without any drugs but some need some kind of medication to relieve the symptoms.

Commonly used drugs are stemetil (real name Prochlorperazine), buccastem – which is the same as stemetil – maxolon (Metoclopromide) and occasionally cyclizine and promethazine (Phenergan). All these are regarded to be safe in pregnancy as there have never been any reports of birth defects associated with their use in pregnancy. Generally, as for all drugs, use is recommended only when necessary.

However, for promethazine (Phenergan) there is a slight worry that it may increase incidence of congenital dislocation of the hip. Evidence to this effect is weak.

Painkillers

Pain can be a major and intractable problem in pregnancy. This could be in the form of lower backache, lower abdominal pain, headache or pain in the lower limbs. What about the use of painkillers?

Paracetamol is generally regarded to be safe at any stage of pregnancy, when taken in normal dosages.

Aspirin's case is slightly more complex. There is certainly no evidence of birth defects associated with use of normal dosage of aspirin in pregnancy. However, prolonged use has been associated with a slight increase in low birth-weight and possibly even an increase in the incidence of stillbirth. There is also the theoretical worry that the baby, especially if premature, could be at risk of bleeding complications. All this means that the use of aspirin in normal or high doses is generally to be avoided in pregnancy. The use of low-dose aspirin at 75 mg daily (1800 mg daily is the recommended dose for pain control) is not associated with these potential problems.

What about codeine?

This is one of the "opioid" painkillers. The most famous member of this family is morphine. On a purely fetal well-being consideration, these drugs are safe in the sense that they do not cause birth defects.

There are several variants of codeine such as dihydrocodeine (also called DF118) and those drugs which are combinations of codeine and other painkillers, especially paracetamol. These combination drugs include co-codamol, codydramol, tylex, solpadol and paramol. There is no evidence of any harm as a result of using normal doses of these in pregnancy.

Does the presumed safety of codeine in pregnancy extend to morphine?

Yes, to a degree. The problem of morphine is that it is addictive, and the dependency and severe withdrawal complications will affect the fetus or newborn likewise. For this reason, it is hard to see any justification of using it long-term in pregnancy. Its short-term use for acute pain should, however, be no cause for concern. The advice for pethidine use is similar.

Constipation and heartburn

Constipation is another common problem in pregnancy. What about medicine used to relieve this?

Any doctor or midwife confronted with this problem should first and foremost proffer a dietary solution. This does help in a lot of cases, though not all. High fibre and fresh fruit should be prominent in the diet. It is only when this does not work that drug preparations should be considered.

- Lactulose is known to be safe in pregnancy. It is contraindicated in people with the rare condition known as galactosaemia (the body's inability to change galactose, a sugar derived from milk sugar, into glucose). It is probably vital for the mother to know that lactulose is not absorbed from the gut and therefore has no chance of reaching the baby.

- Fybogel (isphagula) is one of a group of "bulk-forming laxatives". They need to be taken with plenty of fluids. Other preparations of a similar compound come with names such as regulan, isogel and konsyl. Also related are bran and sterculia (normacol) etc. All these are safe as they do not stimulate the uterus and are not absorbed from the gut, and do not reach the fetus.

- Bisacodyl is one of the "stimulant laxatives". The orally taken stimulant laxatives have no known harmful effect on the fetus. However, there is a theoretical possibility that they could stimulate the uterus and precipitate a miscarriage or preterm labour. They are generally avoided in pregnancy. An exception to this is the rectally administered suppository (glycerine). The action of this is mild and is confined to the rectum. There is no danger of miscarriage or preterm labour.

- Phosphate enema will be used in pregnancy when the situation gets desperate. Its action is local and there is no danger of causing damage to the baby. By its very nature, an enema cannot be used on a regular basis. Use in early pregnancy may cause slight concern of the theoretical risk of precipitating miscarriage. This is highly unlikely but in the presence of several and arguably more user-friendly alternatives, its use at this stage of pregnancy, is rarely justified.

- Picolax represents a group of the powerful laxatives used in preparing the bowel before surgery. It is not used in pregnancy.

Heartburn troubles many in pregnancy. Can a relieving preparation be taken with confidence?

Again, the initial advice for heartburn should be conservative management. This should take the form of small frequent meals, preferably rich in carbohydrates. The expectant mother should also avoid lying flat or prolonged stooping. She may also try to lie in a propped-up position at night. If all these do not work, then medication may have to be tried.

There is lingering concern about safety of antacids (such as magnesium- or aluminium-based preparations) in early pregnancy (the first eight to ten weeks). This is based on reports of occasional congenital defects in the past which have not been fully disproved. In this phase of pregnancy, therefore, they are best avoided.

There is certainly no risk to the fetus in the second or third trimester of the pregnancy and, when required, they can be taken with peace of mind.

Common trade names of these antacids include Gaviscon, Maalox, and Mucogel.

If one has been on specific treatment for peptic ulcers, what then?

The general rule is that peptic ulcers tend to improve in pregnancy. It is exceptionally unusual for peptic ulcers to start or be diagnosed for the first time during pregnancy.

For somebody who has been on specific treatment for the ulcers, the medication is likely to be one of the drugs known as H2-receptor antagonists. These work by inhibiting the secretion of acid in the stomach.

The most common are cimetidine (Tagamet) and ranitidine (Zantac). Other similar drugs include nizatidine (Axid) and famotidine (Pepcid).

There is scant data regarding safety of these drugs in pregnancy, since they are rarely used. They should therefore be avoided unless it is absolutely necessary.

But ranitidine is commonly given in labour or just before a caesarean section in many obstetric units.

This is true. This kind of use is considered perfectly safe and has been used for many years on hundreds of thousands of women about to give birth. No ill-effect on the baby has ever been reported.

Are there any ulcer-healing drugs apart from those mentioned above?

Yes. In some countries, sucralfate (antepsin) is considered ideal for use in pregnancy, since it is not absorbed from the stomach.

Omeprazole (Losec) is another useful drug. Its safety in pregnancy cannot be guaranteed and therefore the advice is to avoid it.

Carbenoxolone is yet another type. It is contraindicated for use in pregnancy.

Malaria

If one is living in or visiting tropical countries where there is risk of malaria, what are the antimalarials to be used in pregnancy?

Malaria itself can precipitate a miscarriage. For those who are not immune (i.e. those who normally live in malaria-free countries), this disease can be quite serious, even life-threatening.

Taking preventative medication will therefore be mandatory if visiting malarious areas.

- Chloroquine: this is considered to be safe and has been used extensively and over many years by pregnant women without any apparent ill-effect. It is, however, not a very effective preventative agent.
- Proguanil (Paludrime): this is considered to be safe but the advice is to take it together with folic acid.
- Mefloquine (Larium): this is contraindicated in pregnancy. The advice is that when used, one should avoid pregnancy for three months thereafter. It is probably safe in late pregnancy but the advice is to use alternatives, even then.
- Halofantrine (Halfan): this is contraindicated in pregnancy.
- Primaquine: while there is no conclusive evidence of ill-effects, the contrary cannot be guaranteed either. For this reason and by virtue of the fact that there are more effective alternatives, the advice is to avoid it.
- Fansidar: this is a pyrimethamine, containing antimalarial. It should be used in pregnancy only when necessary. It is actually not recommended for prevention. When used, folic acid supplements should be taken. The same applies for other pyrimethamine-containing antimalarials, such as metakelfin and maloprim.
- Quinine: the oldest antimalarial still remains one of the most effective. However, in pregnancy, quinine can provoke miscarriage or premature labour. For this reason, it should be opted for with great care. It is not used for prevention. There is no evidence of ill-effect on the fetus otherwise.

Blood pressure

High blood pressure (hypertension) is one of the most common complications of pregnancy. How safe are the antihypertensives?

Methyl-dopa (Aldomet) is one of the most common antihypertensives used in pregnancy. It has been around for many years. It is known to be safe.

"Beta-blockers" is a group of drugs also used commonly in pregnancy. These include propranolol (Inderal), acebutolol (Sectral), atenolol (Tenormin), oxprenolol (Trasicor) and labetalol (a partial beta-blocker). There are many others. Overall, these are regarded to be safe. There is a remote possibility that long-term use in pregnancy could cause intrauterine growth restriction but this is usually outweighed by the potential benefits. Use just before delivery has also been associated with the fall of blood-sugar levels in the baby. The paediatricians therefore need to be informed of the mother's use of these drugs so the appropriate surveillance on the newborn can be maintained.

Hydralazine: this is used only for short-term lowering of blood pressure, usually in late pregnancy. For this, it is known to be safe. Occasionally it has been associated with fall in platelet count in the newborn, but this spontaneously recovers in about two or three weeks.

Nifedipine: this is also used for short-term lowering of blood pressure in pregnancy. For this, it is known to be safe. Regular or long-term use in pregnancy is to be avoided, as safety for the fetus cannot be guaranteed. No adverse effects have been reported, however.

A group of popular antihypertensives are the ones known as "ACE-inhibitors". What about these in pregnancy?

Yes, ACE-inhibitors such as captopril (Capoten), enalapril (Innovace), lisinopril (Carace, Zestril), quinapril (Accupro) and a few others are very effective antihypertensives. However, their use in pregnancy is very much contraindicated. In fact, any woman taking these who is planning to conceive should be weaned off them and put on something else (such as beta-blockers or methyl-dopa).

Some preparations of antihypertensive are combined with a diuretic to make them more effective. Can these preparations be used in pregnancy?

There is no simple answer to this question. However, if hypertension is part of the syndrome known as pre-eclampsia, diuretics (alone or in combination) should not be used. This is because their "drying" effect could worsen the poor blood supply to the baby inherent in this condition.

Chronic hypertension is not associated with this problem. However, pre-eclampsia could superimpose itself on simple chronic hypertension. For this reason, it is probably best to avoid diuretics in pregnancy altogether, especially if their use is to be long-term. As regards their effect on the fetus, the common diuretics (bendrofluazide and frusemide) are probably safe, as there is no evidence of direct ill-effects on the baby.

In summary therefore, diuretics, alone or in combination, should not be used in pre-eclampsia as they can potentially do more harm than good. They can probably be used safely in uncomplicated chronic hypertension but better alternatives are usually available.

Does the above means, where strongly indicated, diuretics can be used in pregnancy?

Yes. If the pregnant woman is in heart failure or has lung oedema, diuretics are indispensable and should be used.

Diabetes

Diabetes is another common complication of pregnancy. How safe are drugs used to manage this condition?

Pre-existing diabetes will almost always be controlled with insulin. The woman will almost always be on this already. If she has used dietary control conception will almost certainly mean a switch to insulin.

Insulin is not only safe, it is actually beneficial in preventing birth defects. Those diabetic mothers whose diabetes had been well controlled before conception reduce the risk of congenital malformation quite significantly. In poorly controlled diabetics, the risk of major malformation in their children is up to three times that of the general population.

Apart from insulin, what drugs are used to control diabetes in pregnancy?

In non-pregnant individuals, there is a place for what are known as "oral hypoglycaemics". These have an effect of lowering blood-sugar levels, to various degrees. Most of them (Chlorpropamide, Glibenclamide, Glipizide and Tolbutamide) cross the placenta and are likely to cause a catastrophic fall in fetal blood-sugar. They are not used in pregnancy.

Metformin (Glucophage) is one oral hypoglycaemic that does not cross the placenta and therefore has no direct effect on the fetus. Even with this known fact, it is not usually used in pregnancy. This is because insulin is infinitely better and more reliable. There has been some debate that in desperate situations – such as with some very obese diabetic expectant mothers – where insulin has failed to bring about the required control, metformin may be supplemented. This is contentious and, fortunately, the need to put it into practice rarely arises.

Systemic Lupus Erythematosus (SLE)

Some people suffering from SLE are maintained on "antimalarials" such as hydroxy-chloroquine (Plaquenil). What is the advice regarding their use in pregnancy?

These drugs are very effective in controlling the disease. Discontinuing their use can cause a flare-up of the disease. Moreover, such a step may increase the risk of miscarriage or fetal death in the uterus quite substantially. It is known for a fact that women suffering from SLE are prone to repeated pregnancy loss. Stopping this medication will therefore not only have an adverse effect on the mother but on the fetus as well. It is also true that there is no evidence that use of this drug in pregnancy has any adverse effect on the baby, short or long-term.

Coughs and colds

There is a wide choice of cough preparations on the market. How safe are these for use in pregnancy?

For coughs, there are two main groups of preparations: the cough suppressants and the expectorants.

Cough suppressants are marketed with a claim that they will reduce the frequency and intensity of coughing. Their effect is modest at best and they may help the person to sleep better. Most of them are based on opioids, especially codeine and sedatives such as diphenhydramine.

Those containing codeine will tend to cause constipation. Constipation is a common problem in pregnancy and if the pregnant woman is already having this trouble, then she should think hard before taking such preparations. They are likely to make the problem worse without really giving her much benefit.

Those cough suppressants based on sedatives will cause drowsiness and may not be ideal for a pregnant women who is working, looking after small children or needs to drive. Their effectiveness, again, is modest at best.

Expectorants are cough preparations which are marketed with the claim that they promote the expulsion of the sputum and secretions produced in the respiratory tract. They are supposed to relieve the symptoms by making one cough less and breathe easier. The reality is that they make little or no difference, and scientific evidence of their effectiveness is lacking. Simple linctus (the most common type) is a citric acid solution (i.e. orange or lemon!).

Some of them are marketed in combination with painkillers (such as paracetamol) and decongestants (see below). Their value, over and above the placebo effect, is dubious.

All these preparations have no direct adverse effect on the pregnancy. Any preparation containing iodine should be avoided. Always read the label.

What about medicines for colds?

The nasal decongestants on the market are mostly made of an active ingredient in the form of pseudoephedrine or similar. Many also contain an antihistamine. Their effectiveness is really unproven and this is probably the biggest gravy-train in the retail trade today. The benefit from most is largely through the placebo effect: you believe it will do something, your mind and body responds to the expectation and you feel better.

Those preparations containing pseudoephedrine and similar drugs need to be used with caution if the mother is hypertensive or has a heart disease. They may also interfere with diabetes control. There is, however, no direct adverse effect on the pregnancy itself.

Preparations containing antihistamines such as chlorpheniramine will tend to make the mother drowsy.

Hay-fever and allergic rhinitis

Many people suffer from 'Seasonal allergic rhinitis' also called hay-fever, or even simple recurrent allergic rhinitis. Is medication for this safe to use in pregnancy?

Nasal allergies of all types are mostly treated with antihistamines. Some of these, especially the newer 'non-sedating' ones, are clearly considerd unsafe to use in pregnancy. It is therefore important for a pregnant woman intending to use any of these preparations to check with her doctor and the enclosed literature about their status vis-à-vis pregnancy. Some of the antihistamines contra-indicated for use in pregnancy include loratadine (Clarityn), mizolastine and astemizole (Hismanal). The contra-indication is based on inavailability of proof of safety in pregnancy rather than any documented adverse effect. The common (older generation) antihistamine chlorpheniramine (Piriton) is considered safe.

Steroidal preparations are also used in allergic rhinitis. These include beclomethasone (Beconase), budesonide (Rhinocort Aqua), fluticasone etc. These are safe to use.

Eczema

What about eczema and its treatment?

This fairly common condition can continue after conception. Treatments to control the lesions commonly consist of an emmolient, a steroidal skin preparation, occasionally oral medication or a combination of any of these.

Emmolients are meant to soothe and re-hydrate the skin. There are many such preparation with many different proprietary names. Common ones include E45®, Oilatum®, Neutrogena®, Vaseline®, aqueous cream, white soft paraffin etc. There is no evidence of adverse effect from their use during pregnancy. Steroidal skin (topical) preparations, when used as recommended, are also regarded as safe to use during pregnancy.

23. Down's syndrome and other chromosomal abnormalities

Introduction

Out of every 700 babies born, one will have the condition known as Down's syndrome. This chromosomal disorder gives the affected individual specific recognizable physical characteristics. However, more significantly, the person will have considerable learning difficulties with an average mental age of five or six years old by the time he or she reaches adulthood. Moreover, a Down's syndrome baby is prone to other major abnormalities of such vital organs as the heart, lungs or gut. It is therefore important that, whatever the opinion of the parents about the merits and drawbacks of antenatal screening for such conditions, they know what the condition is all about. It is only then, from an informed position, that they can rationally decide where they stand.

There are, of course, other (less common) chromosomal abnormalities apart from Down's syndrome, which the screening tests can detect. Some of them are fatal and the baby stands no chance of survival outside the womb.

The screening tests currently used are what are known as the "triple test" and the "double test". They are similar, with equal efficacy in detection. However, the sensitivity is only about 60 per cent, which means, with the blood screening test only, potentially four out of every ten Down's syndrome babies will not be detected. It is also true that there is a significant incidence of false alarms from the test. It is however, the best available non-invasive screening test. This is normally combined with detailed ultrasound scanning to look for the tell-tale features of Down's, where the risk is considered high. However, the only definitive tests, which establish the fact beyond any doubt, are the invasive ones where fetal cells are cultured and the chromosome make-up analyzed in a laboratory.

An established diagnosis moves the issue to a new level of what to do. Many parents who wish to have the screening test and, if the need arises, the definitive diagnostic test, do so because they want termination of pregnancy if the diagnosis is confirmed. A smaller percentage do so simply because they want to know and be prepared. The third group comprises those who decline the screening test altogether because it wouldn't make a difference one way or another.

This book does not pretend to analyze or even give an opinion on these different stances. Those profound questions surrounding the issue of what to do are well beyond the scope of this book. What we have set out to do is to give the facts on the subject of Down's and other chromosomal disorders and clarify them.

Down's syndrome

What is Down's syndrome?

Down's syndrome (or Down syndrome) is a chromosomal disorder where the affected individual will have a number of abnormal physical and mental characteristics. The most significant characteristic is the considerable learning difficulties that the affected person has. A Down's syndrome individual rarely develops a mental age above that of a five-year-old.

What are the physical characteristics of a Down's baby?

The head tends to be flattish, both in the front and the back. The eyes are slanted (hence the older, rather insensitive term "mongoloid", and the ears have a squareish appearance and are rather low-set. The arms may appear slightly short and there may be abnormal creases on the palms of the hands. The tongue tends to appear rather too large for the mouth.

Apart from the external physical features, a Down's baby

may be born with major internal organ abnormalities. Organs particularly affected are the heart and the gut. Some abnormalities could be life-threatening or require major corrective surgery.

What happens when a Down's baby grows up?
Apart from the learning difficulties of variable severity, physically a Down's syndrome individual tends to be of short stature. Most of them attain a maximum height of less than five feet. Many are a lot shorter than this.

What happens to cause the baby to end up with Down's syndrome?
As mentioned earlier, this is a chromosomal disorder.

A normal individual has twenty-three pairs of chromosomes, making a total of forty-six chromosomes. Each and every cell in the body, except for gametes, has forty-six chromosomes. In Down's syndrome, there are forty-seven chromosomes. The extra chromosome is on pair number twenty-one. This means on pair number twenty-one there are three instead of two chromosomes. This is why this condition is also called Trisomy 21. There are other chromosomal disorders where there is an extra chromosome, as we shall see below. Down's syndrome or Trisomy 21 is the most common chromosomal disorder compatible with life.

Are there any predisposing factors?
It is important to know that most Down's syndrome babies are born to mothers who have no known predisposing factors. It means therefore, that without screening tests, all these will come as a complete surprise. However, there are people who are more likely to have Down's syndrome children because of a number of factors. The most important factor is maternal age.

How important is maternal age?
The older the mother, the higher the risk of a Down's syndrome pregnancy. Even though a Down's baby can be born to a mother of any age, the risk increases significantly above the age of thirty-five. The risk to a mother aged twenty is about 1 in 1000, rising to 1 in 600 at thirty years, 1 in 250 at thirty-five and as high as 1 in 70 at forty.

The risk is an extremely high 1 in 20 by the time the mother is forty-four. As can be seen, the risk rises almost fifty-fold at the age of forty compared to the risk of a twenty-year-old mother.

Is paternal age important?

No. There is no evidence that the father's age influences the risk of having a Down's syndrome baby in any way.

Apart from maternal age, are there any other risk factors?

Yes. One or the other parent may carry a potential chromosomal abnormality, even though the parent is normal. Through a complicated chromosome material swap (known as "translocation", in medical language), the parent may produce gametes with extra chromosomal material. If this extra chromosome is on number 21, the resulting fetus will be Down's. If it is the father who is carrying the translocation, the risk of producing a Down's baby is one in ten (10 per cent). If it is the mother who has the translocation, the risk is much higher at one in two (50 per cent). This kind of risk is independent of the age of either parent.

What proportion of Down's syndrome children result from parental chromosomal translocation?

About 2 per cent. When a Down's baby is born to a young mother, it may be worthwhile to check the chromosomes of the parents to establish whether one of them might be a carrier of a translocation. This will help in counselling regarding future pregnancies and estimation of risk of recurrence. Remember, the carrier parent will have no tell-tale features of any kind.

Talking of recurrence, what is the risk of this happening?

Except for those carrying a translocation, a mother who had a Down's pregnancy has a risk of this recurring increased threefold compared to the average. This means, if the mother is going to be thirty at her next pregnancy, while the average risk is 1 in 600 at this age, her risk will be much higher at 1 in 200.

What are the screening tests for Down's syndrome?

Any woman who has been pregnant will be aware of the terms "triple test" or "double test". What the triple test really means is that a small sample of blood taken from the mother is checked for three (hence "triple") different hormones produced by the fetus or placenta. The levels are computed, together with other important factors such as maternal age, gestational age and previous history, to estimate the risk in that particular pregnancy. In the double test, only two of the hormones are checked. The sensitivity of the "double" test in detecting an affected baby is similar to that of the "triple" test. Maternity units tend to adopt one or the other.

Why are those particular hormones checked to screen for Down's syndrome?

It is true that the fetus and the placenta produce many different types of hormones and other chemicals. It is, however, known that some hormones tend to be increased and others reduced in babies with Down's syndrome. By computing levels, therefore, one can have a pretty good impression of which babies are likely to be affected. Two of the most important chemicals are AFP, which tends to be reduced in Down's syndrome, and beta-hCG, which tends to be increased in Down's.

Is there any particular gestational age when the screening test has to be done?

Yes. The screening test is accurate if the blood is taken between fifteen and seventeen weeks of gestation. It is, therefore, important to be very accurate about the gestation. If the dating of the pregnancy is wrong, this will corrupt the calculation of the risk, either making it too high or too low – with all the inevitable consequences.

So, what can the mother do if she is unsure about the gestational age?

An ultrasound scan to confirm or establish the gestational age is easily arranged. The scan in early pregnancy is pretty accurate, with a margin of error of only about three or four days.

How sensitive are the screening tests for Down's syndrome?

About 60 per cent sensitive. That means about 60 per cent of all affected fetuses will be detected and 40 per cent will be left undetected by this standard screening test. It is obviously an unsatisfactory state of affairs but unfortunately, to date, no better screening test is available, though there is a lot of research activity around this area.

For those babies that slip through the screening blood test, is there any other detecting test?

There is still a possibility that an affected fetus can be detected using the detailed anatomy ultrasound scan, usually performed at eighteen to twenty weeks of gestation. As mentioned before, Down's babies have a number of physical abnormalities and organ malformations, which may be detectable by the scan. If a number of those are detected, in spite of a "negative" screening test, the suspicion may be aroused to justify suggesting a definitive diagnostic test. As it happens, not all Down's babies have these abnormalities and therefore a substantial proportion still slip through and are born when not expected.

What are the definitive diagnostic tests?

For all chromosomal disorders, including Down's syndrome, a confirmatory diagnostic test is based on obtaining fetal (or placental) cells which are processed to enable the mapping of the chromosomal make-up of that baby. Once this is achieved, a chromosomal defect – be it an extra chromosome (as in Down's) or deletion of part or a whole chromosome – will be established.

How are the fetal or placental cells obtained?

There are three main ways of getting the cells. The most widely used is amniocentesis, where fluid is obtained from around the fetus and fetal cells isolated from this and then cultured. The second method is chorionic villus sampling (CVS), where a tiny piece of placenta is obtained; and the third is cordocentesis, where fetal blood is obtained from the umbilical cord.

How do the three tests compare?

As can be appreciated, all three are invasive. Amniocentesis is considered to be the least invasive because it avoids both the baby and the placenta. The potential for serious consequences is also considerably less with amniocentesis. The flip side is that it takes between one and a half and three weeks to get the results.

This is a long time for most parents, because of the anxiety associated with it. In addition, since most times the amniocentesis is carried out on the basis of screening test results, it is therefore done at around eighteen weeks. This means the results are obtained at about twenty to twenty-two weeks: rather late if results mean some major intervention.

CVS can be done quite early in pregnancy (at eleven to twelve weeks) or later. The problem is that the miscarriage risk as a consequence of the procedure is about twice that of amniocentesis. However, results are available in two to four days, far quicker than with amniocentesis.

Cordocentesis can be performed only beyond eighteen weeks. The miscarriage rate is even higher than CVS. There is usually little justification to resort to cordocentesis for the sake of chromosomal analysis.

What is the miscarriage rate following amniocentesis?

On average; it is about 0.5 per cent. This means one in 200 mothers who undergo the procedure will miscarry as a consequence. Sadly, some of the babies lost do not have chromosomal defects. It is up to the mother and her partner to decide whether the risk is worth taking.

What is to be done if the diagnosis is confirmed?

It is again up to the parents to decide what to do. In fact, this is an area that should be sorted out well before even the amniocentesis has taken place. Most parents of affected fetuses opt for termination of pregnancy. Others opt to continue with the pregnancy and value the forewarning which prepares them to look after a handicapped child.

In the case of twin pregnancy, what effect does this have on the screening tests?

There are some unique problems here. If the screening blood test is performed before the twin nature of the pregnancy is recognized, as is occasionally the case, the result may be misinterpreted.

The error is recognized with an ultrasound scan, which will establish the status and which is the next test performed in case of any abnormal result. The results are usually recalculated in the light of the new information to take into account the presence of more than one fetus in the womb.

Is the risk of Down's syndrome increased in case of twin pregnancy?

It depends. If the twins are identical, the risk is the same as for a singleton. This is because the chromosomal constitution of the two fetuses is similar. This means, either both will be normal or both will be affected. If the twins are non-identical, the risk is twice that of the norm. This is because the fetuses are two distinct individuals and either of them (or, rarely, both!) can be affected.

If there is a suspicion that one of the twins is affected, how easy is it to verify this?

It is a difficult situation. It requires taking a sample of fluid from each sac and identifying with certainty, which sample came from which sac. If one of the fetuses is confirmed to be affected, the parents may opt to have selective termination of the affected fetus.

How easy is it to do selective termination?

Technically, this is not difficult. However, it means doctors have to be absolutely certain they are terminating the affected fetus. This is not always easy. Moreover, there is the additional concern that by selectively terminating one, the healthy twin may also be lost. The risk of this is of the order of 15 per cent, which is quite considerable. In the UK, this service is available only in specialist centres.

Is there any way round this problem of loss of the healthy twin?

Not entirely. However if, for some reason, the parents seek a diagnostic test in the earlier stages of pregnancy – let's say eleven to thirteen weeks, where a CVS will be used – then if selective termination becomes necessary, the risk of losing the healthy twin is a comparatively lower at 5 per cent. The only risk-free strategy is to opt to continue with the pregnancy as it is.

Talking of earlier diagnosis, is this available if wanted?

This is an area where a lot of research continues to take place and some promising results are starting to emerge.

In the UK, a large study co-ordinated by the Harris Birthright Research Centre for Fetal Medicine has for the last few years looked at offering women early screening for Down's and other chromosomal genetic abnormalities in the first trimester (11–13 weeks). This is by using ultrasound to measure the thickness of the back of the fetal neck (also known as nuchal translucency). This has been used in several hospitals in and around London with promising results. Similar studies are taking place in other countries.

The basis for this screening test is the known fact that, around this gestation, fetuses with a variety of chromosomal defects tend to have increased thickness of the nuchal pad (the skin at the back of the neck). When this is measured and found to be increased (more than 3 mm), it triggers the suspicion of something amiss (which could be Down's or some other condition). This should prompt a careful and thorough search for other physical or organic abnormalities associated with these syndromes.

The mother may then be offered a diagnostic test to definitively establish the truth. The expected benefit of this is that the diagnosis is established much earlier and if the fetus is affected, it is assumed that any decision to terminate the pregnancy will be comparatively less difficult and probably less traumatic.

How much promise does this early screening test have?

The results are promising but it is by no means infallible. Preliminary results indicate it may have a sensitivity of between 65 and 80 per cent, comparing favourably with the established screening (blood) tests. Moreover, it is claimed, if the nuchal pad thickness is more than 6 mm, the possibility of an abnormality (Down's or otherwise) is as high as 93 per cent. These are exciting days but much work still lies ahead. Watch this space.

Is there any prospect of a definitive diagnosis test that is non-invasive?

This is a very attractive idea, since it will eliminate the risk of miscarriage as a consequence of the diagnostic test. Unfortunately, even though much research work has gone into this, so far there is nothing on the horizon. However, this is a fast-evolving field and who knows what we will be telling you in this regard, a few years down the line.

We have discussed Down's syndrome at length; what are the other chromosomal disorders?

There are several chromosomal disorders but Down's syndrome affects one in 700 newborns. However, this figure is fluid and, in the medium- and long-term, is bound to be affected by changes in pregnancy patterns (the proportion of women having babies in their "later" years) and the accuracy of screening tests.

Other less common conditions are Edward's syndrome (Trisomy 18); Patau's syndrome (Trisomy 13), Turner's syndrome (XO) and Klinefelter's syndrome (XXY). We shall discuss each one them briefly below.

Edward's syndrome

What about Edward's syndrome?

This is a chromosomal disorder where there is an extra chromosome on pair number 18; hence it is called "Trisomy 18". It is characterized by a variety of severe physical and organic defects. The baby may die in the womb or could be delivered alive, only to die a few weeks later. It is virtually unknown for an Edward's syndrome baby to survive beyond twelve months. The active advice, when the diagnosis is made during pregnancy, is to terminate the pregnancy. The final decision, of course, rests with the mother.

Is risk of Edward's syndrome associated in any way with maternal age?

Yes. As with Down's, the risk increases with advancing maternal age. At twenty, the risk is estimated at around one in 3600; twenty years later, the risk has shot up to one in 200, an eighteen-fold increase. There is no association with paternal age.

Can the screening tests used for Down's help to detect Edward's syndrome?

Absolutely. The hormones are variably affected in this condition as well, so suspicion could be triggered following a "double" or "triple" test. Even if this does not arouse suspicion, the detailed anatomy scan at eighteen to twenty weeks (which virtually every expectant mother gets as part of routine care) will almost certainly do so. This is because the physical and organic defects associated with the condition are almost always there and relatively easy to detect. An invasive test will be needed to confirm the diagnosis.

Can an Edward's syndrome baby survive into later childhood or even adulthood?

No.

Turner's syndrome

What is Turner's syndrome?

This is a condition that is caused by absence of one sex chromosome. A normal human being has twenty-three pairs of chromosomes, making a total of forty-six chromosomes. One of the pairs is made up of sex chromosomes. The female sex chromosomes are XX and the male chromosomes are XY. A woman is therefore represented as 46XX and a man as 46XY.

A Turner's syndrome person is represented as 45XO (the O standing for a missing chromosome).

Is a Turner's syndrome individual male or female?

Female. There is a normal vagina, a uterus and tubes. The ovaries are, however, streaky and non-functional. This means a Turner's girl cannot ovulate. Nor can she conceive in the normal way.

Apart from the fertility aspect, what are the prospects for a Turner's baby?

Pretty good. In fact, a good number of Turner's syndrome girls are not discovered until their early or mid-teens. However, there are some physical characteristics which may arouse suspicion of something amiss. These may include short stature and a webbed neck. There may also be heart or kidney anomalies, which may lead to investigations for chromosomal defects. Intellectually, they tend to be of average intelligence.

What about diagnosis antenatally?

There are no biochemical or specific ultrasound diagnostic features for Turner's syndrome. There is, however, a lethal form of Turner's, where quite marked physical and heart abnormalities may be detected on ultrasound. Such pregnancies tend to end in miscarriage or stillbirth. This affects only a minority of Turner's syndrome babies.

Does maternal age influence the risk of having a Turner's syndrome baby?

No. The overall risk is estimated at one in 2500 and is constant at any maternal age. Paternal age, likewise, has no influence on the risk rate.

Klinefelter's syndrome

What is Klinefelter's syndrome?

This is a chromosomal disorder where the affected individual has an extra X chromosome. The chromosomal constitution is therefore 47XXY instead of the usual 46XY. Because of the presence of the Y chromosome, the affected child is male.

Can Klinefelter's syndrome be diagnosed antenatally?

Not normally. However, if a diagnostic test is performed for any other reason, the diagnosis of this condition will be established on mapping the chromosomal make-up.

What are the prospects for a Klinefelter's baby?

These individuals have fairly average prospects.

Physically, they attain normal height; they may even be taller than average. However, there is increased incidence of behavioural problems during adolescence.

They may also have mild learning difficulties.

Above-average breast development could pose a problem for an affected young man. More ominous is the fact that, compared to the average male, the risk of breast cancer is increased twenty times.

Is maternal age a risk factor for Klinefelter's?

No. Neither is paternal age.

Klinefelter's is relatively common at one in 500. It is entirely possible for an affected individual to go through life unrecognized.

Patau's syndrome

What is Patau's syndrome?

This is "Trisomy 13", meaning the affected fetus has an extra chromosome at pair number 13.

The occurrence is one in 5000 live births.

Can Patau's syndrome be diagnosed antenatally?

Yes. The screening blood tests for Down's can help detect Patau's as well. In addition, a detailed ultrasound has a good chance of detecting the various physical and organic defects associated with Patau's. There may be facial clefts and increased number of toes and fingers. The scan findings may trigger a definitive diagnostic test.

What are the prospects for a Patau's syndrome baby?

These children have such severe physical and mental handicaps that the majority of them die before the age of two. Less than 3 per cent survive to the age of three and virtually none reach five years of age.

Are there any other chromosomal disorders?

Hundreds. Some of the chromosomal disorders are so lethal that pregnancies never advance beyond the first eight to ten weeks. These are therefore characterized by early miscarriage. Miscarriage will not be recurrent unless one of the parents is a carrier of the defect.

Other chromosomal disorders may be compatible with life, albeit short, but are very rare.

Can a chromosomal disorder be cured?

This is not possible, nor is there any prospect of this being possible in the foreseeable future.

24. *Skin disorders in pregnancy*

Introduction

Skin disorders are not uncommon in pregnancy. In some instances, the problem can be quite difficult and distressing. Many women have had labour induced to rescue them from severe itching that is not relieved by anything thrown at it. However, itching is not the only problem, even though it may be the most common (affecting one in six pregnancies). Other problems include a localized or generalized rash, which may or may not itch.

There may be pre-existing skin disorders such as eczema, psoriasis and SLE. All these may behave in all sorts of ways. Take psoriasis, for example. It could remain the same, improve with pregnancy or get dramatically worse, to the point of necessitating termination of the pregnancy.

Other conditions are specific to pregnancy and are not encountered at any other time. They may actually recur with each pregnancy.

And, of course, there are stretch marks – something that can cause near-panic for prospective first-time mothers.

We have explained all these clearly in this chapter.

Skin changes

How often does one see skin changes during pregnancy?

This is fairly common. Practically every pregnant woman notices some skin changes, either localized or generalized. Most of these are minor and are immediately recognizable as pregnancy-associated changes and therefore cause no alarm. However, some women who have pre-existing chronic skin disorders may notice some changes in these. Others develop skin disorders for the first time in pregnancy. We shall expand on this further on.

Psoriasis

What happens to psoriasis in pregnancy?

Psoriasis is characterized by thickened patches of inflamed red skin; the skin is often covered by silvery scales and the new skin cells are produced about ten times faster than normal. What happens in pregnancy varies. It may worsen, get better or remain unchanged. Some forms of psoriasis may develop for the first time in pregnancy. It is therefore difficult to offer any particular advice to a person with pre-existing psoriasis. The dermatologist should be kept involved in the monitoring and treatment of the condition during the course of the pregnancy. This is mainly because when psoriasis worsens during pregnancy (which is uncommon), it requires prompt and intensive treatment, without which both the mother and baby's life may be imperilled.

SLE

What happens in systemic lupus (SLE)?

SLE causes inflammation of the connective tissues. This condition tends to remain the same in pregnancy. However, as any affected person will surely be aware, it affects other body organs and systems apart from the skin. Because of this, and the antibodies associated with this condition, there is a significantly increased risk of miscarriage, which may become a recurrent phenomenon. Moreover, the baby may have skin lesions when he or she is born, or these may develop in the first few weeks of life.

SLE may be diagnosed for the first time in pregnancy. The rare exacerbation will involve the skin and joints.

Herpes

What happens to herpes?

We are discussing genital herpes here: a sexually transmitted disease that produces a painful rash on the genitals and is caused by the herpes simplex virus. Once herpes infection is acquired, it is there for life. Some people will have frequent recurrence of the painful genital lesions while others have long quiescent periods. Pregnancy does not appear to influence this pattern one way or the other.

The standard advice for people with the primary disease is to avoid pregnancy at that time. For those with recurrent disease, this advice is pointless and symptoms are managed as they appear. Herpes is discussed in more detail in Chapter 6, "Exposure to infection in pregnancy".

Itching

What causes itching in pregnancy?

Itching is the most common skin complaint in pregnancy. It affects one in six pregnant women.

The causes are many and varied and each case calls for careful evaluation by the doctor. The cause could be from a pre-existing skin condition; it could also be a manifestation of a condition affecting the liver, thyroid gland or other body systems, developing for the first time in pregnancy. Itching could also be a result of skin conditions that develop in – and are specific to – pregnancy. In this latter category, there is almost always a rash. It is discussed in more detail below.

Experts acknowledge that there are many cases of generalized itching in pregnancy which do not fit in any of these categories and whose causes therefore remain unknown.

What are the liver conditions causing itching?

There are several liver conditions that cause symptoms of generalized itching, be it in pregnancy or a non-pregnant state. A doctor has to be on the lookout for and always try to exclude the pregnancy-specific cholestasis. It is generally called "obstetric cholestasis". In the USA, it is also called "pruritus gravidarum". Its importance lies in the fact that, if unrecognized, it could lead to loss of the baby through stillbirth. It also makes the woman prone to premature labour. Some specific blood tests are required to establish the diagnosis, after which close monitoring of the disease and well-being of both the mother and the baby has to be maintained. If seen to be progressive, delivery may have to be brought forward. Typically, apart from itching, the mother remains well. Obstetric cholestasis clears up soon after delivery.

How common is obstetric cholestasis?

Uncommon. The estimated incidence is two in every 1000 pregnant women. It is relatively more common among Swedes and some native American tribes. This may mean that there is some genetic susceptibility.

What about the itchy skin eruptions affecting pregnant women?

This is a more common condition. It can occur at any stage of the pregnancy, even though it is rare in the first fifteen weeks of gestation. Some women are affected for the first time in the first week after delivery.

The characteristic rash normally begins on the abdomen, before spreading elsewhere on the body. The face is usually spared.

The itching can be quite severe and distressing.

Apart from the distress caused by itching, the condition is harmless to the mother and the fetus. When the itching is severe, mild steroids in the form of a cream, lotion, even tablets may be used to relieve the symptoms.

It clears up rapidly and totally after delivery.

Does this condition recur in subsequent pregnancy?

Not always, but it may do. When this happens, it is usually milder than the previous time.

Other skin conditions

Are there any other pregnancy-specific conditions?

Yes. The one other dramatic skin condition is the one known as "pemphigoid gestationis". Formerly it was called "herpes gestationis", but the name "herpes" was misleading as it has nothing to do with the herpes virus.

This condition is characterized by the eruption of fluid-filled lesions that then crust. It looks like a water-burn injury, except it itches. The lesions typically start around the navel before spreading all over. Palms and soles are not spared and occasionally the mouth may be affected.

There are no other complications to the mother but the condition has a tendency to recur, with increased severity in subsequent pregnancies.

There is only weak evidence that the baby may be growth-restricted in some cases. A small proportion of babies develop a milder form of the condition after the birth, but this soon clears up.

Is that every skin condition in pregnancy?

Unfortunately not. There are a score more skin disorders which are less common but distinct conditions. In fact, don't be surprised if you have symptoms of a skin condition and your obstetrician throws his or her hands up in horror, out of ignorance. When the diagnosis is not obvious, as is often the case, your obstetrician will liaise with the skin specialist to try to identify the condition and then begin the required treatment.

Should one worry if there is no specific diagnosis?

In general, no. The important issue is to exclude the conditions that may have undesirable effects on the pregnancy. Once this is established and the only complaint is itching, control of the symptoms is all that is required. The disappointment is usually that the normal symptom control measures – with all sorts of fancy and not-so-fancy names – are hardly ever effective.

25. Twins and multiple pregnancy

Introduction

Twins! Triplets! Quads! You find out you are carrying a multiple pregnancy. What is your first reaction?

Stunned! This is almost universal, then soon after the reactions diverge widely. There are those who go into sheer panic and virtual shock and those who cannot contain their excitement. In between, there are those who take it in their stride. "Ah, well, I just have to prepare for one (or two) more."

However, the end result is not the only pertinent question in multiple pregnancy. There are questions such as: what is the experience going to be like? Is hospitalization more likely? Are all of them going to survive? What about screening tests for Down's? Suppose one of them is abnormal on the scan? What about delivery? Is caesarean section more likely or even inevitable?

Here we have answered all these questions and many more, from how it happens through to the point of delivery.

If the prospect of having two, three or more babies at the end of the pregnancy does not make your heartbeat quicken, the prospect of going through the weeks of a multiple pregnancy should at the very least be accorded a slight pause for contemplation. Multiple pregnancy, be it twins or a higher order, is not a low-risk enterprise. As a general rule, all the potential pregnancy complications are commoner in multiple pregnancy, except perhaps for prolonged pregnancy; and then there are those problems which are unique to multiple pregnancy. Having said all that, a multiple pregnancy can be an enjoyable and fulfilling experience and often is. It does not hurt, however, to know what it can and often does entail.

Twins

I am carrying twins; how unique am I?

It depends on your ancestry. If you are Caucasian, 1 per cent of all of pregnancies will be twins; if you are of black African origin, the rate is slightly higher, at 1.5 per cent, and if you are of Japanese or other oriental origin, then the rate is lower at about 0.7 per cent. These rates apply to naturally conceived twins.

Fig 7 Twins in the early trimester with two separate sacs and separate placentas. It is impossible at this stage to tell if they are identical or not. If they are of different sexes – something that can be established in the mid-trimester – this will confirm that they are non-identical; otherwise the question remains unanswered throughout the pregnancy.

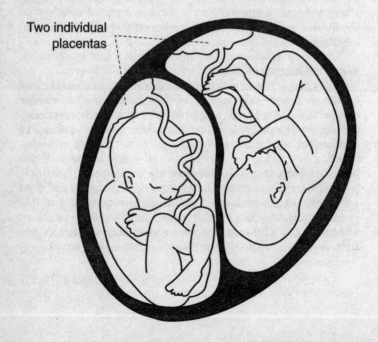

Two individual placentas

What if I am using clomiphene (clomid) to help with ovulation?

The chances of having twin pregnancy with use of this ovulation-inducing medication shoot up several-fold, to around 10 per cent. With clomid, when multiple pregnancy occurs, it is usually twins rather than triplets or other higher-order multiples.

Are there any factors that make one prone to multiple pregnancy?

Yes; family history is a strong factor. If you are a twin yourself (non-identical), then you have a higher than average chance of having twins yourself. The same applies if you have first-degree relatives who are twins (non-identical).

The chances of having a twin pregnancy also increase with age and the number of pregnancies.

What about identical twins?

The rate of this kind of twins is constant throughout the world and is not influenced by age, race, family history or the number of pregnancies.

If you are an identical twin yourself, your chances of having a twin pregnancy is the same as the average.

What if the father is a twin?

If he is an identical twin, then there is no increase in the chance of twin pregnancy. If he is a non-identical twin, then there is some increase in the chance of a twin pregnancy, though not as high as when the family history of twins is maternal.

What causes multiple pregnancy?

With identical twins (doctors call them "monozygotic"), it is the result of the division of an already fertilized egg.

With non-identical twins (also called "dizygotic" or "fraternal"), it is because of fertilization of two separate eggs that happened to be released at the same time. Most twins are non-identical.

Virtually all higher order multiples (triplets and so on) are non-identical.

What about twins resulting from fertility drugs?

These drugs work by promoting ovulation. It therefore follows that twins or higher-order multiples will be non-identical, as they result from fertilization of two (or more) separate eggs.

When multiple pregnancy follows the use of clomiphene (clomid), as happens with about 10 per cent of users, it is mostly twins. When it occurs as a result of IVF treatment, rates are higher at 25 to 30 per cent; the chances of higher-order multiples such as triplets or quads are significantly increased.

The occurrence of identical twins among fertility treatment users is the same as in the general population, i.e. about one in 250 births.

Can doctors tell whether twins are identical before they are born?

Only if they share the placenta or the sac. To establish with an acceptable degree of certainty whether or not twins share a placenta, an ultrasound scan needs to be performed rather early, probably before sixteen weeks of gestation. Later on, two placentas, which are close together, may appear to be virtually continuous and one cannot say with absolute confidence whether they are separate or not.

A single sac with two fetuses is a sure certainty that they are identical and can be confirmed at any stage of the pregnancy by ultrasound scanning. Only about 1 per cent of identical twins share the same sac. Non-identical twins never share a placenta or gestational sac.

Does the presence of two separate placentas therefore indicate that twins are non-identical?

Not at all. All non-identical twins have separate placenta but so do 30 per cent of all identical twins. If the division of the egg occurs early, say within three days of fertilization, this division is total and the two fetuses will have separate placentas and sacs. This is why establishing whether twins are identical or not is not a straightforward affair before they are born. Of course, if the twins are of different sexes, this confirms that they are non-identical.

What about Siamese twins?

The proper term is "conjoined twins". The mechanism is still the same and it is all to do with the timing of division. If this occurs very late, at about the twelfth day or later after fertilization, the division is incomplete and the twins will be joined and will share some parts of their bodies.

Conjoined twins are therefore identical twins, where division occurred rather late and was therefore incomplete.

Can Siamese twins be diagnosed before they are born?

In virtually all cases, yes. It is, however, possible to miss the diagnosis if they only share a thin pliable piece of skin, as this may not be immediately apparent on the ultrasound scan.

Is there anything of clinical importance in establishing the kind of twins that one is carrying?

Yes. Those twins with separate placentas (all non-identical twins and 30 per cent of identical twins) always fare best. They have the least number of complications.

Identical twins sharing a placenta have a potential of developing complications that never occur with those having separate placentas. These can be quite serious for both twins. Twins sharing a gestational sac fare worst and up to 50 per cent of these may be lost. Fortunately, these are the least common, accounting for about 1 per cent of identical twins and less than 0.3 per cent of all twins.

What are the problems unique to twins sharing a placenta?

Of most importance is the so-called "twin-to twin transfusion syndrome". This results from the fact that the twins may share some vessels and this may lead to one twin losing its blood to the other. Both the recipient (who is overloaded) and the donor (who is drained) are at peril. If this complication occurs early in pregnancy (before twenty-four weeks of gestation), virtually all twins will be lost. The first to die is usually the recipient. When this problem manifests itself late in pregnancy, the situation can be salvaged but preterm delivery cannot be avoided.

What are the other problems associated with identical twins?

Twins sharing the same sac are prone to cord accidents, resulting from tangling of the cords. This accounts for the increased death rate of these twins.

Birth defects are more common with identical twins, and they suffer more from growth restriction in the womb when compared to non-identical twins.

Are there any other problems associated with twins in general?

Any multiple pregnancy, by virtue of this fact alone, is at increased risk of practically every potential pregnancy complication when compared to a singleton pregnancy.

Premature delivery is certainly commoner with twins or higher-order pregnancies. Only between 50 and 70 per cent of twin pregnancies reach term, compared to about 90 per cent of singleton pregnancies.

Prematurity is the single most common cause of death among these babies. Perinatal death statistics (which include those babies lost through stillbirth and those who die within days of delivery) show that up to 10 per cent of all twins are lost. This is several times the death rate among singletons.

Even the rate of spontaneous miscarriage is several times higher than for singletons.

Complications such as pre-eclampsia, anaemia and bleeding in pregnancy are also significantly more common.

What does a "vanishing twin" mean?

It has now been established that only a proportion of twins starting off as such actually continue as twins to delivery. If all twin pregnancies were identified early enough by ultrasound scan (at six to ten weeks), it is estimated that one twin will subsequently be lost in between 30 and 50 per cent of all.

Twins delivered therefore represent only a proportion of pregnancies that started as such and a substantial proportion of babies born as singletons started off as twins. The other twin, by implication, vanished. The twin that is lost, usually with such minimal symptoms and at such a very early stage of the pregnancy that the mother hardly notices, is known as a 'vanishing twin'.

Antenatal care with twins

What do I need to do to maximize the chances of a good outcome with a twin pregnancy?

As the expectant mother, your role in improving outcome is pivotal.

- Ensure you are getting appropriate and adequate diet. Do not hesitate to ask for dietary advice from your midwife or obstetrician, if you are unsure. The dietician may be involved, although this is rarely necessary.
- Allow yourself adequate rest and avoid unnecessary physical and mental stress.
- Never ignore any physical symptoms. Contact your midwife or hospital immediately: it may be an early warning of a complication.
- Keep all your antenatal appointments. You may be amazed at the amount of incipient problems detected at these seemingly routine reviews.

What should I expect from the antenatal care?

Various centres will have different management policies. Any policy will be geared towards early detection of problems and timely intervention.

You are likely to be seen frequently in the antenatal clinic – probably every two weeks after twenty-four weeks of gestation. This is likely to be flexible, depending on the progression of your pregnancy. If you develop any major complication, such as twin-to-twin transfusion syndrome (rare) or pre-eclampsia (not so rare), you are likely to be admitted into hospital. Premature delivery is virtually inevitable in such a case.

You are likely to have serial ultrasound scans after every two to four weeks to keep track of growth or any restriction. The situation will cause more concern if only one twin appears to be affected. Ultrasound scanning will also detect other problems.

Suppose I am carrying a higher-order multiple, such as triplets?

You are likely to have an even closer follow-up. Many obstetric units operate a policy of routine admission of all mothers expecting triplets at some point in the pregnancy, e.g. twenty-four or twenty-six weeks. This is even in the absence of apparent complications.

If you are carrying quadruplets or more, expect to almost certainly be in hospital from somewhere around twenty weeks to the time of delivery.

Why would I be admitted at twenty weeks when the chance of survival is nil if they were born at that stage?

The aim of hospital admission is to maximize rest, which is crucial in such pregnancies. This is meant to allow optimal blood supply to the womb. In addition, it means if you develop problems such as vaginal bleeding (which can be very severe), these can be managed promptly if you are in hospital.

The higher the number of fetuses you are carrying, the higher the incidence of complications.

Can I expect home-leave for weekends if I am to have a long admission in hospital?

It will depend on your circumstances. However, many people find the idea of home-leave illogical as it defeats the purpose of admission and goes against the primary reason for admission – which is the unpredictability of the complications.

If I develop pre-eclampsia while carrying twins, what should I expect?

Expect early delivery. Attempts will be made to keep the condition under control for as long as it is safe to do so. Valuable time may be bought to give your babies a better chance of survival. Remember, pre-eclampsia is only treated by delivery and whatever measures are instituted while you are pregnant, they are meant just to keep the lid on. If the condition gets worse, in spite of everything thrown at it, delivery becomes inevitable. Most obstetricians would prefer to get to thirty weeks of gestation or beyond. However, nobody tries to achieve this at any price. Delivery will be carried out when it becomes necessary. In such a situation, a balancing act is essential but maternal well-being remains paramount.

What is the likely method of delivery in such a situation?

It depends on a number of factors. If there is no contraindication to vaginal delivery, this will be aimed for. Labour will be induced. If, however, you are too remote from term – let's say below thirty weeks of gestation – induction of labour may be considered not feasible as it is unlikely to succeed in reasonable time. In such a situation, a caesarean delivery is the logical option.

What if I am developing twin-to-twin transfusion?

This is a serious problem and you will need to be admitted in hospital.

If this happens early in pregnancy (before twenty-four weeks), the chances of saving either baby are practically nil. Difficult as this may be, you may be advised to terminate the pregnancy.

If it develops later, say, after twenty-six weeks (twenty-four to twenty-six weeks is a "grey" period), endeavours are made to prolong the pregnancy to achieve viability.

The main plank of the management is likely to be frequent draining of fluid from the womb. This is because there is a tendency in this condition for the recipient twin to accumulate excessive amounts of fluid. This is actually the earliest sign of the complication. If left unchecked, it almost inevitably leads to premature labour, as well as being extremely uncomfortable for the expectant mother.

Is there anything else that can be done to contain the situation?

Some people advocate use of a medicine called indomethacin. This is meant to reduce the production of excess fluid and also prevent premature labour by inhibiting uterine contractions. Not everybody agrees. The argument against it is that it hardly works, has the potential to cause heart complications in the fetus and may well cause kidney damage to the donor twin as it works by reducing urine output.

Recently, some centres have been trying surgical treatment in the form of laser coagulation of the rogue blood vessels in the placenta. There is mixed opinion about its place in the management of this condition because, with the little data available, it appears not to work too well and fetal loss immediately after the treatment is upward of 50 per cent, i.e. unacceptably high. It is still being perfected, however.

Fetal death

How often does fetal death of one twin occur?

Nobody knows for sure as figures from different countries; even different centres in the same country seem to differ widely. The lowest quoted figures are 0.5 per cent (that is, one in 200 twin pregnancies), while the highest available claim a 5 per cent rate, which is ten times the former. Either way, it is pretty uncommon. These figures do not include deaths occurring in twin-to-twin transfusion.

What are the consequences of fetal death?

Apart from the inevitable parental distress over the loss of one of the babies, it may also have adverse effects on the surviving twin. This twin may be found to have birth defects affecting the brain, skin or kidneys. Various other organs may be affected. Long-term, the surviving twin may have cerebral palsy or mental retardation and learning difficulties. Fortunately, only a minority of twins are affected thus.

Is there anything that can be done to prevent these consequences for the surviving twin?

No. In most cases by the time the demise of one twin is discovered – which is often more than twenty-four hours later – the die is cast. If the surviving twin is to be affected, the damage is already done. This should therefore not be an indication for delivery unless there are other relevant obstetric indications. Even then close monitoring of the surviving twin is necessary to ensure its continued well-being.

Can the dead twin cause infection in the womb if left there?

No. As long as the membranes around the baby are intact, there is no such risk. If the membranes are ruptured, prompt delivery is the only option.

Is death of one twin an indication for caesarean delivery?

No. Caesarean delivery will be considered for the usual obstetric indications. Death of one twin is not one of them.

If I have higher-order multiples, with evidence of increased risk of complications and unfavourable outcome, how can I be helped?

There is no question that both expectant mothers and obstetricians find the idea of killing one or more of the fetuses quite distressing. However, it is being increasingly acknowledged that this is sometimes a necessary evil. When the number of fetuses is more than four, severe prematurity is inevitable. Unfortunately, most do not survive and those that do are at increased risk of ending up with debilitating brain damage. This sort of situation calls for a hard-headed decision which may boil down to performing a fetal reduction. When this is opted for, the number left should not be more than three. It should be done early (at or before twenty weeks of gestation), to avoid complications.

The common method is to inject a chemical into the fetal heart, which will make it stop beating. The surviving twins or triplets will therefore be left with enough room to allow growth to a viable gestation. The injection is done under ultrasound guidance.

Can fetal reduction be offered for twins or triplets?

This is a matter of opinion. There is consensus however that there is no obstetric indication to perform fetal reduction in normal twins. It is also very difficult to justify the procedure – for obstetric reasons – for triplets.

Are twins at increased risk of chromosomal anomalies such as Down's syndrome?

The answer should be no. The fact that they are twins (or more) in itself is not a risk factor. However, if you are carrying non-identical twins, it means the chance of having an affected baby is doubled (and tripled for triplets, and so forth).

For identical twins, it is an all or nothing principle. If one is affected, the other one will be; conversely, if one is normal, the other one will also be normal. This is because they are genetically identical.

If I am carrying non-identical twins and one is found to have Down's syndrome or some other chromosomal disorder, can I have a partial termination?

If this is what you wish, this is technically possible. However, what will be done is – strictly speaking – not termination but fetal reduction, where the only affected fetus is killed.

The practical difficulty is in identifying the affected fetus and this may be a stumbling block. It can be extremely difficult to know for certain which of the twins is the one with a chromosomal defect and which is normal.

Delivery

How are twins delivered?

That depends on a lot of factors. If the pregnancy has been problem-free and you have gone to term or close to term, you will discuss the delivery plan with your obstetrician.

Of primary importance is the way the twins are lying. Normally, there is a leading twin, commonly termed "twin I". If twin I is leading with the head, in the absence of contraindications, the accepted mode of delivery is vaginal. This is the case whether twin II is leading with the head or breech.

The consensus probably ends here. Most experts agree that if the first twin is breech then, regardless of the presentation of the second twin, delivery is best achieved by caesarean section. There is a substantial minority of dissenting voices, however.

You will best be advised to discuss the situation with your obstetrician to see where he or she stands on the issue. Nobody has a monopoly of truth on this matter and each school of thought has powerful arguments and evidence to back it. Obstetrics is never an absolute science, a fact eloquently demonstrated by the management of twin delivery.

What is locked twins?

This is a rare complication (historical incidence 0.1 per cent) which may occur if twin I is breech and twin II is leading with a head. It is probably only of historical importance, as virtually all twins presenting as such are delivered by caesarean section nowadays.

If I am carrying triplets, what is the likely method of delivery?

Caesarean section. There are some countries in continental Europe and Africa where vaginal delivery in some selected cases of triplet pregnancy is advocated and practised. In the UK and most other parts of the world, the only accepted method of delivery for triplets – and indeed other higher-order multiples – is caesarean section. This is because they have a higher incidence of prematurity and growth restriction. This makes them more prone to such problems as fetal distress. It is, however, not possible to continuously monitor all three during labour and therefore distress in one or more of them may go unrecognizd.

What is the acceptable interval of delivery between twin I and II in vaginal delivery?

One hour. Most will be delivered within thirty minutes of each other. Beyond this it may be necessary to stimulate the uterus to expedite delivery of the second twin.

However, the operative word here is "acceptable" and it applies to the obstetrician. Most obstetricians feel that after one hour, vaginal delivery of twin II is unlikely and probably waiting longer poses a small risk to this baby. It is also true, however, that in the presence of satisfactory monitoring of the baby's condition and if the mother so wishes, a much longer interval can be allowed. Twins have been known to be born several hours apart with no undue consequences to twin II. The most famous is the pair born on two different days of two different years, twin I on 31 December and twin II on January 1.

There is no hard and fast rule in this, as long as safety measures are not flouted.

Are there any potential complications after delivery?

Mothers who have delivered twins are at an increased risk of heavy blood loss (postpartum haemorrhage) after delivery. Measures will undoubtedly be taken to minimize this risk.

Twins sound like a catalogue of bad news

It tends to come across as such but it is not. Try to see the bigger picture. Over 85 per cent of mothers with twin pregnancies go home with not one, but two perfectly normal bundles of joy.

26. Weight and pregnancy

Introduction

Ideally, if there is a weight problem – be it underweight or over-weight – this should be tackled in the pre-pregnancy period to optimize conditions for pregnancy. Ideally.

Since we do not live in an ideal world, we need to deal with situations where women conceive while having a significant weight problem at each end of the spectrum. General measures will be to give appropriate dietary advice and monitor its effect on the mother and the pregnancy. This may even be a multi-disciplinary measure involving a midwife, dietician, obstetrician, physician and sometimes a psychologist. It is important that each case is individualized.

In between these two groups are those women whose body-weight is within the normal range but who may be concerned about the aftermath of pregnancy on their bodies.

Weight gained during pregnancy, which roughly averages 12 kg (just under two stone), is relatively easy to shake off in the weeks after delivery.

If you think of the fact that a third or more of this weight is the baby, water and the afterbirth – which is instantly wiped off at delivery – you can breathe a little easier. Most of the remainder is actually retained water; adjustment in the body's physiology after delivery will lead to this water being lost through urination in the few days following delivery. The only part that may require active input from the mother is the fat mostly deposited under the skin on the abdomen, upper thighs and lower back. This is well under half a stone (2–3.5 kg). Exercise in the period after delivery will take care of this. Breast-feeding may facilitate the overall strategy.

Of course, the weight gain and speed of loss differs from one individual to another and even from one pregnancy to the next. However, the general picture is similar. Here, we answer specific questions on this important subject.

Risks in pregnancy

Is there any pre-pregnancy weight that is regarded to be a risk factor?

Both very low and overweight states are regarded as risk factors in pregnancy. There are, however, no standard cut-off points.

Many maternity units use 45 kg as the lowest border of normal, below which the woman will be regarded as underweight. The upper border of normal is 80 kg for some units and 85 kg for others. Weights above these cut-off point put the woman in the overweight category.

Some units use a calculated Body Mass Index (BMI). This is scientifically regarded as more objective. A BMI of less than 20 is too low and over 30 represents obesity. It is calculated by dividing the body-weight (in kg) by the square of the height (in metres). For instance, if the woman weighed 70 kg and her height was 1.72 m (5 ft 8 inches), her BMI will be $70/1.72^2$ which works out at 23.64, within the ideal range. If, on the other hand, her height was 1.47 m (4 ft 10 inches), her BMI will be 32.4 which is classified as obese.

Underweight

How does underweight come about?

In the Western world, this problem is mostly a result of eating disorders such as anorexia nervosa and bulimia. These conditions mostly affect young women from the affluent social classes, and in themselves make it difficult for these young women to conceive, but some do.

Another group of underweight women are those who are chronically abusing drugs. These are likely to be underweight simply as a result of under-nourishment. Food becomes a minor priority in their lives.

In some poorer countries in the developing world, underweight may be a direct result of poverty and consequently poor nutrition.

Why is underweight a risk factor in pregnancy?

Underweight women are likely to cope poorly with pregnancy. The primary causes of their underweight are likely to become more complicated and could worsen. As far as the baby is concerned, there is increased possibility of restricted fetal growth and birth of an underweight baby, whatever the gestation at delivery. These underweight babies are at risk of several early life complications (such as hypothermia, low blood-sugar, feeding difficulties and viral infections) and the risk of losing the baby in the perinatal period is significantly increased.

Is maternal underweight a risk factor for miscarriage?
There is no evidence to this effect.

What about premature delivery?
Again no evidence exists that underweight on the part of the mother may in itself lead to premature delivery.

Can such women receive any help?
Ideally, a woman suffering from eating disorders – such as anorexia nervosa or bulimia – should be treated before they become pregnant, to allow for a normal or near-normal weight at the time of conception. However, if the problem comes to light when she is already pregnant, treatment of the underlying problem goes hand-in-hand with general antenatal care. The management is multi-disciplinary for eating disorders – including obstetricians, a physician and a psychiatrist.

Those with a drug habit will also require a multi-disciplinary management, which will include, among others, the midwifery team, obstetrician and a social worker.

Central in all management regimes will be a plan to achieve appropriate nutrition.

Are there any special measures required in labour if the expectant mother is underweight?
Not really. If the fetal growth has been unsatisfactory during the pregnancy, then continuous electronic monitoring of the fetus will be necessary. Of course, intrauterine growth restriction increases the possibility of intervention in labour and delivery by caesarean section. Apart from this, the labour will be treated as any other.

Will there be any special measures after delivery?

The management of the underlying causes of the problem will most likely need to continue beyond delivery.

Overweight

Is obesity a risk factor in pregnancy?

Obesity is without doubt a risk factor, as far as various pregnancy complications are concerned. These include an increased risk of hypertensive disorders (including pre-eclampsia), gestational diabetes, large babies with consequent difficult delivery, postpartum haemorrhage and urinary tract infections. There is some evidence, albeit inconclusive, that the risk of thrombosis and thrombophlebitis may also be increased.

What about pregnancy care with obesity?

There is no doubt that examining an obese pregnant woman's abdomen can be quite difficult; it may even be impossible to make out what you are feeling. Naturally this means there is an increased likelihood of missing potentially risky situations such as a breech presentation or reduced fluid around the baby. It may also create anxiety on the part of the mother, especially if the midwife spends what appears to be an eternity searching for the baby's heartbeat, always a reassuring sound to a prospective mother.

Does this difficulty extend to technological aids such as ultrasound?

Unfortunately, yes. When there is marked obesity, the image on ultrasound can be very poor and the technician may fail to get all the required information – a situation which can cause anxiety because of questions left unanswered.

What about delivery?

Obese women, because of an increase in antenatal problems, are at increased risk of ending up with a caesarean delivery. This is not a simple matter of an alternative method of delivery.

Overweight women are more risky anaesthetic subjects. Inducing anaesthesia – both general and spinal or epidural – is more difficult.

Moreover, such potentially serious post-operative complications as thrombosis are more likely to occur among the overweight.

Even when all seems to pass off without a hitch, excess weight still has a sting in the tail. Wound infection following surgery is much more common among the obese.

Should an overweight woman booking for antenatal care be encouraged to lose weight?

Not at all. If a woman conceives while overweight the issue of losing weight should and must be put on hold until after delivery. Of course, she may be overweight because of poor eating habits in the first place, in which case dietary advice will be given. Sensible exercise, not to lose weight but to keep healthy, will be encouraged as well.

Is there anything that needs to be actively done to minimize complications?

It is important for the service providers (i.e. midwife or doctor) to be aware of potential problems associated with obesity in pregnancy and to look for them. Surveillance for raised blood pressure, urinary tract infection and diabetes will be meticulously maintained. In case of a caesarean delivery, preventative antibiotics – and, in most cases, heparin, to try to prevent thrombosis – will be administered. Heparin will normally continue until the mother is on her feet again; getting up and walking about will be actively encouraged.

If delivery is vaginal, what are the potential problems?

In general, obese women give birth to large babies; consequently they tend to have comparatively more difficult deliveries (but not necessarily so).

If a newborn is found to be large for his or her gestational age, close monitoring of his or her blood-sugar will be done in the first few hours of life. This is done even if tests for gestational diabetes on the baby's mother were negative.

Weight gain during pregnancy

For a woman of "normal" weight at conception, how much weight should she expect put on during pregnancy?

On average, it is about 12 kg (26 lb, or just under two stone). The range is quite wide, from as little as 8 kg to 16 kg, sometimes more. These figures refer to singleton pregnancies. Those with multiple pregnancies, such as twins, are likely to put on more.

What are the factors that determine the amount of weight gained?

As with most circumstances in life, a dietary habit is the most important factor. However, other factors are important too.

The weight before conception is crucial in that the higher the pre-pregnancy weight, the bigger the potential weight gain. Age is another factor, as an older mother will tend to gain more weight. Parity is also a factor: for each subsequent pregnancy, the weight gained tends to go down.

Is there any particular phase of pregnancy when weight gain is maximal?

Weight gain is not constant throughout the course of pregnancy. In fact, in the first ten weeks of pregnancy, weight put on is minimal, averaging no more than 1 to 1.5 kg for that entire period.

After about fourteen weeks, the average weight gain accelerates to about 0.4 to 0.5 kg weekly. This is almost 2 kg (4.4 lb) every month. After about the thirty-weeks mark, the rate of weight gain is again reduced. In the last weeks of pregnancy, there may be little or no weight gain at all.

It is important to remember that much of the weight gained is retained water and also that the uterine contents (fetus, placenta and amniotic fluid) account for a lot of the weight, which is going to be lost instantly at delivery.

But surely there is weight gained in the form of fat?

Yes. Some fat is laid on under the skin in the back, abdomen and thigh areas. This occurs mostly in the first half of pregnancy. The propensity for this differs among individuals but, in most cases, it is only little or modest. Proper exercises, started a few days after delivery, almost always succeed in eliminating this.

What happens after delivery?

As mentioned before, a substantial proportion of the weight gained during pregnancy is retained water. This phenomenon is promoted and maintained as a direct effect of pregnancy hormones. Within ten days of delivery, all the excess water will have been lost. At this stage, the mother will be only about 3 kg above her pre-pregnancy weight, provided she has had a sensible diet. This remaining weight is mostly the fat and, to a small extent, protein gained during pregnancy.

How can the fat be shifted?

A woman who is generally physically active and who maintains this lifestyle after delivery may not need to do anything extra and the excess fat will be lost, even though it may take up to ten weeks for her to reach her pre-pregnancy weight. Breast-feeding, preferably when not mixed with bottle-feeding, helps in accelerating the process of weight loss. This is because of the extra calorie requirements on the body. For a woman who is in a hurry to lose the weight, appropriate exercises will help.

Is there anything to worry about if a woman is not putting on weight during pregnancy?

There can never be any justification to encourage or ignore total lack of weight gain or sustained weight loss in pregnancy. The body physiology in pregnancy is geared towards weight gain and reversal of this has to be investigated. Sometimes the explanation is obvious, as in excessive vomiting. In the absence of such an explanation, dietary habits should be looked it. It normally boils down to diet.

Sustained lack of weight gain risks leading to intrauterine fetal growth restriction, with all the consequent potential problems.

Dietary restriction is rumoured to reduce the risk of pre-eclampsia. Could this be true?

There is no truth whatsoever in this.

27. Sport and exercise in pregnancy

Introduction

Exercise or a physically active lifestyle is known to be good for one's general health. This is still true during pregnancy. However, there may be certain considerations because of the special nature of pregnancy: questions as to the type of exercise, extent of physical exertion, what is safe and what is not. As a general rule, a pregnant woman should be encouraged to be physically active, which does not necessarily mean a formal exercise regime. A regular walk, a swim and using the stairs at work instead of a lift may do just as well.

For those who engage in sport, pregnancy does not necessarily mean having to give up, unless it is a contact sport (such as boxing or wrestling) where there is a theoretical risk of injury that may imperil the pregnancy. Most amateur and professional sportswomen engage in non-contact sport, and most of these are quite compatible with pregnancy. In fact, even those engaged in competitive sports can still carry on, especially if this falls in the early part of the pregnancy. Exercise and sport have several benefits for a participating pregnant woman, as we have detailed below. There are those who, by virtue of pre-existing medical conditions, may be unable to engage in active physical exercises. These are very much in the minority and specific advice regarding this is usually given.

The benefits of exercise

Is exercise good for a pregnant woman?

There is no doubt that a pregnant woman who exercises regularly accrues significant psychological benefits from the activity. All other things being equal, she will be more relaxed, more energetic and feel good about herself, more so than her sedentary counterpart.

Are there any physical benefits?

Yes. There is reduction in things such as bloatedness, backache, fatigue and headache – all common problems in pregnancy.

Women who exercise have also reported significant reduction in shortness of breath and constipation.

Does exercise have any benefit regarding weight gain in pregnancy?

One has to be careful here. Weight gain in pregnancy is no bad thing and one should never set out to try to prevent this. However, several things account for the weight gained. These include the growing uterus and its contents; increase in the blood volume; retained water (an effect caused by the progesterone hormone) and fat – usually on the abdominal wall and thighs.

Most of this weight requires little or no effort to get rid of after delivery. The exception is the deposited fat. Exercise in pregnancy, even in moderation, limits the amount of fat deposited under the skin. This, in turn, reduces the effort required after delivery to shift this weight.

Are there any risks associated with exercising during pregnancy?

Yes. That is why it is important that only the appropriate types of exercise are carried out. The progesterone hormone softens the ligaments that hold the various joints together and keep them stable. The softening effect will therefore make the joints somewhat unstable. The wrong kind of exercise could quite plausibly lead to injury of some of these joints, such as those in the spine, the pelvis, knees and ankles.

So what sort of exercises are ideal for a pregnant woman?

We would not attempt to give an ideal exercise programme here. It is important that such a programme is individualized, according to the woman's state of health, the existing level of activity and what she enjoys doing. It is important that an expert is involved in formulating such a programme and all maternity units will have such people available, if and when needed.

If a woman has been exercising regularly pre-conception, what should she do?

She should ideally carry on. However, before doing that she should seek advice regarding the type of exercise she should and should not do.

Any programme of exercise should observe some or all of the following:

- A warm-up period lasting several minutes, an exercise session of fifteen to thirty minutes, then a slowing down period, again lasting several minutes, before stopping. She should avoid sudden physical exertion as well as sudden stopping.
- Adequate fluid as well as calorie intake.
- The correct kind of sportswear, including comfortable sports shoes, clothes and a purpose-built support bra. The clothes should preferably be loose-fitting comfortable ones.
- If a device to continually monitor the pulse rate is available, she should aim to keep the rate below 140 per minute. If the rate creeps above this, it is time to wind down.
- The exercise area must be well-lit and allow good air circulation. This will prevent over-heating.
- Avoid exhaustion. A well-planned exercise programme should allow her to finish short of this point.
- The exercise should allow her to carry on a conversation. If she cannot, it is a reliable sign that she is doing too much and it is time to slow down.

Short of proper exercise programmes, what other activities can a pregnant woman engage in to try to get some of the benefits?

Swimming, cycling, walking and jogging are excellent and considered safe to pursue during pregnancy. Golf, due to the walking involved, is also good.

Unsafe exercise and worries

Are any activities considered unsafe?

Skiing – including water-skiing – contact sports such as basketball and hockey, and such activities as gymnastics, ice-skating and scuba-diving are considered unsafe. The risk increases as the pregnancy advances.

What sort of exercises should be avoided during pregnancy?

Avoid full sit-ups, hopping and skipping and double-leg raising. Any exercise which involves prolonged lying on the back should be avoided, particularly after the half-way stage of pregnancy. This is because the heavy uterus presses on the major blood vessels, interfering with blood-flow.

What about stretching?

Anybody who has attended an aerobics class will be aware of the stretching exercises used for the build-up and wind-down. These exercises are positively encouraged during pregnancy. Most antenatal classes will include these.

Suppose there is concern about the fetal growth. Should the pregnant woman carry on exercising?

The standard advice in such situations is to "take it easy". However, this is based on an unproven hypothesis. There is absolutely no evidence that exercise in moderation will have any deleterious effect on such a pregnancy.

The effects of exercise on pregnancy and labour

What advantages does a woman who has been exercising regularly have over one who has not bothered, when it comes to labour?

There is no doubt that a woman who has been active goes into labour with more energy and better reserves to cope with labour.

Experiences of labour differ widely among individuals and whether they have exercised or not is only one factor among many that will influence this. It is very difficult, if not impossible, to quantify the benefits of this aspect.

Does exercise during pregnancy have any influence on the length of labour?

There is no evidence that exercise status will make labour shorter (or longer, for that matter).

Back stretches

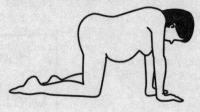

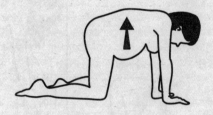

Legs stretches

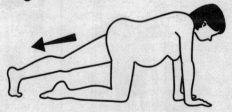

Fig 8 Gentle stretching exercises a woman can do in late pregnancy. Evidence that continued physical activity confers benefit both physically and psychologically is strong. Exercise does not have to be formalized. A regular walk or swim is just as good.

Fig 8 continued.
More stretching exercises for women in
late pregnancy

Trunk stretches

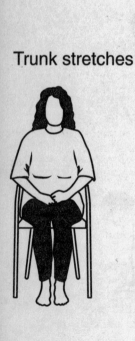

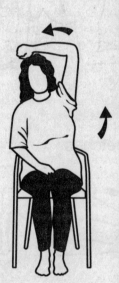

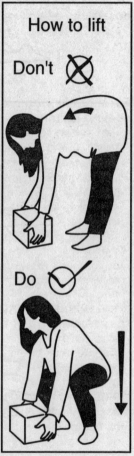

How to lift

Don't

Do

What about exercise and the requirements for pain relief in labour?

There is no evidence that exercising during pregnancy will help reduce need for pain relief in labour.

Does exercise during pregnancy reduce the possibility of ending up with a caesarean section?

No evidence to this effect exists.

Specific sports

For women who engage in endurance sports such as long-distance running: what sort of advice is given when they conceive?

There is no doubt that they can continue engaging in their sport for as long as they feel able to, as long as there is regular and adequate antenatal care. There is no evidence whatsoever that this will affect the course or progress of the pregnancy.

If such an athlete develops any of the pregnancy complications which can affect any woman, then the appropriate advice will be given. Studies carried out have shown that such athletes continue to be actively engaged in their sport to well beyond the half-way mark of the pregnancy, with no noticeable effect on their performance.

What will be the condition of such athletes when they resume training after delivery?

Many such women go back to their sport several months after delivery. Normally there is no noticeable effect on the performance level that they eventually achieve post-delivery.

What is the advice regarding women boxers?

Boxing is one of the sports that have crossed the gender barrier in recent years. The advice is to stop during the course of the pregnancy. There is no evidence that even the protective gear that is sometimes available is sufficient in eliminating the risk entirely.

Resuming exercise after the birth

How soon should a woman who has had an uncomplicated delivery resume exercising?

If she had a vaginal delivery without any problems, two weeks or thereabouts is a good enough interval to start aerobic exercise. There is no harm in starting a few days earlier with light exercise, if she feels like it.

What about swimming?

Swimming has special constraints, because of the inevitable vaginal discharge that follows delivery and may continue for several weeks.

If using communal pools, one should avoid swimminguntil this has stopped. This may take four to six weeks.

What about exercise after caesarean section?

In this case, it is wiser to stay off exercise for at least four weeks. After this, the build-up to the previous level of activity should be slow and steady.

Does this advice include pelvic floor exercises?

No. These can be resumed even before leaving hospital if one is able. However, a woman who had a caesarean section may find that the soreness from the surgical scar limits even these.

What if one has had an episiotomy?

An episiotomy (a cut made to increase the birth passage in vaginal delivery) heals quite fast: in most cases, in less than a week. However, lingering soreness in the area may mean that pelvic floor exercises may have to wait.

Suppose the new mother has opted to breast-feed. Will exercise or sport have any effect on this?

They should not. In fact, moderate exercise does not alter any of the essential ingredients of breast-milk. Nor does it have any effect on quantities produced. Extreme exercise may alter the pH of the milk making it slightly more acidic. The effect may last for sixty to ninety minutes post-exercise. Overall, exercise has no significant effect one way or another on breast-milk. The advice regarding adequate fluid replacement remains the same for a breast-feeding exercising mother.

28. Stillbirth

Introduction

Stillbirth is a profoundly tragic event in any prospective parent's life. The sense of utter hopelessness is usually overwhelming. Mercifully, this is an uncommon event.

In the vast majority of cases of stillbirth, it is completely unexpected and therefore unpredictable. This obviously adds to the weight of the tragedy.

Many parents' anguish is not helped by the fact that, even after the event, extensive investigations that are carried out do not yield the important answer: the cause. This is true in roughly half the cases of stillbirth.

Getting an explanation does at least have the effect of allowing them to try to come to terms with the loss. It also helps the doctors to give credible and informed advice about the future.

So what do we known about causes of stillbirth?

As we shall see in answers to specific questions below, the identifiable causes can be divided into three broad groups. There are maternal illnesses that are usually known before the event: examples include diabetes or pre-eclampsia. There is therefore room to institute measures to prevent this eventuality. Sometimes the measures fail. The second group constitutes fetal problems which may include viral or bacterial infections (usually silent and unrecognized) and cord accidents. The third group is where the problem is in the placenta (afterbirth).

Any one of the mentioned potential causes of stillbirth is relatively easy to identify after the event. It is therefore possible to give informed advice to the parents.

There are many support groups which parents in this situation find very useful. Medical science has advanced to a stage where any further reduction in the rate of stillbirth is an unrealistic prospect. Efforts are therefore appropriately concentrated on trying to ensure that this sad event does not affect the same mother more than once.

Stillbirth and miscarriage

How would you describe stillbirth as opposed to miscarriage?

It may surprise many that the medical fraternity does not appear to agree as to what stage of pregnancy fetal loss becomes technically a stillbirth.

In the UK and most other countries, survival outside the womb is considered realistically possible only after twenty-four weeks of gestation. If the fetus dies in the womb before twenty-four weeks and delivery subsequently occurs; this is regarded as a miscarriage, albeit "late" if it was beyond sixteen weeks.

In the USA, however, fetal death occurring after twenty weeks is regarded as "mid-trimester stillbirth". This is because, in the United States, a fetus of twenty weeks' gestation is regarded as potentially viable even though, to date, there has been no proven survival of a baby delivered at this gestation.

To the affected mother however, all this may be pointlessly academic and the gestation at which the baby is lost may have little or no bearing on the intensity of her grief.

How common is stillbirth?

In developed countries of Western Europe, stillbirth occurs in three to four in 1000 live births. This merely means that for every 1000 babies born alive, there will be three or four stillborn babies. In the USA, where the gestational cut-off point is lower, the rate is seven in 1000.

In some cases, the mother will not know the gestation age of her pregnancy, only to have a fetus that is no longer viable; how will this be classified?

In such a situation, the weight of the fetus will determine whether it is to be classified as a late miscarriage or a stillbirth. If the fetus weight is more than 500 grams (1.1 lb), this will be a stillbirth and be registered as such. If it is below this weight, it will be classified as a miscarriage (500 grams is the average weight at twenty-four weeks of gestation).

Causes of death

How often is the cause of death identifiable?

There is a whole battery of tests, which feature in most obstetric units' protocols for investigating stillbirth. Depressingly, most of them almost always come back negative. Depressingly – because most parents would want to know what caused the death of their baby. In the best centres, about 50 per cent of stillbirths are adequately explained. This leaves half of all stillbirths with no conclusively established cause.

How often is stillbirth predictable?

This is a very difficult question to answer. From time to time, an at-risk pregnancy is identified but a doctor makes an error of judgement regarding timing of delivery and the fetus dies.

Occasionally, the mother may be reluctant to heed advice on early delivery and tragically loses the baby. Evidently, such incidences are rare and form only a very small part of stillbirth statistics. Most stillbirths nowadays are completely unexpected. In other words, stillbirth is rarely predictable.

What are the fetal causes of stillbirth?

The fetus may carry a serious chromosomal anomaly which has not been suspected following the standard screening blood tests or ultrasound. Alternatively, the fetus may have a serious neurological or structural condition which leads to death in the womb. These conditions are rare and many of them are identifiable, or at least can be suspected as a result of screening tests and/or ultrasound in mid-trimester or later.

Are there any maternal conditions that may lead to stillbirth?

Yes. The readily identifiable condition is what is termed as anti-phospholipid syndrome. In this condition, the mother carries antibodies in her circulation, which attack small vessels in the placenta, seriously compromising its function. This may lead to early miscarriage or, if the pregnancy survives till late, a stillbirth.

People with SLE are quite prone to this problem. However, the majority of women who are eventually found to carry these antibodies are otherwise healthy and there would have been no cause for concern prior to the miscarriage or a stillbirth. Every woman who experiences the tragedy of stillbirth is investigated for presence of these antibodies.

Can a woman identified to carry anti-phospholipid antibodies be helped to avoid a similar fate in subsequent pregnancies?

Certainly. There is treatment to prevent the effects of the syndrome, even though the underlying condition cannot be completely eliminated.

An appropriate treatment regime (which lasts the entire course of the pregnancy) has a potential for a successful outcome of about 75 per cent, as opposed to a possibility of less than 25 per cent of babies surviving if no treatment is used.

Are there any other maternal causes of stillbirth?

Conditions such as chronic kidney failure and people with rare clotting abnormalities may lead to fetal death in the uterus. The latter condition, if identified, can be successfully managed in subsequent pregnancies.

Infections are sometimes blamed for stillbirth. What are they, and can they be avoided?

Every protocol for investigating stillbirth will include screening for possible viral infections. The known rogue viruses which may infect the fetus and lead to its demise include parvovirus, CMV, Rubella and a few other less common ones. Non-viral infections which may cause stillbirth include toxoplasmosis and syphilis.

Bleeding inside the womb may lead to stillbirth. How?

Sometimes – in most cases inexplicably – the placenta detaches, either partially or wholly, from its base. This leads to bleeding which could be so severe that it leads to fetal death. The bleeding may actually remain concealed with no visible outward blood loss. This condition is almost invariably associated with abdominal pain. When the placental separation is extensive, fetal death is so rapid as to be practically unsalvageable. This condition is called abruptio placenta or "placental abruption".

Are there any factors associated with abruptio placenta?

Yes. Cigarette smoking is a risk factor and cocaine drug abuse is a definite cause.

Does standard antenatal care have any role to play in preventing stillbirth?

Most definitely. Not infrequently, a pregnancy may be identified where progress is unsatisfactory.

Growth may be noted to be slow and an ultrasound scan may confirm this as well as identifying reduced amniotic fluid volume. The latter is often a sign that all is not well with a pregnancy. All these features may be identified when the mother feels nothing is amiss.

Naturally, when such a pregnancy is identified, close monitoring measures will be initiated and this may culminate in hospital admission or even intervention in the form of early delivery. This kind of scenario is usually a case of obscure placental insufficiency. There could be other potential risky conditions which can only be identified through regular antenatal care. These include such conditions as diabetes or pre-eclampsia. All these have a potential to lead to fetal death with little or no warning.

A mother has a duty to herself and her unborn baby to play her part by regular attendance at the antenatal clinic.

Are there any environmental causes of stillbirth?

There is no concrete evidence that any environmental pollutants (except massive radiation) can lead to stillbirth. This state of affairs may change in future as we gain more knowledge of the effects of environmental pollution. After all, about half of all stillbirths go unexplained.

What happens after stillbirth

What should a woman expect, once a diagnosis of fetal death has been established?

This is usually a very difficult time. There is an initial explanation and counselling is offered. Ideally, the mother should have her partner or another person who is close to her with her. Plans of delivery will be discussed and normally this will be vaginal unless there is a contraindication to this, where a caesarean section may have to be undertaken.

The process of investigating the cause of death may begin soon after the diagnosis. This may be in the form of amnio-centesis (taking fluid from around the baby). This is done early to maximize the chance of successfully culturing the fetal cells, if investigating possible chromosomal abnormal-ities. Other (blood) tests will normally be deferred until later.

Options will normally be given as to the time and day of labour induction and some mothers opt to go home first for a day or two before being admitted for induction of labour.

What about a post-mortem?

Unless the cause of fetal death is definitely known, the parents will be advised to have a post-mortem examination done on the baby. This quite often comes up with an explanation as to the cause of death.

Is breast-milk produced, in spite of stillbirth?

Yes. The extent of milk production will depend largely on how advanced the pregnancy was. If the baby is lost late in the third trimester, there is full lactation and breast engorgement is a problem which will need to be addressed. This could be conservatively managed or medication can be given over a course of two weeks, sometimes longer, to suppress lactation.

What happens to the baby?

It is believed to be a good idea to encourage the mother to hold her baby. Pictures will be taken and if the mother does not want them immediately, they will be kept safe in case she changes her mind later. If, a few months after the event, she still does not want them, then they may be destroyed.

The parents are also encouraged to name the child. A dis-cussion with parents is held on the subject of the kind of ceremony they would want for disposal of the baby's body. They may opt for a formal funeral or probably cremation.

So what follows for the parents?

Most hospitals have dedicated counsellors to deal with such a situation. In the immediate aftermath, a counsellor will be available to explain things and answer questions.

On discharge from hospital, the parents will normally be put in touch with the various support groups within their locality. An appointment to see their obstetrician will be made, usually within six to twelve weeks. It is at this visit that the parents will have an opportunity to know the results of the various tests and to have their many questions answered.

What is the likelihood of a stillbirth recurring?

Unlike miscarriage, stillbirth is fortunately a rare occurrence. A recurrence – although possible, in theory – is exceedingly rare.

However, it is the duty of the attending obstetrician to counsel each affected woman on the basis of the evidence relevant to her particular case. If the cause of death was not established, then all the doctor can offer is reassurance on the basis of statistics.

Statistics undoubtedly show that recurrence will be extremely unlikely. None the less, the subsequent pregnancy will be classified as "high risk" and antenatal care will be intensive.

If the cause of stillbirth is identified, what then?

The advice is simpler then, because it will be based on what is known about the specific cause of death.

If it was a one-off freak occurrence, then reassurance will be given on this basis.

If it is a residual problem such as anti-phospholipid syndrome, then the mother will be made aware of the steps to be taken next time round, to maximize the chances of a successful outcome.

If it is a treatable condition (such as syphilis), then treatment will be given.

How soon should a woman try to conceive, following a stillbirth?

For the vast majority of cases, the advice is to try whenever and as soon as she feels psychologically and emotionally ready. Physically, there is usually no contraindication for another pregnancy.

The rare exceptions are in situations where a serious maternal condition such as chronic renal failure led to the stillbirth. The advice then may be to defer until the condition has been stabilized, or she may be advised to abandon the idea altogether. Such cases are the exception rather than the rule.

29. Preterm rupture of membranes

Introduction

When "waters" go prior to reaching term (thirty-seven weeks and beyond), the event can cause acute anxiety and even panic.

There is little doubt that nature meant the membranes to rupture either just before the onset of labour or during labour.

The further from term the event occurs, the higher the risk of complications for both mother and baby. In fact, if this happens at or around twenty weeks of gestation (the halfway mark), the prognosis for the baby is, in all honesty, quite dire. On the other hand, if this takes place closer to term – let us say at around thirty-four weeks – unless the cause was something very serious, the baby will usually emerge relatively unscathed. This is regardless of whether delivery follows a few days after or much later.

You will see in the following section that there are areas where obstetricians do not appear to agree on the best strategy when membranes rupture. Mothers, quite understandably, hate this. Unfortunately, this is one area where you do not have a clear black and white picture. The apparent dithering is because there is, in reality, no scientific evidence to say which strategy is superior to the other. It is therefore not unusual to hear one advising immediate delivery because it is his or her preferred strategy, while the other advises conservative management "to await events". This is usually the case when "waters" rupture in the so-called grey period between thirty-four and thirty-seven weeks. There is virtual consensus when it is before this, as we shall see in the following section.

Rupture of membranes at term, even before the onset of labour is not regarded as a problem. It just means labour is imminent, even though the waiting for the actual event may stretch from an hour to two or even three days. This is unless the doctors decide to intervene to encourage things along, as they may do, with the mother's consent.

Frequency of rupture

How common is it for membranes to rupture before term?

It is fairly common in the sense that it affects about 8 per cent of all pregnancies. Overall, 10 per cent of all pregnancies will be affected by membranes rupturing before labour. The difference (2 per cent) is accounted for by rupture at term but before the onset of labour.

What is the difference between membranes rupturing before term and before labour?

If membranes rupture before the onset of labour then this is termed "pre-labour rupture of membranes", regardless of the gestation. If this occurs before thirty-seven weeks of gestation, then it is further qualified by the term "preterm pre-labour rupture of membranes". The significance is in the prematurity in the latter case.

When should membranes ideally rupture?

Amniotic fluid membranes (or "waters", in popular terms) should stay intact until the onset of labour. The waters will go at any stage of labour. This may be spontaneous or they may be artificially ruptured, if this is seen to be useful or necessary. This is what happens in 90 per cent of all pregnancies.

What does "premature rupture of membranes" mean?

This has been mentioned here in case it is a term that has been used by your midwife or doctor. It is in fact an old term which is both inaccurate and misleading. The original meaning of the term was a situation where waters broke before the onset of labour, even at term. This, as you can see, can create confusion. It is a term that has been largely abandoned but old habits die hard and old medical habits probably die hardest. You may therefore encounter somebody using it. In this text, we shall stick with the currently used terms, i.e. preterm rupture of membranes and pre-labour rupture of membranes, which are self-descriptive.

What happens when membranes rupture?

What happens when membranes rupture before labour?

You will notice a gush or trickle of fluid from the vagina. It is usually clear and feels warm. It can be – and often is – confused with urine incontinence, especially when it is only a trickle. The tendency is for the leak to continue and it is normally made stronger by actions such as laughing, coughing or sneezing. There is usually no pain.

What do you need to do when the waters break?

Regardless of the gestation, the mother should be seen in a maternity unit promptly. One of the not infrequent statements that obstetricians and midwives hear with a sinking heart is, "Oh, I have been wet for the last three days or so." This, frankly speaking, is irresponsible on the part of the mother. The plan of management needs to be put in place immediately after any pre-labour rupture of membranes, regardless of whether it is term or preterm.

Why should one worry about the waters breaking if the pregnancy is already at term?

There are immediate concerns such as cord complications. Pre-labour rupture of membranes could be complicated by prolapse of the cord, which may then be compressed, effectively cutting off the blood supply to the fetus. By the time the mother is alerted – by, let's say, loss of fetal movements – it is really too late.

Delayed complications of pre-labour rupture of membranes at term include infection, especially if labour is delayed for a number of days. The baby may be born in poor health and could suffer from severe pneumonia or other serious infections as a result.

Most obstetric units operate a policy of inducing labour after twenty-four hours if it has not happened spontaneously. Even those units which observe a more conservative policy will take measures to exclude infection or to monitor for any signs of this, so that timely appropriate action can be taken.

What about preterm pre-labour rupture of membranes?

This is a different ball-game. There is the added dimension of prematurity as a problem to contend with. The outlook for the pregnancy will therefore be heavily dependent on the gestation, i.e. the degree of prematurity.

It is important to be aware that once waters break, four out of five pregnancies will conclude within a week, whatever measures are instituted. In cases where the membranes rupture before twenty-six weeks of gestation, the outlook is rather bleak. For the 20 per cent where pregnancy continues successfully, there are still other problems which plague the mother and baby. These are discussed below.

How the mother and baby are affected

If the pregnancy continues after preterm rupture of membranes, what are the potential risks to the mother?

For the mother, the feared complication is infection, a condition called "chorio-amnionitis". It simply means "inflammation of the membranes". This is a potentially serious problem and can even lead to septicaemia (infection of the blood).

It is estimated to affect up to a third of all pregnancies with prolonged rupture of membranes, the vast majority of cases being only mild and treated in time.

Preterm rupture of membranes also increases the chance of a caesarean delivery.

We should not forget that this complication of pregnancy is managed wholly in hospital and the prolonged hospitalization, sometimes lasting several weeks, could be severely disruptive on the home front.

How is the baby affected by preterm rupture of membranes?

This depends on the extent or degree of prematurity. Again, remember, once the waters break, delivery will occur within a week in 80 per cent of cases. If the rupture occurs as early as around twenty-four weeks, one is facing a spectre of delivering a tiny baby with hardly any lung development.

The outlook is then very poor indeed, unless the pregnancy can be prolonged for several weeks. Even when this is achieved, it is not all light and sunshine. These babies face multiple problems as a result of developing in the womb where there is no water. If the rupture occurred very early, lung development – which is dependent on the presence of adequate fluid – will be severely impaired.

This may be a difficult problem to overcome even after delivery and the baby may not survive. Other problems caused by lack of fluid in the womb include limb deformities (which are positional and correctable), facial deformities (usually mild) and growth restriction. In any case of prolonged rupture of membranes, there is the ever-present risk of infection, which will normally force delivery. Once infection is detected, there is no option but to deliver the baby.

Poor lung development appears to be the most serious potential complication of preterm rupture of membranes. Can anything be done to overcome this?

Precious little, if any. If the membranes rupture relatively late – let's say after twenty-eight weeks – the problem is either mild or does not occur. If it is as early as twenty-two or twenty-four weeks, it is potentially very serious. One management strategy which is not quite established in mainstream practice and whose value has yet to be fully established is the so-called "amnio-infusion". In this, sterile fluid is infused into the womb every few days to try to create a "normal" environment for the fetus. Results so far have been variable but the procedure is still in its infancy.

What is the role of steroid injections?

Any woman who has had an episode of threatened or real premature labour will probably know that steroid injections are offered, as is generally described, to "help mature the baby's lungs". It is important to know that the problem that we try to correct using steroids is not the same as the one created by lack or deficiency of water.

Lack of water impairs structural development of the lungs and therefore there is insufficient lung tissue development in such a situation. Steroids are meant to stimulate lung tissue to produce a chemical which facilitates normal lung function. It therefore means that, for the steroids to be useful, there has to be a sufficient amount of lung tissue there in the first place. Steroids facilitate lung function and not lung development.

What should a mother-to-be expect, faced with such a complication?

The primary aim of the doctors is to evaluate the situation and explore the possibility of a favourable outcome. They will then give thorough counselling to the prospective parents. It is very important to be honest. In cases where preterm rupture of membranes occurs before twenty-six weeks of gestation, the chances of the baby surviving are probably less than 40 per cent.

Even for those who survive, well over half will have some degree of handicap. Prematurity is the main problem. For gestation of over twenty-seven weeks, the outlook is more favourable, but prematurity and its complications still cause considerable havoc. (For more detail see Chapter 30, "Preterm labour".)

After thirty-one weeks of gestation, the outlook is good and nine out of ten babies survive without problems.

What is the standard advice in preterm rupture of membranes?

There is no standard advice. Each case must be evaluated and managed individually. If, for instance, there is infection already involving the membranes, delivery will be made promptly, regardless of the gestation.

The method of delivery will also depend on the circumstances, even though the chances of having a caesarean section are increased considerably because of such potential problems as cord compression or fetal distress. Rupture of membranes in itself is not an indication for caesarean section.

Late and pre-labour ruptures

What if the preterm rupture occurs rather late in pregnancy?

If membranes rupture between thirty-four and thirty-seven weeks of gestation, worry about the baby's well-being has receded and many obstetricians will just wait for things to happen (as they will do in the majority of cases) within twenty-four to forty-eight hours. This is on the proviso that both the mother and the baby are well. This policy is adopted mostly because the alternative is to induce labour. This may not be easy, increasing the chance of an otherwise unnecessary caesarean section.

If delivery was going to be by caesarean section anyway, for other reasons, and preterm rupture of membranes occurs, then delivery will be brought forward, because there is no conceivable benefit in waiting at this gestation.

The conservative approach is not favoured by everybody, however. Some obstetricians start the process of induction of labour as soon as the mother is admitted with ruptured membranes at this gestation. Still others try to compromise by putting a limit to the waiting time. After this time has elapsed (without labour), induction of labour is commenced. All the facts will be put to the mother-to-be, explaining the options and allowing her to make an informed decision on how she would like to proceed.

What happens in cases where membranes rupture pre-labour at term?

If the gestation is over thirty-seven weeks, it means the pregnancy is effectively at term. If the waters break before the onset of labour in this period, most obstetricians advise a waiting approach, as labour will ensue in well over 80 per cent within twenty-four hours. Because of this fact, most units operate a policy where induction of labour is done for the few who have not gone into labour after twenty-four hours. There is evidence that leaving such cases for longer than forty-eight hours increases the risk of infection for both the mother and the baby.

Others, however, have a more interventionist approach, where assessment is made at the time. If the neck of the womb (cervix) is found not to be favourable for labour, the process of induction of labour is commenced immediately. If, on the other hand, the cervix is favourable, nothing is done. This is on the assumption that spontaneous labour onset is likely to happen in a matter of hours.

There is no scientific evidence to suggest that one approach is superior to the other.

In preterm rupture of membranes, are there any additional measures to improve the outcome?

The main measure is a close surveillance to detect the development of infection at the earliest possible stage. These measures will include monitoring the mother's own vital signs, including temperature and serial blood tests. Some will add vaginal swabs every few days, but this is controversial.

The other measure is monitoring the fetal well-being.

Is there room for outpatient management of this problem?

You will have to search long and hard to find an obstetrician who will consider outpatient management.

Most obstetricians consider such an approach insufficient and probably irresponsible. There are, however, a few who argue quite vigorously that it could be adopted in a few well-selected cases. This will probably remain a very controversial approach in the foreseeable future.

Is there room for use of antibiotics to prevent infection in such cases?

This is another controversial area. Many studies have shown that antibiotics are ineffective in preventing the development of infection in such cases. Most obstetricians will therefore not use antibiotics for the sole purpose of trying to prevent infection. There is an argument, however, that antibiotics may help to prolong the pregnancy and therefore add a few more precious days to it. This is unproven, at least for now.

The only undisputed use of antibiotics is in cases where there is already evidence of infection, where treatment is commenced, together with putting delivery plans under way.

Are there any likely complications after delivery?

Yes; the most important one is the oft-mentioned problem of infection.

Also, there is increased incidence of excessive haemorrhage (or blood loss).

What causes these complications?.

The causes are poorly understood. In some cases, they have been associated with vaginal infection. Cigarette smoking is considered a risk factor.

In the vast majority, no cause or associated factor can be identified. This is one area where medical research is very active.

Does preterm rupture of membranes recur?

Yes. In just over 20 per cent of women, the problem will recur in a subsequent pregnancy.

Do membranes ever reseal if they rupture early in pregnancy?

This probably never happens. There is certainly no hard evidence that such an occurrence has ever taken place.

30. Preterm labour

Introduction

Preterm labour, also called premature labour, is a fairly common pregnancy complication. Sometimes there are identifiable causes but, in most cases, the trigger remains a mystery. A small minority of women are prone to preterm labour and therefore will tend to have it as a recurrent phenomenon. For most, however, it is a one-off.

There are a great deal of false alarms and some studies have estimated that, in up to 80 per cent of instances, there is really nothing significant going on. However, it is absolutely imperative that any uterine activity occurring before term is investigated. It is also crucial that any such suspicion is reported promptly because, if it turns out to be true preterm labour, time is a critical factor in the eventual outcome. In this case, quite literally, "every minute counts". We shall see why this is so, in the following section.

A few myths need to be exploded up front. There is no such thing as an effective treatment for preterm labour. The best on offer can only curtail labour for hours, at most. If perceived "contractions" stop after some form of "treatment" and do not recur again, there is strong evidence that this simply means they would have stopped without the treatment anyway.

Another myth is that inactivity in the form of bed-rest may arrest preterm labour. There is no evidence that this is ever the case.

There are claims appearing in the popular press from time to time that, even as early as twenty-two or twenty-three weeks, the baby should survive, if given the maximum benefit of modern medical technology. This is a cruel hoax perpetuated by sensationalist down-market journalists. Any expert or caregiver who spends his or her life in the highly charged and very intense atmosphere of a special care baby unit will tell you that, for every perceived triumph of a healthy baby painstakingly retrieved from the jaws of severe prematurity, there are dozens who never make it or survive with profoundly severe cerebral palsy. However, it is fair to state that the care of prematurely born babies has advanced so much over the years that prospects for these children are, in modern times, infinitely better than only a few years ago. The degree of prematurity is, however, still a critical factor.

Preterm labour and its causes

What is the meaning of "preterm"?

Obvious though this might seem, it is not clearly understood by everyone and that might include some of those providing obstetric care. "Preterm" describes the gestation period between twenty-four weeks and just under thirty-seven weeks.

If symptoms appear before twenty-four weeks of gestation, this is a threatened miscarriage and not preterm labour. Thirty-seven weeks onwards is term and labour at any stage thence is in order. After forty-two weeks, it becomes post-term. "Term" therefore spans a period of five weeks from thirty-seven to forty-two weeks. It is not a fixed date.

So what is preterm labour and how can it be recognized?

When there are uterine contractions, usually regular and painful (and occasionally painless), accompanied by changes to the cervix (it becomes thinner and starts to open or dilate), then this is preterm labour – that is, if it is happening during the described gestational period.

Other symptoms include low backache which may be quite distressing, a feeling of pressure in the pelvis and occasionally the passage of a mucous bloodstained discharge, popularly called a "show".

Does preterm labour inevitably lead to delivery?

No. In fact, in about 50 per cent of expectant mother who have symptoms suggestive of preterm labour, examination reveals no cervical change whatsoever. Technically, this is not preterm labour, and almost all will resolve without any action. However, when symptoms are there even in the absence of supporting clinical evidence, observation in hospital is the preferred form of management.

In those cases where the cervix is found to be already thinning and dilating, the outlook for continuation of the pregnancy is less favourable and many – probably the majority – will go on to deliver within hours and, at most, days.

What causes preterm labour?

In the vast majority of cases, the cause remains unidentified. To be realistic, one has to talk of factors that may predispose to preterm labour rather than causes of preterm labour. There are a good number of risk factors that predispose to preterm labour. These include:

- fetal abnormality
- abnormalities of the womb or cervix
- multiple pregnancy – the greater the number of fetuses, the greater the likelihood of preterm labour
- excessive amounts of amniotic fluid
- extremes of maternal age – the very young and the older mother (late thirties onwards) are more prone
- serious infection, not necessarily of the genital tract
- urinary tract infection (UTI)
- rupture of membranes
- fetal death. Death of the fetus is usually followed by the onset of labour within days.

Are there any maternal habits that might predispose to preterm labour?

Yes. Smoking and drug abuse increase the risk of preterm labour. Anybody who has threatened preterm labour or has had actual preterm labour and delivery in a previous pregnancy and is using either should be strongly advised to quit. Of course, those patients who are abusing heroin are not asked to stop during pregnancy but are switched to a safer and better-controlled drug – methadone. Cocaine increases the risk of placental abruption, which is associated with preterm labour and a very high rate of fetal loss.

Is there any risk of recurrence of preterm labour?

Yes. A previous preterm labour should be regarded as a risk factor for preterm labour. If the factor that predisposed to preterm labour in the first instance is unidentified, the risk of recurrence is considered to be considerable.

Many experts now recommend regular (weekly or fortnightly) vaginal swabs from about twenty-four weeks of gestation for women at risk in order to detect any low grade asymptomatic genital tract infections (i.e. those that do not cause symptoms to alert the mother or caregivers). These are considered to be legitimate risk factors. This may be done if there is a history of previous preterm labour and an absence of any identifiable risk factor.

Is there anything that can be done to influence things in preterm labour?

It depends on the gestation and other factors present, as will be discussed below.

If the preterm labour occurs after thirty-four weeks, most experts agree that there is no need to interfere. Assessment of the labour and maternal and fetal conditions will be made. Labour will be allowed to proceed, unless there are obstetric contraindications (for labour or vaginal delivery), when delivery may be made by caesarean section.

If the preterm labour is before thirty-four weeks, efforts may be made to stop or – more realistically – postpone labour, to achieve a few more valuable days or, if lucky, weeks.

Suppressing labour

What is used to stop (or postpone) labour?

There are a number of medications that can be used to suppress contractions and therefore stop labour. These are not always successful and have a number of side-effects. There is evidence, albeit weak, that any one of them can prolong pregnancy for a maximum of forty-eight hours. In fact, most experts agree that if the pregnancy continues for more than a few days, it would have done so anyway, with or without the medication. It is, however, very important to understand that the forty-eight hours or so that may be gained as a result of using these drugs could be extremely crucial for the baby's prospects, once he or she is born. This is explained further below.

How can twenty-four or forty-eight hours gained by suppressing labour help a baby that is going to be born prematurely?

One of the most feared problems of prematurity is immaturity of the lungs. After twenty-six weeks of gestation, an administration of steroids – usually in the form of two injections, twelve or twenty-four hours apart – significantly improves the functional capacity of the baby's lungs, thus improving its chances of survival and the chances of survival without handicap.

Are there any circumstances where suppressing labour is not a good idea?

Yes. However preterm the labour might be, no attempt to suppress it will be made in the presence of:

● placental abruption
● severe vaginal bleeding
● severe pre-eclampsia or eclampsia
● infection affecting the pregnancy itself (chorioamnionitis)
● fetal distress
● fetal abnormalities incompatible with life.

As has been mentioned before, if the gestation is over thirty-four weeks, in most instances labour won't be suppressed. However, there is room for flexibility here and assessment may lead to a decision to try to prolong labour if it is perceived that the fetus is likely to benefit from this.

What are the potential side-effects of the drugs used to suppress labour?

There are various types of drugs used to suppress labour. The most popular type by far are the group known in medical parlance as "beta-agonists". The side-effects of these include palpitations, lung congestion and occasionally chest pains, rising blood-sugar levels (hence great care is needed if the patient is diabetic), and lowering blood pressure. Of these, the most common and most vexing, as far as the patient is concerned, is palpitations. The most serious (and fortunately rare) one is lung congestion (oedema). Labour-suppressing drugs are collectively called "tocolytics".

Delivery and post-delivery

If delivery was inevitable, what would be the method of delivery?

As with all deliveries, term or preterm, the method of delivery is dependent on a lot of factors, and preterm labour in itself does not dictate this one way or the other.

As a general statement, in the absence of contraindicating factors, the aim will be for a vaginal delivery in preterm labour. If the baby is in the breech position, this general plan may have to be reviewed. This does not mean preterm breech babies are not delivered vaginally. It only means a careful evaluation on the best method of delivery needs to be done by the obstetrician.

Will forceps be used to deliver the baby, if it is a vaginal delivery?

This is no longer considered to offer any advantage to the premature baby and will therefore be used only if there are any of the usual indications for using forceps. The ventouse is not used, certainly not before thirty-four weeks, after which it can be used for the usual indications.

Do any potential maternal complications result from preterm delivery?

There is a slight increase in the risk of retaining the afterbirth, thus requiring surgical removal in theatre.

Probably the potential problem which creates most concern among prospective or new parents is the interruption in the mother-baby bonding as the baby, if needing intensive care, will be transferred to the special care baby unit. In some cases, if facilities are inadequate or unavailable at the local hospital, the baby may have to be transferred to another hospital further away. Efforts are usually made to maximize access of the parents to the baby. Breast-feeding, when and if possible, is encouraged.

What kind of problems does the newborn face in the short and long term?

It all depends on the degree of prematurity: the lower the gestation, the more severe the complications.

The immediate problem the baby faces is usually respiratory. Infant respiratory distress syndrome (also called "hyaline membrane disease") affects virtually all babies born before twenty-six weeks of gestation. Between twenty-six and twenty-eight weeks of gestation, four out of five babies will be affected by this condition, but at thirty-two to thirty-four weeks, the figure falls to only about one in ten and is less severe.

Other short-term concerns include brain haemorrhage and bowel inflammation, both of which could lead to loss of the baby.

Long-term, there is the potential of developing chronic lung disease, eye complications (which, in some cases, lead to blindness) and general or localized handicap, resulting from brain haemorrhage. Again, the risk is higher the severer the degree of prematurity.

Of all the above-mentioned, the most frequent and greatest cause of illness and death is the respiratory distress syndrome.

31. Prolonged pregnancy

Introduction

The concept of prolonged pregnancy means different things to different people. It is an indisputable fact that most pregnancies labelled as such are not prolonged. Not that blame for this can be apportioned to anybody in particular: it is just a consequence of the doctors' attempts at meticulous management of pregnancy.

To practically every pregnant woman, if the pregnancy continues beyond the calculated expected date of delivery (EDD), it is prolonged. Pure and simple.

The expected date of delivery or EDD is calculated from the date of the onset of the last period and falls on the fortieth week from that point. This concept presupposes that a human pregnancy is supposed to last forty weeks exactly. This is, of course, not the case. In fact, those who have conducted surveys to see what proportion of women actually deliver on their calculated EDD will tell you it is less than 1 per cent. This means 99 out of 100 women will deliver either before or after their calculated EDD. Most will deliver before. The formula also assumes that all women have a 28-day cycle, which is clearly not the case. For a woman with a shorter cycle, the gestational age will be underestimated and for those with long cycles, the reverse is true. All this is clarified further in this chapter.

It is now an accepted fact that term pregnancy is not a fixed point. In fact, there is world consensus that "term" (i.e. mature pregnancy) spans a total of five weeks. Over 80 per cent of all women will deliver, spontaneously or otherwise, during that phase. If no intervention is made, anything between 3 and 10 per cent of all women will go beyond the forty-two weeks mark. In this era of meticulous antenatal care, this happens rarely. This is because most women go for induction of labour either just before or at the forty-two weeks mark. So, while most women regard anything beyond the forty weeks mark to represent prolonged pregnancy; in truth, this does not begin until two weeks later. For descriptive purposes, the period beyond the forty weeks mark (EDD) is known as "post-dates" and if it goes beyond forty-two weeks, then it becomes "post-term". Postmaturity means the same as post-term.

So, are there any potential problems associated with prolonged pregnancy? This and other related questions are answered in this section.

Term and dates

What does prolonged pregnancy mean?

Although this may seem a straightforward question, many mothers do not know the right answer to it. It actually reflects rather badly on the quality of antenatal care, because every pregnant woman should have this concept explained and discussed at her booking-in visit.

Prolonged pregnancy means a pregnancy that has extended beyond forty-two weeks of gestation. This is counting from the onset of her last menstrual period, unless adjustment has been made following an ultrasound scan within the first twenty weeks of pregnancy.

Prolonged pregnancy, "post-term" and "postmature" mean exactly the same thing.

"Post-dates" has a different meaning and is less significant.

If "post-term" refers to the period beyond forty-two weeks of gestation, what is "term"?

It is very important to be clear that term does not refer to a specific date. In fact, "term" refers to the five-week period from thirty-seven weeks to forty-two completed weeks of gestation. Over 80 per cent of women deliver within this period and their babies are physiologically mature. The date that is given as the "Expected Date of Delivery" (EDD) is a forty-week mark which is within this period. It has no sanctity of any kind.

What is the significance of the so-called expected date of delivery (EDD)?

Frankly speaking, this is only a reference point within the "term" period. It is a point to focus on for both the mother and the attending midwife or doctor. The baby can arrive any day around the EDD. It could be three weeks before or two weeks after, and this will be of no consequence. It will still be term.

Only a tiny minority of babies arrive spontaneously on the calculated EDD. When someone last bothered to check what proportion of women actually deliver on the so-called expected date, they came up with a figure of 6 per cent: that is, less than one in sixteen. This study actually included those induced and those who had elective Caesarean sections. Most studies have actually shown much lower figures (in the region of 1 per cent) representing only those going into spontaneous labour.

Is there any reason to panic if pregnancy continues beyond the EDD: that is, the forty weeks mark?

Absolutely not. If the pregnancy is categorized as low-risk or minimal risk, there is absolutely no reason to panic. Of course, a midwife or doctor will have followed up the progress of the pregnancy to ensure that it remains low-risk. If there have been any factors or developments which move the pregnancy out of that category to moderate- or high-risk status, then advice will be given accordingly. This could take the form of early delivery.

What proportion of pregnancies become prolonged, i.e. continue beyond forty-two weeks?

About 3–10 per cent of all pregnancies will reach the forty-two weeks mark.

Causes of prolonged pregnancy

What causes the pregnancy to be prolonged?

This is unknown. In a very small proportion of affected mothers, some factors have been identified which could explain the phenomenon. These may include some forms of fetal abnormalities (easily ruled out by an ultrasound scan), certain placental enzyme deficiencies and low thyroid hormone levels.

These, however, constitute an exceedingly small proportion of those women with prolonged pregnancy. Of more significance is a group of women where dates may have been wrong from the start, where no verification of the gestation was made in the first half of the pregnancy.

It is by no means uncommon to find a pregnancy over-estimated by up to four weeks, following a routine eighteen to twenty weeks ultrasound scan. If such a pregnancy slips through the net at that stage of the pregnancy, it is practically impossible to correct the error in late pregnancy. At a supposedly forty-weeks visit, when she will actually be thirty-six weeks, she will be expected to deliver within two weeks. If this does not happen, she will be categorized as post-term. Lesser errors of one to two weeks are even more common.

Surely an ultrasound scan performed in late pregnancy should be able to correct the error?

Unfortunately not. At about twenty-eight weeks and beyond, the boat has been well and truly missed. The ultrasound scan is too inaccurate at dating pregnancy at this late stage.

This is not due to the weakness of the technology itself. It is rather the nature of pregnancy. Babies will grow to quite different sizes because of a variety of factors. These differences are usually quite marked in the third trimester. Any attempt to date a pregnancy for the first time at this stage is futile.

Risk factors

What factors will move a pregnancy from the category of low-risk?

There are various factors that may make the pregnancy regarded as no longer being low-risk. These may include:
- unsatisfactory growth rate
- reduced amniotic fluid around the baby
- vaginal bleeding in pregnancy (antepartum haemorrhage)
- hypertensive disorders, including pre-eclampsia
- diabetes.

This is why proper antenatal care is important, in order to detect factors that may increase risk to a pregnancy and to have them dealt with in good time.

Apart from recognized risk factors, what could prompt intervention before forty-two completed weeks?

The expectant mother's wishes. The obstetrician will try to allay unfounded worries as much as possible. This is not always possible and if a woman is beside herself with worry, however baseless her fears may be, there is little justification to deny her induction of labour, just to prove a point. It is, however, important that she is made aware of a small but definite increase in the risk of caesarean section associated with induction of labour, especially if associated with an unfavourable cervix.

Fetal well-being

Are there any measures to check fetal well-being in the period leading to forty-two weeks of gestation?

Strictly speaking, there is no need to carry out any measures up to forty-two weeks. This is because the baby is no more at risk in the forty-first or forty-second week compared to, let's say, the thirty-seventh, thirty-eighth, thirty-ninth or fortieth week. If there was no reason to monitor in those weeks leading to the EDD, there should be no need to monitor in the two weeks after.

However, most obstetricians agree that some form of monitoring should be carried out: one, because there may be a risk factor that has been missed in the weeks leading to the EDD and two, to give peace of mind to all concerned, especially the expectant mother. When this monitoring should start depends on each obstetrician's opinion. Some start at forty weeks, most at forty-one weeks and a few will only monitor at forty-two weeks. Based on evidence accumulated over the years, in a low-risk pregnancy, all this monitoring is unlikely to influence any decision on the timing of delivery.

How is the fetal well-being assessed?

This will include monitoring the fetal heart activity using a cardiotocograph (CTG) and an ultrasound scan, which will be used to assess several factors, including amniotic fluid volume and fetal activity.

What is the role of Doppler ultrasound in assessing fetal well-being?

It has no role in low-risk pregnancy. Even in high-risk pregnancy, its usefulness remains limited and uncertain.

After forty-two weeks

What is to be done once the pregnancy has reached the forty-two weeks mark?

Beyond this point, the pregnancy is prolonged. Most obstetricians will advise a plan for delivery at this stage. This could be induction of labour or caesarean section. The latter is used where induction of labour is considered risky – such as where the baby is in breech presentation or lying in an abnormal position (e.g. oblique or transverse). Ultimately, once she has been given all the information, the mother's wish is to be respected. A few mothers will still want to wait for spontaneous labour beyond forty-two weeks.

Is there a risk to allowing pregnancy to continue beyond forty-two weeks?

The post-term period (i.e. beyond forty-two weeks) is not a fully understood area. Very few women are allowed to go beyond forty-two weeks by more than a handful of days. In the few truly scientific observational studies of what happens in the forty-third week of pregnancy, there appears to be an increased risk of fetal loss. Some studies have claimed that by forty-three weeks, fetal loss may go up threefold compared to term. It is assumed that placental function deteriorates rapidly about this time. It can only be assumed that beyond forty-three weeks, the risk will be higher. This is uncharted territory.

If the mother is keen to wait for spontaneous labour after forty-two weeks, close fetal monitoring – probably every other day – will be offered. This is reassuring but does not offer an absolute guarantee of continued fetal well-being. The truth is, even though CTG and ultrasound monitoring may be accurate for the here and now, in prolonged pregnancy, its predictive value is reduced and things could be radically different within hours of an excellent score on the monitoring.

Labour

How is labour induced?

This may be by using some form of a prostaglandin preparation – usually a gel – vaginally. This is to prime the cervix, allowing it to open easily in labour. If the cervix is already favourable, induction will be in the form of breaking the waters (membrane rupture). This, in itself, may be sufficient to trigger contractions. More often, an infusion of an oxytocin hormone is required to bring about contractions. *See* Chapter 35, "Induction and augmentation of labour", for more details.

If an expectant mother requests a caesarean section for prolonged pregnancy, can this be granted?

Most obstetricians frown upon caesarean section on demand, and rightly so. Prolonged pregnancy per se is not an indication for caesarean section and the obstetrician will be within his or her rights to decline such a request. In fact, by declining to perform a caesarean, he or she will be doing the expectant mother a favour, even though it won't be perceived that way at the time. After all, the obstetrician is acting in the patient's best interests.

How likely is prolonged pregnancy to recur?

It appears that this mostly happens in first pregnancies. The majority of mothers will not get it again. It is estimated, however, that up to a third will have a similar experience in a subsequent pregnancy.

Can prolonged pregnancy be predicted in the antenatal period?

No.

Is there any natural way of expediting the onset of labour if prolonged pregnancy is threatening?

Sexual intercourse to bring about the onset of labour is the stuff of folklore. There may be something in the claim, considering that semen is rich in prostaglandins, but this has never been proven scientifically – probably because setting up such a study would be rather tricky.

Amniotic fluid

Is there anything special about amniotic fluid volume and prolonged pregnancy?

As a general rule, amniotic fluid volume starts to decline around the thirty-eighth week of pregnancy. In prolonged pregnancy, reduced amniotic fluid volume is common. This, combined with ever-increasing fetal size and weight, means there is less and less room in the uterine cavity. Because of this, movements may be perceived less during this time. More importantly, the risk of cord compression is increased. If, during the routine fetal surveillance at around forty-one weeks, the amniotic fluid is found to be significantly reduced, intervention in the form of labour induction will be advised by many obstetricians.

What is an amniotic fluid index (AFI)?

It is a way of estimating the fluid volume, using an ultrasound. It is a standardized way of measuring the volume which has been found to be reasonably objective, though it is not infallible.

Is labour after a prolonged pregnancy in any way special?

Yes. Labour after a prolonged or post-term pregnancy is no longer low-risk. Because of this, many obstetricians would prefer to have continuous electronic fetal monitoring (cardiotocograph). However, in the absence of other detectable risk factors, others will be content with intermittent monitoring, provided the first hour or so at the establishment of labour has shown a satisfactory trace of the baby's heartbeat and the expectant mother wishes to have this kind of monitoring. When this is adopted, the monitoring will be performed for about thirty minutes every two hours or so. There are no strict rules about this.

What is the significance of meconeum staining of the amniotic fluid in labour in cases of prolonged pregnancy?

Passage of meconeum in the uterus for babies, who have stayed beyond term is a common occurrence. It is therefore, never surprising to see stained fluid (at this juncture called "liquor") on breaking the waters. However, if the meconeum appears fresh and thick, it may reflect distress on the part of the fetus. This should trigger immediate electronic fetal monitoring. If the cardiotocograph shows suspicious features at an early stage of labour, a caesarean delivery will most likely be made.

The passage of fresh thick meconeum before or at the onset of labour, signalling distress, is not the preserve of post-term pregnancy. It is also seen in labour occurring at term or occasionally preterm.

Is labour after prolonged pregnancy likely to be more difficult?

There is no evidence to this effect. Delivery is probably marginally more difficult because, on average, these babies tend to be bigger.

What is amnio-infusion?

This is mentioned here for completion's sake. This is a practice where sterile fluid – usually warm saline – is infused into the uterine cavity using a catheter. The aim is to counter the effect of severely reduced amniotic fluid and reduce such occurrences as cord compression. Where this has been used, results have been reported as encouraging. However, it is by no means mainstream obstetrics and, at this juncture, it remains an experimental technique.

32. Pain in pregnancy

Introduction

Discomfort or even pain are, unfortunately, not uncommon features of pregnancy.

The causes are quite often directly related to the pregnancy. These may include an over-exuberant fetus, pressure effects from the fetal head or limbs, and over-distension of the abdomen because of large fluid volume, a big baby or both. There are several others, as we shall see shortly.

Other causes of pain in pregnancy are only indirectly related or even incidental.

The attending doctor needs to be able to discriminate between the miscellaneous pregnancy-related discomforts and pathological causes of pain, which may require specific remedial action. It is after this that all forms converge under a common denominator, that of pain: hence requiring relief.

Modes of pain relief during the course of pregnancy are limited and in many cases not as effective as the expectant mother – or her doctor – would like. However, establishing the cause of her discomfort or pain and confirming the absence of any serious illness does go a long way in enabling the mother-to-be to cope.

Sometimes, though this is uncommon, the pain is so severe as to prompt induction of labour. This decision should never be taken lightly, not least because it has a tendency of assuming a slippery-slope phenomenon. Induction of labour, especially if remote from term, can be a protracted affair and psychologically and physically traumatic. The success of the procedure is also far from being a foregone conclusion and may very well lead towards a caesarean section.

The various aspects of pain in pregnancy are discussed here.

Physiological pain

Are all types of abdominal pain in pregnancy something to worry about?

Not really. A majority of cases of mild and moderate abdominal pain in pregnancy are described as "physiological". This means that they are a result of the changes brought about by the growing pregnancy. The expectant mother needs to give her doctor a good and precise history of the pain. The doctor will then distinguish between physiological pain and pain resulting from an underlying disease requiring specific action.

What are the common causes of the so-called physiological pain?

This diagnosis should be made by exclusion.

It is important that conditions such as urinary tract infection, kidney stone, appendicitis or pregnancy complications (such as placental abruption) are excluded. Once this is established, then the pain may be caused by:

- stretching of ligaments
- Braxton-Hicks contractions
- heartburn
- constipation
- mild torsion of the uterus.

We shall expand on these below.

How will the expectant mother know whether the pain is only physiological, or whether there is an underlying condition?

A mother should never try to make a diagnosis herself. If she has any pain, it is imperative that she consults her doctor to verify the symptoms. It could be dangerous to ignore any symptoms, however mild they may seem to her.

What is this "ligament stretching" business?

On the front of the womb there are two ligaments, one on either side. These are called "round ligaments" and they run from near the fundus of the womb to the pelvic wall. As the womb grows, the ligaments inevitably stretch. In some people, this stretching is believed to cause considerable pain, although there is no cast-iron evidence of this being a cause of pain. Strong subjective evidence exists to show that up to a third of all pregnancies may be affected by ligament stretching to varying degrees. For most, it appears to be only a mild discomfort over the lower abdomen, usually midway through the pregnancy.

Are Braxton-Hicks contractions supposed to be painful?

In most cases they are not, but there is a substantial proportion of women who find them uncomfortable, even painful. They very rarely start before twenty-eight weeks of gestation. Any painful contractions, however remote from term, should be taken seriously, as these might be a sign of preterm labour. A vaginal examination is frequently required to rule out labour.

What about heartburn and constipation?

Both heartburn and constipation are common in pregnancy. Most people will have no trouble in recognizing heartburn, by virtue of its symptoms and location (in the upper part of the abdomen). In very late pregnancy, near term, this may not be straightforward and, if in doubt, an examination will distinguish uterine fundal pain from heartburn.

Pain resulting from constipation is usually colicky and confined to the left side on the lower part of the abdomen. Again, it may be wise to have an examination to establish or confirm whether the pain is indeed due to constipation. Constipation is easily cured but is notorious for recurring again and again in pregnancy.

What is torsion of the uterus and what causes it?

For torsion to be regarded as physiological, it has to be mild. When it is severe – which is rare – it becomes pathological and that is a serious condition which may require an emergency operation. Mild rotation of the uterus is in fact quite common, probably occurring in the majority of pregnancies. Because a pregnant uterus is much bigger on the upper part (fundus), it is not unusual for it to rotate on its axis, usually towards the right. When this rotation (or torsion) goes beyond a certain degree, which happens from time to time, it may be perceived as discomfort or pain. This usually occurs late in the pregnancy, normally well beyond the halfway mark. It could possibly occur earlier, in the presence of predisposing factors such as fibroids or uterine abnormalities.

Mild torsion does not require any specific measures.

What causes severe torsion of the uterus?

We have discussed mild torsion of the uterus as a "physiological" cause of pain and said this is not uncommon. Fortunately, severe torsion is extremely rare. The causes are not always immediately apparent but the presence of benign tumours, such as fibroids or large ovarian cysts, are predisposing factors.

Torsion is usually quite difficult to diagnose before operating and exposing the uterus.

Even though it is usually quite painful, it does not always affect the well-being of the fetus and can be managed conservatively, as long as painkillers are effective. Remember, this is a rare condition, and rare things happen rarely.

Pathological pain

So what are the pathological causes of pain in pregnancy?

Pathological pain is caused by a disease, as opposed to physiological pain, which is caused by the changes to the body brought about by pregnancy. There are several potential causes and no list can by any means be exhaustive. Here we can try to highlight the more common ones.

The pregnancy-specific causes of pain include:
- preterm labour
- placental abruption
- severe torsion of the uterus
- uterine rupture
- pain over the liver in severe pre-eclampsia
- ectopic pregnancy
- uterine fibroids
- miscarriage.

Preterm labour as a cause of pain?

Yes. Preterm labour is one of the most common causes of pain in pregnancy. Contractions of the uterus are painful at whatever stage of the pregnancy they occur. Labour can only be known as such after twenty-four weeks of gestation. If contractions occur before this stage of pregnancy and if the mother goes on to lose the baby, this is a miscarriage. The process of miscarriage is also painful but the degree of pain, as with labour, is widely variable.

What is placental abruption?

The placenta – or afterbirth, as it is commonly known – could detach prematurely in the course of a pregnancy. This is a serious condition which could lead to the loss of the baby. It is usually painful but again, the degree of pain varies between individuals and depends on the extent of the abruption. It is normally, but not necessarily, accompanied by vaginal bleeding. This is discussed further in Chapter 19, "Bleeding in pregnancy".

What about ectopic pregnancy?

The vast majority of pregnancies establishing outside the womb will be in one of the fallopian tubes. The tube, even though it can swell from pressure inside it, is a very small organ compared to the womb and, as the pregnancy increases in size, the tube will distend, causing pain. Bleeding into the pelvic cavity will also occur, irritating the inner surface and increasing the pain felt inside the pelvis.

The pain is normally but not necessary localized on one side in the lower part of the abdomen. The area will also be tender to the touch. If the pain at this stage has not aroused the mother's concern as to there being something amiss, the tube will go on to rupture, which usually causes quite severe acute pain, even shock.

Most ectopic pregnancies reveal themselves well before ten weeks of gestation. This is therefore a cause of pain in early pregnancy.

Can ectopic pregnancy exist without pain?

Yes, but this is extremely rare. Occasionally a patient may only have symptoms of vaginal spotting in early pregnancy, without any pain. The first inkling as to the probable diagnosis is when an ultrasound scan reveals an empty uterus in the presence of pregnancy symptoms and a positive pregnancy test. Remember, an ectopic pregnancy is not always identifiable on the scan. In fact, the majority are diagnosed by exclusion.

What will cause uterine rupture and how common is this?

There has to be an inherent weakness in the uterine wall for it to rupture spontaneously. Even in labour, when the uterus is subject to stresses and strains, this remains a rare occurrence. Before labour, the main (and probably only) predisposing factor for this complication is a previous operation on the uterus. This could have been a caesarean section or surgery to remove fibroids.

In labour, rupture may be caused by weakening of uterine muscles as a result of multiple pregnancies (and deliveries), or overstimulation of the uterus.

How do uterine fibroids cause pain in pregnancy?

If a woman has fibroids, pregnancy usually makes them prone to undergo some kind of degeneration, which may cause pain. The pain is usually moderate, but occasionally may be severe enough to require admission into hospital and the use of strong painkillers. It usually clears up in time.

What causes pain in pre-eclampsia?

In severe pre-eclampsia, liver complications may cause pain on the right border of the ribcage (where the liver is situated). It may also have symptoms similar to heartburn. This is frequently a warning of impending eclampsia and, more often than not, emergency delivery will be made. Of course, there have to be other supporting features to reach this diagnosis.

Non-pregnancy related pain

Now that we have covered probable causes of pain that are pregnancy-related, what are the other causes?

As we mentioned before, no list can be exhaustive; below, we cover the causes encountered more commonly. Pathological conditions which are incidental in pregnancy (i.e. which may have similar symptoms in a non-pregnant state) include:

- appendicitis
- kidney stones
- urinary tract infection
- gallbladder infection
- peptic ulcer
- torsion of ovarian cyst
- pancreatitis
- bowel obstruction
- inflammatory bowel disease.

It looks like a long list of causes!

Yes, and this is by no means everything: all the more reason why an expectant mother should refrain from making her own diagnosis. It is important that any pain in pregnancy is assessed by an expert, to rule out disease. Some causes – such as appendicitis or urinary tract infection – will require immediate treatment, while others (such as gallstones) may be managed conservatively in pregnancy.

Pain in pregnancy is, in most cases, innocent. In other cases, it is not, and an expert should be allowed to make the distinction.

How common is appendicitis in pregnancy?

The susceptibility is neither increased nor decreased by pregnancy. One in every 2000 pregnancies will be complicated by appendicitis. A correct diagnosis is very important, as fetal loss is quite high if the appendix perforates. The mother's life is also endangered by this.

How common are gallstones in pregnancy?

Gallstones are generally uncommon in the teens and twenties. The condition becomes more common from the mid-thirties. Obesity is a predisposing factor even at a younger age. Pregnancy clearly makes pre-existing gallstones worse and symptoms may appear for the first time in pregnancy. Moreover, this may be complicated by infection of the gallbladder, a condition seen in 0.1 per cent of all pregnancies. As mentioned before, gallstones in pregnancy are usually managed conservatively, but sometimes an operation becomes necessary. It is important to be aware of the fact that gallstones predispose to acute pancreatitis, another important – albeit uncommon – cause of pain in pregnancy.

What about peptic ulcers?

If one does not have a pre-existing peptic ulcer, it is extremely unlikely that this condition will develop for the first time in pregnancy. Moreover, peptic ulcer patients almost always experience improvement in their symptoms in pregnancy. Having said all that, perforation of a peptic ulcer has been known to occur during pregnancy.

Surely backache should rank among the types of pain in pregnancy?

Yes. Backache after the midway stage of the pregnancy becomes increasingly common. The not-so-good news is that it tends to worsen as the pregnancy advances and it responds poorly to the common painkillers based on paracetamol and/or codeine. The good news is that there is almost always nothing wrong with the pregnancy and the backache tends to clear up soon after delivery. The main cause is usually strains to the spine by the increasingly heavy uterus.

Poor posture, physical exertion and wrong sleeping positions could worsen backache. The attending midwife should be able to advise on this. It is however important to remember that pathological conditions such as kidney infection could cause symptoms of backache, although there are almost always other symptoms. If left untreated, kidney infection worsens rapidly.

What about pelvic girdle pain?

This is one of the causes of intractable and progressive pain in pregnancy. It usually starts late in pregnancy, rarely before the twenty-eight weeks mark. It is usually felt around the pubic area and the side joints of the pelvis. Movements and especially rolling from side to side in bed exacerbate the pain. Climbing stairs can be torture.

The cause is partial separation of the joints under the influence of pregnancy hormones, especially progesterone.

The truth is, painkillers hardly touch this pain but a special brace worn around the pelvis to stabilize the joints may help control the exacerbation caused by movements. It is not the most comfortable of devices. The pain clears up completely a few weeks after delivery.

Persistent pain is virtually unknown but recurrence in a subsequent pregnancy is common. This condition is known by the fancy name of "pelvic osteo-arthropathy".

So, what type of painkillers are recommended for use in pregnancy?

Paracetamol usually suffices for most types of pain in pregnancy and is perfectly safe for the baby. If a stronger painkiller is required, then most obstetricians will recommend preparations based on a combination of paracetamol and codeine (or dihydro-codeine). There are several such preparations. The most common side-effect of these is constipation. The taking of painkillers is dealt with in greater detail in chapter 22, "Taking medicines in pregnancy".

33. Breech presentation

Introduction

While anything between a quarter and a third of all fetuses are "breech" (that is, positioned in the womb so that the bottom will emerge before the head) around twenty-two to twenty-four weeks of gestation, only one in twenty will be in that position at term (after thirty-seven weeks). Breech presentation is therefore not a normal feature in pregnancy and is regarded by doctors as a risk factor.

The structure and function of the body mean that a longitudinal lie with the baby's head coming first is the ideal and safest position for delivery.

The breech position does not confer any disadvantage to the fetus while it is still in the womb. Delivery is a different matter. This is why a considered decision has to be made before the onset of labour as to the best method of delivering such a baby. In general terms, the decision will be made on the basis of the absence of any contraindicating factors, parental wishes and the availability of the necessary expertise.

There is, of course, the option of manually turning the baby (a procedure known as external cephalic version or ECV) before labour, to allow it to come head-first. All these issues are discussed and explained in detail in this chapter.

There is unfortunately an element of lottery in management of breech presentation, depending on where the unit is. This will influence the advice given and will in turn be influenced by the doctor's own opinion and the expertise available on the unit. However, an informed mother-to-be can significantly influence how her pregnancy is managed, a factor that is ultimately crucial in the overall experience of the pregnancy.

Breech presentation – the types and how it happens

How common is breech presentation?

Towards the end of pregnancy, the overwhelming majority of babies will be lying in the womb with the head as the leading part. This is called "cephalic presentation". Less than 5 per cent or one in twenty have the bottom as the leading part at this stage and this is what is known as breech presentation.

What about earlier on in pregnancy?

The leading part is of no significance in the first half of pregnancy and normally it would not be sought for.

At around twenty-four weeks of gestation, approximately a third of all fetuses (33 per cent) will be found to be in breech presentation; the figure drops to about 15 per cent by thirty weeks and is 4–5 per cent at thirty-seven weeks. It is said to be even lower (2–3 per cent) at forty weeks. It is therefore quite obvious that most babies will be leading with the head at term, regardless of the position earlier on in pregnancy.

Remember, "term" refers to the period of pregnancy after thirty-seven weeks of gestation.

What are the predisposing factors for breech presentation at term?

In many cases, no explanation can be found for the baby's persisting breech presentation. However, there are some known predisposing factors that make some women more prone to have a baby presenting with breech.

These include:

- uterine abnormalities
- presence of masses or tumours in the pelvis, such as fibroids and ovarian cysts
- fetal abnormalities
- excessive or reduced amniotic fluid.

Are there different types of breech presentation?

Yes. The mother will often hear her doctor or midwife describing the type of breech that the fetus is in.

The least common breech presentation is what is known as "complete breech" (or flexed breech). In this type, the baby is in a sitting position and both the hips and knees are flexed (squatting).

The second type is "footling breech" where a foot is leading just below the baby's buttocks. Very rarely, both feet may extend below the buttocks.

The most common type of breech is "frank breech" (extended breech), where the knees are extended and therefore the legs lie alongside the body, with the feet adjacent to the baby's head.

Is there any significance to this classification of the type of breech presentation?

Yes. It influences the plan of action regarding the method of delivery, as we shall see shortly.

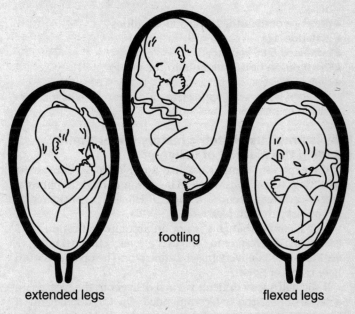

footling

extended legs   flexed legs

Fig 9: The three main types of breech presentation where the legs are extended alongside the body, the legs are bent at the knee (squatting) or one leg is straight and the other is bent. The findings on the scan influence the decision about the method of delivery.

Delivery

What should be the method of delivery in breech presentation?

This is the big question and the bottom line is that there is no single answer.

Each case needs to be thoroughly evaluated and a decision on the method of delivery made on its own merit.

There are many factors that will influence the decision, and each has to be considered individually before reaching a conclusion on the best way forward. These factors include:

- the previous obstetric history of the mother
- the presence or absence of uterine abnormalities or pelvic masses
- presence of identified fetal abnormalities
- gestation age
- estimated fetal weight
- the position of the placenta in the womb
- type of breech.

As everybody will appreciate, it is not a light or easy decision to make.

Why is previous obstetric history important in deciding the method of delivery?

If the expectant mother has had a caesarean section in the past, then this is considered to be reason enough to opt for a repeat caesarean section. A vaginal delivery is considered to be too risky in such a case.

Bear in mind that this is not an absolute indication for a caesarean delivery and, in exceptional circumstances, a vaginal breech delivery may be aimed for. The operative word here is "exceptional".

If she had a very difficult vaginal delivery in the past, again a caesarean section is recommended. On the other hand, if her previous deliveries had been smooth – and in the absence of any other contraindicating factors – vaginal breech delivery will be recommended.

What about estimated fetal weight?

In breech presentation, most obstetricians agree that an above-average weight fetus should best be delivered by caesarean section. If, on an ultrasound scan, the baby is deemed to weigh 4 kg (8 lb 10 oz) or more, then the majority will advise a caesarean section. In fact, for a first pregnancy, the cut-off point is lower for most obstetricians: 3.5 kg for some and 3.75 kg for others. The ultra-cautious obstetrician will perform a caesarean section for all first-time mothers with a breech presentation, a stance that is bound to remain quite controversial.

How does the type of breech influence the decision on the method of delivery?

We have seen that there are three main types of breech presentation: frank (where the legs are extended), footling and complete (flexed leg).

The most common type of breech, which is frank, is considered the most ideal for vaginal delivery, as it is the one least associated with cord prolapse. On the other hand, about one in ten footling breech presentations will be complicated by cord prolapse. The figure is about one in twenty-five for complete breech.

Many obstetricians consider footling breech reason enough to recommend a caesarean section as soon as it is recognized. Again, this is only a relative indication and there is room for alternative opinions.

Cord prolapse

What is cord prolapse?

This is a state where the "waters" break and the umbilical cord protrudes through the cervix. The cervix is normally incompletely dilated, and consequently the cord is compressed, causing acute fetal distress.

Cord prolapse requires immediate caesarean section to save the baby – unless it occurs when the cervix is fully dilated and vaginal delivery can be achieved almost immediately. This is rare.

Can the cord prolapse accident be prevented?

In managing labour in breech presentation, the membranes ("waters") are left intact for as long as possible.

This helps to dilate the cervix and reduces the risk of a cord accident (prolapse). Unfortunately, sometimes the membranes break spontaneously, and these are the circumstances where footling breech is particularly risky.

It appears as if obstetricians prefer to deliver breech babies by caesarean section.

It is not a question of preference but of being realistic.

It is a known fact that the risk of vaginal breech-delivered babies dying just before or after the birth is almost ten times as high as those presenting with the head. Even illness is five times higher. Admittedly, most of this is influenced by prematurity and the major abnormalities that these babies tend to have. With that in mind, most obstetricians would want to err on the side of caution. This is why most breech-presenting babies are delivered by caesarean section. This should not be used as an excuse on the part of the obstetrician to deliver all breech babies by caesarean section.

Are congenital abnormalities more common in breech-presenting babies?

Yes. In any cases where the fetus remains persistently breech, an ultrasound scan is performed, to search for possible congenital abnormalities as a potential explanation for the presentation, among other things

The overall rate of major congenital abnormalities among newborns is 2.5–3 per cent. Among breech-presenting babies, the figure is almost four times higher. This is one of the main reasons why death and illness just before or after the birth, whatever the mode of delivery, is significantly higher among breech babies than in those presenting with head first.

Alternative deliveries

Is there any alternative to breech vaginal delivery and caesarean section?

Yes, there is a third alternative and that is "external cephalic version" (ECV).

What is external cephalic version?

This is where a manoeuvre is performed to turn the baby inside the womb from breech to cephalic presentation (head first).

An experienced doctor in hospital performs this manoeuvre usually after thirty-six weeks of gestation. It lasts about five to ten minutes and has a success rate of about 50 per cent.

The manipulation is performed only in the absence of contraindications such as:

● multiple pregnancy
● previous caesarean section
● vaginal bleeding
● low lying placenta (placenta praevia)
● pre-eclampsia or any hypertensive disease
● intrauterine growth retardation.

The presence of any one of these precludes use of this manoeuvre.

Is "external version" painful?

No, it should not be. Most practitioners use an injection of a drug to relax the womb to facilitate manipulation. The manipulation may cause discomfort but is not painful. Generally, if it is to succeed, it happens very quickly before you are aware of what is happening. Most experienced practitioners will tell you that, if it hasn't worked in the first three to four minutes, it is unlikely to do so, and hence most will give up at this stage.

Can't this manoeuvre be performed under a general anaesthetic?

The majority opinion is that this is unwise, because it allows for the risk of trying too hard. The amount of discomfort that the woman feels is considered a useful safety factor. With a general anaesthetic, this will be abolished, potentially putting the fetus in peril in the process.

Is the manoeuvre safe?

Very safe. It is estimated that fetal death as a result of ECV is about two or three per 1000. The safety checks are both simple and effective. After every manipulation, whether it succeeds or fails, the baby is monitored for at least thirty minutes. If the manoeuvre has caused anything which could lead to fetal distress, this will be immediately apparent and the necessary action will be taken promptly.

What are the potential complications of ECV?

External cephalic version is generally a very safe procedure. Potential complications include induction of labour as a result of the manipulation, placental abruption (partial detachment of the afterbirth) and cord entanglement.

If there is placental abruption or cord entanglement, the fetal monitoring performed immediately after will give clear evidence of fetal distress and, in such a case, an immediate delivery by caesarean section is carried out.

The fact that this manipulation can provoke labour or trigger delivery is one reason why earlier manipulation (before thirty-six completed weeks) is not advocated. This is to prevent the possibility of premature labour or delivery.

Can ECV be performed in labour?

No.

When external cephalic version is carried out after thirty-six weeks of gestation, does the presentation stay cephalic (head) thereafter?

In the majority, yes. The rate of spontaneous reversion back to breech is estimated to be less than 3 per cent.

If this happens, repeat ECV is not advocated. If ECV is performed earlier than thirty-six weeks, the possibility of reversion to breech is significantly higher.

If a breech-presenting baby is left alone after thirty-six weeks, what are the chances that it will spontaneously convert to cephalic (head) presentation?

About 2–4 per cent. That is, over 96 per cent of babies that are found to be breech at thirty-seven weeks will persist as breech thereafter. Some studies have claimed that up to 15 per cent of breech presentations will convert to cephalic after thirty-seven weeks. Evidence of this is lacking in most centres.

Is the timing of delivery of any importance in a breech presentation?

It depends on the method of delivery.

If it is to be an elective caesarean section, in the absence of any compelling factors to do it earlier, delivery will be at thirty-nine weeks (give or take a few days). This is ideal because the baby is then certainly mature. There is no point in going beyond the calculated expected date of delivery as nothing can be gained.

If the planned method of delivery is vaginal, one cannot influence the timing of delivery. Spontaneous labour is awaited and if this does not happen by forty-two weeks of gestation, a review of plan is called for. This will mean reverting to caesarean section. Induction of labour is not considered safe by most obstetricians in a case of breech presentation.

If a woman goes into labour prematurely with a breech presentation, what will be the method of delivery?

Again there is no straightforward answer to this question.

For one, it depends on whether there are factors that rule out vaginal delivery from the outset. In the apparent absence of any such factors, the extent of prematurity will influence the method of delivery.

It is generally accepted that in mild to moderate prematurity (thirty-two to thirty-six weeks of gestation), caesarean section confers no advantage over vaginal delivery.

In severe prematurity (below thirty weeks), a debate still rages on the best and least traumatic way of delivering these tiny babies. Most obstetricians still opt for caesarean section, but evidence to its superiority over vaginal delivery is weak. Regardless of the method of delivery, these babies do not fare very well.

Is vaginal breech delivery more difficult?

Not for the mother. However, for the person assisting in the delivery, it requires special skills and experience. It will always be conducted by a senior midwife or doctor. Most mothers find breech delivery easier than delivery of a head-presenting fetus.

Is there special advice for labour in breech presentation?

Breech labour is managed actively. Labour is expected to proceed smoothly without any undue delay or other problems. The special advice advocated by most is epidural analgesia. This facilitates the smooth progress of labour by preventing the severe backache which characterizes breech labours. More importantly, it prevents premature maternal efforts (pushing), an urge to which these mothers are prone.

The risk associated with this is that if the mother feels these strong urges to push, the lower limbs and body of the fetus could be pushed through an incompletely dilated cervix, leading to head entrapment. This is a serious but fortunately rare complication.

Effective epidural analgesia virtually eliminates this risk.

How many of those who attempt breech vaginal delivery actually succeed?

About a third to half of those embarking on breech labour end up having a caesarean section, for a variety of reasons. The most common is unsatisfactory labour progress (velocity). This means over half of breech labours have a successful conclusion. Most of these mothers will tell you it was worth every minute.

What about breech presentation in twin pregnancy?

This is common, especially for the second twin. Vaginal delivery of a breech-presenting second twin normally poses no problem.

If the first twin is breech-presenting while the second is cephalic (head down), most obstetricians will advocate a caesarean section.

If both twins are breech-presenting, an assessment will be made to consider all factors and decide on the best method of delivery.

It could be either of the two and there is no one preferred method.

It is said, in breech vaginal delivery, the use of forceps is necessary. Is this so?

It is certainly common but by no means necessary. There are various methods of delivering a breech vaginally and not all of them involve the use of forceps. If the mother has a particular antipathy to forceps, she should feel free to express her reservation to the doctor assisting the delivery. The doctor will try to avoid the use of forceps unless this becomes necessary. In some cases – such as premature delivery – forceps have an additional important function, which is to protect the still-delicate head (that is, the brain). The doctor is duty-bound to explain all this well in advance.

Is breech presentation recurrent?

No, unless these is an unchanging predisposing feature, such as uterine abnormality, where breech or another form of abnormal lie of the fetus may feature in every pregnancy.

34. Labour monitoring of fetal well-being

Introduction

The word "normal" has the unattractive but ultimately necessary connotation of being restrictive. For labour, what is normal encompasses a broad and quite varied picture. A woman whose contractions start and then she goes on to deliver after four hours without needing pain relief or an episiotomy has had a normal labour. Her opposite number could have four hours of latent labour (with nothing tangible happening, other than increasing low backache and irregular contractions), ten hours of first-stage labour and two hours of second-stage labour. This will also be normal labour. In the process, she may also have covered the gamut of pain relief, from using entonox ("gas and air") through multiple doses of pethidine, culminating in the "epidural" being inserted. At delivery, the midwife may have applied an episiotomy. This is still a very normal labour. Needless to say, the experiences of labour narrated by the two women will be very different.

The aim of this chapter is to describe broadly what labour involves and to define the acceptable degrees of departure from that picture which will still fall within the confines of normality.

Starting labour

What are the factors that trigger labour?

This may surprise many people but the truth, is we do not know how labour is triggered!

What is known – and this is incomplete – is the fact that prostaglandins (which are natural chemicals) play a crucial role in the initiation of labour.

What triggers the release of prostaglandins at the crucial moment is not clearly known. To date, it is practically impossible to predict when labour is going to start.

Why is it that some women go into labour prematurely every time and others go into labour at various stages of pregnancy each time?

For the same reason as above, nobody can answer this question succinctly – at least, not yet. The intricate mechanism of labour onset remains largely a mystery.

Where are the prostaglandins produced?

Mainly in the uterine muscle, the lining of the uterus and the fetal membranes.

There is what is described as spurious labour or false labour. What does this mean?

Normally, in late pregnancy, the uterus tends to go into mild painless contractions, on and off. These are known as Braxton-Hicks contractions. If these contractions become painful, the woman may erroneously assume that she is in labour. Sometimes there is an unrelated but concomitant low backache, which reinforces the impression of being in labour. Vaginal examination will reveal that there is no evidence of labour.

Spurious labour can be quite distressing and can continue for several days before the onset of true labour.

How is spurious labour managed?

No specific treatment is required. The doctors and midwives will explain the situation patiently to the mother-to-be. Painkillers may be prescribed, to take the edge off the pain. A mixture of light domestic activities, long warm baths and plenty of rest will help to alleviate the discomfort. Labour will eventually start.

Head engagement

What is "head engagement" and what is its significance?

What engagement means is that most of the baby's head has descended into the mother's pelvic cavity and only a small part can be felt abdominally (or not at all). The significance varies. If there are known potential problems – such as a uterine abnormality, pelvic abnormality or a pelvic mass – lack of engagement in late pregnancy (beyond thirty-eight weeks) or at the onset of labour may signify potential problems. The same may be the case if the fetus has been noted to be very large.

The attending obstetrician may then re-evaluate the planned method of delivery and if there are other strong indicators of potential problems in labour, then the relevant advice will be given. It is, however, very unusual to advise against labour or vaginal delivery simply on the basis of head engagement or lack of it.

Is early engagement of the head of any significance?

Not really. It may be reassuring to have the head engaging early but this does not guarantee a successful vaginal delivery. When everything is normal, early or late head engagement does not make any difference. In fact, in black women, engagement before the onset of labour is unusual, except in a first pregnancy, when it is slightly more common.

Latent phase of labour

What is the "latent phase" of labour?

This is the time when changes in the body start occurring in preparation for labour. The latent phase differs so widely among individuals, both in character and duration, that it almost defies description. Doctor will define this phase as that time when irregular and painful contractions start and continue to build up both in intensity and frequency. This may last anything between one and twenty hours, occasionally more. It tends to be long in the first pregnancy. Some women find the pain in this phase so mild that they can hardly believe that actual labour is imminent. Others are so distressed by the pain in this phase that hospital admission and repeated pain relief with strong painkillers is necessary.

The latent phase tends to blend imperceptibly into the first stage of labour and one should not expect to experience anything specific to signify the true onset of labour. Professionals are also caught out, occasionally. This may happen when a woman with very mild pains in the latent phase is admitted. A midwife may continue to believe that labour has yet to establish, only to be confronted by an imminent delivery a few hours later. This, fortunately is uncommon.

So, what is really taking place during the latent phase of labour?

The uterus is contracting irregularly and the various chemicals necessary for labour are being produced. Some of these are acting upon the cervix, causing it to soften, thin out and become more pliable. It then starts to open. For purely descriptive purposes, it is said that once the cervix has dilated beyond 3 cm, true labour is established and the latent phase has passed.

The three stages of labour

What are the stages of labour?

There are three main stages of labour.

Stage one starts at the end of the latent phase to the time the cervix is fully dilated (open).

Stage two starts at full cervical dilatation to the time the baby is delivered.

Stage three is from the time the baby is delivered to the delivery of the placenta (afterbirth).

How long does the first stage of labour last?

This is the longest part of labour and the one most women remember vividly. It is the time when contractions get stronger and stronger in an endeavour to build up sufficient expulsive force to get the baby out. The cervix is also continually dilating, to enable the baby to pass through to the outside world. All this time, she is experiencing such excruciating pain that she wonders again and again how she could be so crazy as to let herself in for this (unless she has effective pain relief such the as an epidural – in which case she is likely to be blissfully oblivious of the titanic struggle in her pelvis). The whole process will last between six and ten hours. It could be much shorter for the lucky ones. It is usually longer in the first pregnancy and, in most cases, shorter in subsequent pregnancies.

How long does the second stage last?

This is the culmination of it all. The pain is at its pinnacle. This is where the pushing has to be done. All the swearing is done during this stage. This is when women invariably swear that there is no way they are going to survive this and some take it out on anybody of acquaintance in the vicinity – usually the partner – swearing how passionately they hate him. Others demand to go home. And then suddenly it is over! The baby is delivered. The transformation of the woman in this instant from one writhing in extreme pain to one wreathed in the most wonderful smile is one of the incredible wonders of childbirth. All this takes between thirty minutes and two hours. Epidural analgesia, though very effective in pain control, could cause prolongation of this stage of labour. This is thought to be a direct weakness of its effectiveness. As the woman feels no pain, so she gets no urges to push and is really not motivated. Nature is cheated!

How long does the third stage last?

Once the baby is born, in most cases an injection of ergometrine or oxytocin (or a mixture of the two) will be administered to facilitate detachment of the afterbirth. This is then eased out within about five minutes of the baby being delivered. There is no need to push at this stage.

Some women prefer "natural" childbirth and do not want any of these drugs administered for the third stage. Here, the delivery of the placenta may take a bit longer.

Either way, the third stage rarely lasts more than fifteen minutes and is certainly not allowed to last beyond thirty minutes. If the placenta is not detached by then, steps are taken to have it removed manually, usually in the operating theatre under an effective anaesthetic. It is usually a general anaesthetic, but a spinal or even an epidural could suffice.

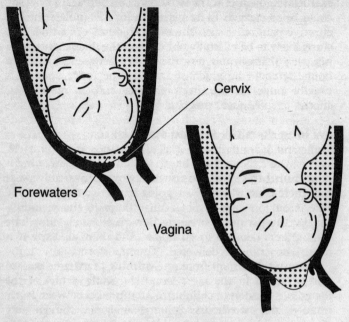

Fig 10 Cervix dilated at 3 cm and then at 10 cm

Progress of labour

How is the progress of labour monitored?

To ensure that labour in the first stage is progressing smoothly – i.e. the cervix is dilating and the head of the baby is descending down the birth canal – vaginal examinations have to be performed. Different units operate different polices and the length of the intervals between examinations makes little difference, provided appropriate action is taken whenever necessary.

The intervals between examinations could be two, three or four hours. Sometimes, the intervals are tailored to suit the particular individual and examinations may be performed more frequently if this is deemed necessary. The examinations are never left for longer than standard, however.

What is the expected rate of progress?

As mentioned, two of the main things that are assessed during a vaginal examination are cervical dilatation and descent of the baby. Regarding dilatation, which is the main yardstick of labour progress, the cervix is expected to dilate a minimum of 1 cm per hour.

If the initial examination shows the cervix to be 4 cm dilated, an examination three hours later should reveal a dilatation of at least 7 cm. Remember, full dilatation is 10 cm, so a woman at 7 cm cervical dilatation should expect to come to the end of the first stage in three hours or less.

If it is found that the labour is not progressing as expected, what then?

The main focal point of a slow labour is whether the contractions are strong enough. More often than not, in such cases, they will not be. If this is suspected to be the case, two courses of action are possible.

Firstly, if the membranes are still intact, the waters may be broken. This may have the effect of increasing stimulation of the uterus, resulting in stronger contractions.

The second alternative is to give the mother an intravenous infusion (drip) with the hormone oxytocin. This directly stimulates the uterus to contract more strongly.

It is important to remember that weak contractions are not the only cause of poor labour progress and it is up to the attending obstetrician to make correct analysis and institute the right corrective measure.

If, in spite of corrective measures labour still does not progress, what can be done?

If labour stalls in the first stage, in spite of corrective efforts, then the doctor will have to resort to a caesarean delivery. He or she may then investigate postnatally why labour never progressed. Even then, the causes may remain a mystery.

There is a widespread belief that using pethidine or diamorphine may actually cause contractions to weaken or stop altogether. Is this true?

There is no truth in this. Weakening of contractions is usually a figment of the imagination, brought about by the blunted perception of the pain and the sedative effect of these drugs.

Does epidural analgesia weaken contractions?

No, it does not. It is still true, however, that the second stage may be prolonged because of blunting of the urge to push.

Is there any merit in remaining mobile during the first stage of labour?

Yes. There is evidence that walking about may somewhat reduce the distress of the pain in the first stage, by giving the mind something else to concentrate on. The shortening of labour is an unproven benefit.

Can one have an "epidural" and still be mobile?

This is occasionally possible. However, this will have to be a "light" epidural, so as not to deaden the limbs. Another prerequisite is the continuous presence of an assistant – be it a midwife, the partner or another responsible adult – whenever the mother is walking. This is to ensure her safety.

Can I have a meal or at least a snack in labour?

This is not a good idea. Firstly, the labouring woman is unlikely to benefit from eating, because hardly any absorption is taking place from the stomach. Secondly, vomiting is rather common in labour and this can be quite distressing, especially after a meal. This takes on particular significance if a surgical procedure under a general anaesthetic (such as a caesarean section) becomes necessary. Vomiting of semi-solid food can be dangerous in this state of unconsciousness as the stomach contents may be aspirated into the airway, creating a dangerous complication. Sips of plain water or sucking on ice is OK to relieve mouth and throat dryness.

Pushing

When should the pushing start?

This should be at a stage when the cervix is fully dilated and the head (if this is the leading part) is reasonably down in the pelvis. This is the second stage of labour.

Surely, the earlier pushing is commenced, the shorter the labour?

This is a bad idea. If pushing is commenced before the cervix is fully dilated, it can cause all sorts of problems. The cervix itself is likely to swell up and may be pushed out of the vaginal canal, with serious risk of damage to it, and bleeding. The efforts themselves will not hasten delivery; instead, this will help to exhaust the mother, running the risk of her being unable to push when the appropriate moment arrives. This may mean an instrumental (forceps or ventouse) delivery which was otherwise unnecessary.

Why is it then that sometimes the mother feels such strong urges to push when she is not ready?

This is true. The reason is partly because the birth canal is right next to the rectum and back passage. Pressure from the leading part is inevitably transmitted across to this area and this produces the urge to bear down. Sometimes these urges are extremely strong.

Is there any way of avoiding this premature urge to bear down?

As part of parentcraft classes, which are widely available, expectant mothers are taught breathing exercises, which might help in this regard. Epidural analgesia is, of course, much more effective in preventing premature pushing.

When the right moment comes, what is the right way of pushing?

Again, this is taught in parentcraft classes. It is important to push only when there is a uterine contraction. Pushing at any other time is ineffective and only serves to sap precious energy.

The push should be as hard and as long as possible during the contraction.

As the mother feels a contraction building up, she should take a deep breath, hold it (this is very important) and bear down. It is OK to take snatches of breath very quickly in the middle of a push without relaxing. A good "push" lasts thirty to forty seconds.

Shouting, screaming or expressing an opinion during a push may be irresistible but does no good. All it does is blunt the effort and in effect prolongs the second stage. It should be resisted.

In between pushing, the mother should try to "let go" and relax as much as possible – breathing deeply in and out, preparing for the next contraction and effort.

Sometimes, there is a strong feeling of an imminent bowel motion. What should I do?

This is quite common. Again, it is the effect of the pressure of the baby in the birth canal transmitted to the rectum, which is immediately adjacent. Even when the rectum is empty, a strong feeling of an imminent emptying of the bowel may be there. Many women find this hard to cope with because, culturally, opening the bowels is a very private thing. It should really never be a worry because midwives and doctors are used to it and half-expect it to happen anyway. Ideally, she should go in labour with an empty rectum but this does not always happen and should never be a cause for worry.

Sometimes, when a woman is seen in the latent phase of labour and is examined vaginally, a loaded rectum may be felt. Since there is still time, a suppository or even an enema may then be administered, to facilitate a bowel movement before the establishment of labour.

Sometimes a midwife uses a catheter to empty the urinary bladder; is this really necessary?

Yes, sometimes this is necessary. A full bladder may impede both contractions and the descent of the baby down the birth canal. In the first stage of labour, normally the woman will be encouraged to pass urine herself from time to time. If an epidural has been used, then she may lose the sensation and therefore a catheter will be left in place to continuously drain the urine.

In the late first stage and in the second stage, it is usually impossible for the woman to pass urine herself. If her bladder is rather full, then a catheter may need to be used for the reasons explained above.

Episiotomy

Is an episiotomy always necessary?

An episiotomy is the incision or cut that is made on the perineum to increase the size of the opening, thereby facilitating delivery. It is not always necessary. To do or not to do an episiotomy is one of the most important (and quick) decisions the person assisting delivery has to make.

An episiotomy will prevent a perineal and/or vaginal tear and also hasten delivery. It is also believed to prevent future urinary problems, to some extent, by protecting the pelvic support muscles from damage that may be caused by over-stretching.

It is, however, unnecessary to perform an episiotomy where progress in the second stage is smooth and the risk of a tear is deemed minimal.

It is impossible to be precise every time in this assessment and sometimes the judgement is wrong and a tear occurs where it was least expected.

It is said an episiotomy is mandatory in the first pregnancy (vaginal delivery). Is this true?

It is never wise to be dogmatic in these things.

The truth is, most first-timers will have an episiotomy, but there is a significant minority where this will be correctly judged to be unnecessary. It is up to the midwife or doctors assisting in the delivery to make that decision rather than hide behind a blanket policy. By the same token, some mothers who have had a previous baby may require an episiotomy.

With forceps delivery, an episiotomy is necessary, regardless of the number of past deliveries. This is because the risk of a tear is quite high with this method of instrumental delivery.

Just before the head is delivered, it is common for the woman to be asked to pant. Why?

The head is quite considerably compressed in the birth canal. Because the woman at this stage will be trying to get the baby out, there is a risk of sudden decompression of the head if the expulsion is forceful and sudden. Panting removes this risk, as the assisting person can gently ease the head out. Sudden decompression of the head could cause brain damage.

What happens after the head is delivered?

In most cases, another single push will help facilitate delivery of the shoulders. After that, the rest of the baby is eased out without the need of any maternal contribution. In fact, delivery of the shoulders does not necessarily require a uterine contraction.

What is shoulder dystocia?

This is a difficult but fortunately rare complication of delivery. With a big baby, sometimes the head is delivered but the broad shoulders are stuck above the pelvic brim, with the neck stretched in the birth canal. This requires quick action where the mother will be put in a special position, a large episiotomy (if not already there) is applied and special manipulations of the baby are made to allow delivery. This can be quite difficult and fractures of some of the baby's bones may result. Most vulnerable are the collarbones and the bone in the upper arm (humerus).

It is virtually impossible to predict shoulder dystocia.

The third stage of labour

What happens in the third stage of labour?

Moments after the baby is born, the uterus contracts, allowing the placenta to detach from its base. The midwife will wait for the telltale signs of this and then deliver the placenta by applying gentle traction on the cord. The mother does not have to do any pushing. In most cases, this happens within minutes of delivering of the baby. Occasionally, the placenta does not detach and it has to be manually removed. This requires adequate pain relief, such as an epidural, spinal or general anaesthesia. It is not done under a local anaesthetic.

What happens after the third stage is complete?

If there was an episiotomy, this is repaired. Labour is then complete and the new mother can rest and savour this very special moment.

How is the episiotomy repaired?

Normally a local anaesthetic will have been injected before the cut is made. Some more local anaesthetic may need to be injected or, if there is an epidural in place already, this may be sufficient. The repair is done using suture material that dissolves with time. There is therefore no worry about having the stitches taken out.

The area will inevitably be sore when the local anaesthetic wears off after a few hours. Painkillers are sometimes necessary. This soon resolves and the new mother is likely to be perfectly comfortable within three or four days. Complete healing may take a couple of weeks or so, even though she will not be aware of it.

Fetal monitoring

How effective are the fetal monitoring methods in labour?

Pretty effective but they are not infallible. It is, however, extremely unusual to be unable to detect a baby in trouble. The one charge against the current monitoring methods that will stick is the fact that, as a result of them, there is over-intervention.

How is a baby monitored in the uterus?

In the Western world, the standard is electronic fetal monitoring. It is what is known as a "cardiotocograph" or CTG.

A CTG continually monitors the activity of the fetal heart (hence cardio-) and also monitors the contractions (toco-). A trained person, on looking at a trace made by the machine, will be able to distinguish a normal from an abnormal pattern.

How does CTG monitoring cause over-intervention?

A CTG is excellent in telling a normal pattern. This means, when it indicates that things are normal, they almost certainly are.

Unfortunately, an abnormal pattern cannot be taken at face value. Its positive predictive value is rather poor. Some experts quote a figure of 30 per cent. This means, about 70 per cent of the seemingly abnormal traces will be from babies that are perfectly happy. A doctor, therefore, has a duty to analyze each apparently abnormal pattern and take the necessary steps.

So what kind of intervention is available if the CTG trace raises suspicions?

The doctors need to make a critical assessment of the situation. If the pattern is benign enough and there is no other evidence of possible fetal distress, then waiting and watching for developments is the logical option.

If the pattern is causing sufficient concern, then there is a way of objectively verifying the situation. This is by taking a tiny sample of blood from the fetus and having it analyzed by a special machine to check the acid-base balance and oxygenation of the baby's blood.

If the pattern looks alarming and if there is little doubt that the baby needs bailing out, then it is up to the doctor to move fast and deliver the baby by the quickest means feasible. This could be by instrumental delivery (such as forceps or ventouse) or by caesarean section.

How is a blood sample obtained from an unborn baby?

As mentioned above, a fetal blood sample may be required to verify whether an abnormal CTG truly reflects a fetus in trouble.

This is obtained by making a tiny scratch on the fetal scalp (or the buttock, if the baby is breech-presenting). A sample is made up of about two small drops of blood. Usually, two samples will be taken, to ensure a correct reading has been obtained. The whole procedure takes about three minutes from beginning to end, and the results are available within two minutes of taking a sample. It is a truly remarkable piece of technology which has saved millions of mothers from an unnecessary caesarean section. In addition – and probably more importantly – it has allowed timely intervention where this is required. This is because the results do not only show where there is distress, they also show the actual degree of distress and therefore guide the speed of intervention.

How good is the CTG in monitoring contractions?

The conventional CTG will tell you how frequently the mother is getting contractions, how regular they are and how long each contraction lasts. It also allows the doctors to analyze what effect the contractions are having on the fetal heart pattern. It does not tell how strong the contractions are. This still requires the ever-dependable hand of the midwife – by feeling. Of course, in some cases, even this does not work very well. Markedly obese women are a case in point.

So, how can contraction strength be objectively monitored?

For some years now, there have been gadgets available which can be placed inside the womb itself to monitor the strength of contractions. They are supposedly useful in cases where there is a perceived risk of uterine rupture – such as in cases where there was a caesarean section or surgery on the womb in the past.

Unfortunately, they have been rather disappointing in the sense that, while they monitor uterine contraction strength very well, they do not seem to confer any tangible benefit over the conventional CTG. They are also expensive, delicate and cumbersome. Their place in mainstream labour ward practice is uncertain.

Is there any alternative to a CTG?

Before the advent of electronic fetal monitoring, a simple device called a pinard fetal stethoscope was the standard equipment in monitoring the fetal heartbeat. It is still used in some labour wards in conjunction with a CTG.

Is there any newer technology on the horizon?

The one development that seems to hold promise is the impressive-sounding "near-infrared spectroscopy". This involves attaching a soft pad on the fetal scalp, from which a special light is beamed into the fetal brain. The pattern of absorption of this light by the blood can be analyzed to identify which babies are getting insufficient oxygen to the brain and therefore in need of rescue. The technology has been undergoing tests to perfect it for a few years, now. As with all new developments, it is best to wait until it is squarely on the table before applauding (or otherwise).

Most labouring women appear to be monitored continuously. Is this necessary?

This is quite controversial. There is strong evidence that continuous monitoring is not for everyone, yet many units continue to do this. In a labour where there is no apparent risk factor (low-risk pregnancy), intermittent monitoring is just as good. It has the advantage of not curtailing the woman's mobility for hours on end. Of course, those women whose pregnancies have some risk factors (such as fetal growth restrictions, pre-eclampsia and diabetes) need continuous monitoring. It remains a fact that the majority of pregnancies are low-risk and the restriction of continuous monitoring for them is unjustified.

How difficult is it to monitor twins in labour?

Not difficult, as long as the position of each baby is known – and it is easy to confirm this, using ultrasound. Monitoring transducers are then put on the appropriate positions and each baby's heartbeat is monitored. Twins are almost always monitored continuously.

If the second twin shows features of distress, how can one gain access to it to take a blood sample for analysis?

It is not possible. If a CTG shows worrying features for twin II, the only solution is to perform a caesarean section and deliver them. Quite often it turns out to have been a false scare but most people will agree that it is better to be safe than sorry.

What is a fetal scalp electrode?

Part of the failings of the conventional CTG is the weakness inherent in monitoring the fetal heart remotely, with the probe on the maternal abdomen. It is not unusual to fail to pick up the heartbeat or to pick it erratically. Sometimes one ends up with the maternal heartbeat. A fetal scalp electrode is a simple device, which is a significant improvement on this state of affairs. The small probe is attached to the skin of the fetal scalp and it directly monitors the heartbeat. It is more accurate and more reliable.

In twins, it is normal practice to monitor twin I with a scalp electrode and twin II with an abdominal transducer.

Of course, calling it "scalp" electrode is a slightly restrictive term. In breech presentation, the electrode can be placed on the fetal buttocks and it functions as usual.

35. Induction and augmentation of labour

Introduction

Sometimes it becomes necessary to bring about labour for a variety of reasons. In most cases, it is a result of concern for the fetal well-being if it continues to stay in the womb. This is compounded by the fact that there are good but no foolproof methods of monitoring the well-being of the fetus in the uterus. In such circumstances, it very occasionally becomes necessary to expedite delivery and, unless there are contraindications, induction of labour (aiming for vaginal delivery) is the preferred method.

Occasionally, the induction of labour is done as a result of concern for maternal well-being, for example to allow the treatment of a serious unrelated illness diagnosed during pregnancy. In some instances, such as pre-eclampsia, there is concern for both the mother and the baby and labour may be induced.

Induction of labour for social reasons ("I am moving house", "I want it before Christmas", "my partner has a business trip" and the like) sits firmly albeit uncomfortably along all these possible indications.

Induction of labour is ideally done as close to term as possible.

Contrary to what many a woman believes, induction of labour is not always a routine affair. It can be a protracted and very unpleasant experience indeed. This is uncommon but the possibility should never be ignored. Moreover, induction can and does occasionally fail. Which leads inevitably to the question of "what next"? The answer may very well be a caesarean section, which in the cold light of day may be seen to have been unnecessary.

There are only a few methods of labour induction of proven efficacy. All these are discussed in detail below.

Are there any DIY methods for labour induction? Not at present, nor in the foreseeable future. However, many midwives could give you tips on how to encourage things along. All are of unproven value but at least they are harmless and may even be fun. We discuss these as well here.

What induction and augmentation are

What does labour induction mean?

This is the process of starting off labour by initiating uterine contractions. The process may include the initial preparation of the cervix to facilitate its dilatation (opening) in labour.

How does this differ from labour augmentation?

Labour augmentation is carried out when the woman is already in labour but where the progress of labour has been unsatisfactory. It is therefore an act of accelerating the process and never involves cervical preparation.

When induction is considered necessary

When is labour induction considered necessary?

Indications for inducing labour are many and varied.

It may be deemed necessary to intervene and bring about labour and delivery for fetal reasons and, less commonly, for maternal reasons. If there is sufficient concern about the fetal well-being, labour may be induced. This may be because of growth restriction, recurrent vaginal bleeding (antepartum haemorrhage), maternal diabetes or infection.

Are there any other fetal indications for inducing labour?

Yes. Prolonged rupture of membranes is regarded as a risky state, as infection may ascend into the uterine cavity and affect the baby. It may be decided therefore that the baby will fare better outside the womb.

In the case of a Rhesus negative mother who is carrying antibodies, if the fetus is seen to be affected by the antibodies, delivery may be deemed to be the best way forward and labour could be induced.

In multiple pregnancy, labour may be induced because one or the other twin is not doing too well.

"Unstable lie" is another indication. If the baby is changing position all the time, labour may be induced as a "stabilizing" procedure to try to prevent an otherwise unnecessary caesarean section.

What about a prolonged pregnancy?

This is one of the most common indications for labour induction. When the pregnancy continues beyond the expected date of delivery mark (forty weeks), most obstetricians will adopt a conservative wait-and-see policy while monitoring the well-being of both the mother and the fetus. If all remains well, most obstetricians will advocate no intervention until at some point ten to fourteen days after the "due date".

Induction of labour is advised at or soon after this point. A few obstetricians are prepared to advise leaving well alone up to forty-three weeks before intervening.

Why is maternal diabetes an indication for inducing labour?

If for any reason, insulin-dependent diabetes is not well controlled in pregnancy, the fetus is clearly at risk and fetal demise is a real possibility. Labour may be induced when doctors are confident of fetal survival outside the womb.

Diabetes that starts during pregnancy (gestational diabetes) is normally not an indication for inducing labour.

Well-controlled insulin-dependent diabetes is also a less clear-cut indication. Many experts argue that, in such cases, intervention in the form of labour induction is not necessary, at least not before the due date.

Is a large fetal size an indication for induction of labour?

This is another controversial indication. Some obstetricians argue that after thirty-seven weeks, when the fetus is mature, labour may be induced before a large baby gets bigger. The argument is that you will prevent a potentially difficult delivery and probably a caesarean section. Evidence that this is true is lacking.

Is breech presentation an indication for labour induction?

No: at least, not in its unchanged form.

Some practitioners will convert a breech presentation into a head-down presentation. Once this is achieved, some will consider inducing labour to prevent the fetus flipping back to breech, which is always a possibility, albeit a slim one.

Does previous obstetric history have any bearing on deciding to induce labour?

It could. In tragic cases of previous unexplained stillbirth late in pregnancy, it may be decided to induce labour, probably at thirty-seven to thirty-eight weeks, when the chances of success are good and the baby is mature enough not to need any special care after birth.

Talking of chances of success, does it mean induction of labour can fail?

Yes. This happens occasionally. A rough guide to the chances of success is the gestational age. The more advanced the pregnancy, the better the chances of success. This, however, is not a black-and-white situation. Labour induction at forty-two weeks of gestation has been known to fail.

What are the maternal indications for inducing labour?

If the mother has a medical condition that is deteriorating because of pregnancy or which needs treatment urgently but only after the end of pregnancy, labour may be induced. Such conditions include pre-eclampsia (which is always confined to a pregnant state), kidney failure and cancer.

Is pain an indication for induction of labour?

It can be. Of course, pain is subjective and it is difficult for the doctor to objectively judge what pain justifies intervention to bring the pregnancy to a premature conclusion. It is true, however, that sometimes pregnancy is associated with severe debilitating pain, usually in the pelvic region. This may justify induction of labour as a rescue measure.

Are there any indications that are neither fetal nor maternal?

Yes. In the tragic event of fetal demise late in pregnancy, labour will be induced.

Induction of labour is also advised in a case where a lethal fetal condition has been diagnosed late in pregnancy. Such conditions as anencephaly (where there is no brain), chromosomal disorders (e.g. Edward's Syndrome) and the absence of kidneys are incompatible with life outside the womb.

Most of these are diagnosed early in the second trimester and termination of pregnancy is offered. However, a few do inadvertently escape detection till late in pregnancy, where induction of labour will be offered.

People talk of "social indications" for induction of labour. What are these?

This term simply refers to a situation where induction is carried out for no obstetric or medical indication. In other words, it is labour induction requested by the parents for their convenience. The most common reasons include to allow a partner or another family member to be present at the birth, to avoid certain dates and occasionally to allow the baby's arrival before Christmas or the New Year!

How labour is induced

How is labour induced?

There are really two principal ways of inducing labour. One or both may be used in each case.

Prostaglandins are the chemicals used specifically to prime the cervix for labour. They also have an "oxytocic" effect in that they stimulate the uterus and may bring about contractions.

The second method of labour induction is that of amniotomy. Amniotomy simply means rupturing the membranes or "breaking the waters". Both methods are, in most cases, supplemented with an oxytocin drip.

What do the prostaglandins do?

During pregnancy, the cervix or "neck of the womb" is firm and closed because its main function is to maintain the ever-increasing size and weight of the uterine contents inside the womb cavity. At term, before labour, the cervical function changes to facilitate smooth and safe birth.

To be able to do this, the cervix undergoes profound changes, whereby it becomes softer, thinner, shorter and distensible. These acquired characteristics allow it to open (dilate) when uterine contractions start.

Prostaglandins are used to bring about these changes to the cervix.

How are the prostaglandins administered?

The most popular method of administration is vaginal. It is mostly given in the form of a gel but also, less commonly, it could be administered in the form of vaginal pessaries. Some obstetricians use prostaglandin oral tablets, but these are known to be less effective.

Also available are slow-release devices, which are also inserted vaginally and can be retrieved instantly if the need arises. They are more expensive and less popular with obstetricians.

There is no place for intravenous prostaglandins in induction of labour.

What does induction using vaginal prostaglandin involve?

To begin with, a vaginal examination will be performed. This is to assess the state of the cervix and to determine whether the prostaglandins will be required and at what dosage. This will be followed by administration of the gel. This is followed by fetal monitoring for anything up to one hour – longer, if necessary. The monitoring is essential because sometimes the uterus responds abnormally to the stimulus of the prostaglandins and causes fetal distress. Monitoring is therefore an essential precaution. Fetal distress is, however, a rare complication.

How many times do prostaglandins have to be administered before the cervix is "ready"?

Most women will need one or two administrations, given

four to six hours apart. In a few instances, more administrations of the gel may be required because of poor cervical response to the prostaglandins.

Rarely, no response occurs and the cervix remains obstinately unchanged. This is a failed induction.

What happens after the cervix is ready, following prostaglandin administration?

The next step will be amniotomy or "breaking the waters". Once the waters are broken, uterine contractions are expected to follow. Some practitioners will start the oxytocin drip straight away after "breaking the waters", while others advocate giving some time (one or two hours) to allow the uterus to start contracting spontaneously before considering the drip.

Can the mere administration of the prostaglandin gel (or pessaries) cause the membranes to rupture?

This occasionally happens. Following instillation of the prostaglandin gel, changes take place to the cervix. As a direct result of this, probably combined with low-grade uterine activity, rupture of membranes may occur.

Can labour commence after prostaglandins without need for the other steps in the induction process?

This frequently happens. Besides the cervix, the uterus itself may respond as well, with contractions following shortly after the prostaglandin has been instilled. This means labour is established and will be managed like any other labour.

What happens if the cervix does not respond to prostaglandins?

This is a difficult situation and the attending obstetrician has to weigh up the options. One will be to try and go ahead with amniotomy (rupturing the membranes) and an oxytocin infusion. Such a strategy has a high chance of failure, especially if the cervix is in a very unfavourable state. It simply won't open.

The second option is to postpone the procedure for a few days and try again later. This is only possible where there is no concern for the baby's well-being by the continued stay in the womb.

The third option is to abandon the failed induction and deliver by caesarean section.

What kind of side-effects can occur, following the use of prostaglandins for labour induction?

Many women complain of an aching pain that is persistent in the lower back and abdomen, following prostaglandin administration. Sometimes this is bad enough to require anti-pain medication,

Hyperstimulation of the uterus is another potential side-effect. This may cause fetal distress. Using drugs called tocolytics, which allow the uterus to relax, can effectively counteract hyper-stimulation. They are given intravenously but the inhalational route has also been used with success.

Nausea, vomiting, headache, flushing and dizziness are rare and usually mild side-effects.

Is the use of prostaglandins contraindicated anywhere?

There are a few contraindications, including:

- where there has been significant antepartum haemorrhage (vaginal bleeding during pregnancy) or where there is confirmed placenta praevia, with or without bleeding, prostaglandins are not used
- when the fetus is lying in an abnormal position, e.g. transverse or oblique
- in the ocular (eye) condition known as glaucoma
- when there is an infection in the birth canal.

What if the membranes have ruptured and the waters are draining?

This is not a contraindication to using prostaglandins.

What if the previous delivery was by caesarean?

This in itself is not a contraindication; however, many obstetricians are not comfortable with the idea of using prostaglandins in such circumstances. Of course, if the indication for the previous caesarean section is still there, the need for inducing labour will not arise as delivery will be by a repeat caesarean section.

In which circumstances is the use of prostaglandins not necessary?

If, on assessing the cervix, it is found to be favourable, then prostaglandin use will be unnecessary. The doctor will proceed to rupture the membranes and probably use the oxytocin drip to stimulate contractions.

If the membranes are already ruptured, then all that remains is to initiate contractions. The oxytocin infusion is used for this.

What are the potential side-effects of oxytocin?

Oxytocin is actually a natural chemical which is produced by the pituitary gland in the brain for the same purpose – to stimulate the womb to contract.

If the oxytocin drip becomes excessive, the uterus may be over-stimulated.

Over-stimulation in a woman who has had a number of children in the past could cause rupture of the uterus. There is also the risk of fetal distress as a result of over-stimulation. This effect can be readily reversed by stopping the infusion or, if deemed necessary, by stopping the drip and administering a tocolytic drug. These complications are uncommon.

How is the oxytocin drip administered and controlled?

Most labour ward units use either an infusion pump or a syringe driver. With these methods, one can very accurately determine the rate at which oxytocin is being administered. The rate can therefore be adjusted upwards or downwards, according to need and response.

How does oxytocin differ from syntocinon?

There is no difference. Oxytocin is a generic name and Syntocinon, is the commonly used brand name (in the UK and Europe). The other common brand name is Pitocin. They are the same thing.

What about syntometrine?

This is a combination of Syntocinon (oxytocin) and ergometrine. It has no role to play in induction or augment-ation of labour. In fact, its use is contraindicated in pregnancy. It is used after delivery to facilitate expulsion of the afterbirth (placenta) and to produce sustained uterine contractions, which are essential in preventing excessive blood loss.

Are there any other methods of induction, apart from those already discussed?

Some hormones and chemicals, including oestrogen, have been tried and found to be either very slow or ineffective. These are therefore not in use for this purpose.

Mechanical preparation of the cervix, using what are termed as "laminaria" (vaginal pessaries made from a kind of starch, extracted from seaweed) and some chemically impregnated cervical "sponges" were once tried, especially in the United States. All these methods have not taken hold because of their inferior effect and the potential risk of infection.

What about anti-progestogens?

There is considerable interest in these chemicals. They are already in widespread use for second trimester termination of pregnancy. If the concerns about their safety can be conclusively allayed, they are bound to have a place in induction of labour.

Augmentation

Regarding labour augmentation, when does this become necessary?

If labour has commenced – i.e. the cervix has started to open and the uterus is contracting regularly – but the progress is unsatisfactory, labour augmentation is indicated.

When is labour progress deemed unsatisfactory?

Progress is judged by what is found to be happening to the cervix and the presenting part of the baby. Vaginal examination is the only way of verifying labour progress. The cervix should dilate progressively and the minimum acceptable rate of dilatation is 1 cm per hour. The leading part of the baby should descend continually down the pelvis.

If serial examinations reveal that cervical dilatation is not taking place at the acceptable rate, it may be time to consider augmenting labour.

Head descent has been mentioned above; what if the leading part is a breech?

Most obstetricians contend that labour augmentation has no place in breech presentation. Poor labour progress in breech presentation is regarded as a warning sign of a possible difficult delivery and hence an indication for caesarean delivery. There are a few obstetricians who disagree. This is probably one of the genuinely grey areas of obstetric practice where no clear-cut answer should be expected. An experienced obstetrician will usually use his or her judgement on how best to proceed in each individual case.

The use of oxytocin drips in breech presentation is certainly a contentious issue.

Does labour augmentation always succeed?

No. In some cases, in spite of prolonged use of an oxytocin drip at high concentrations, labour progress remains sluggish, even stagnant. The reason for this is not always clear. In any case, that is an indication for caesarean delivery.

Is oxytocin infusion the only method available for labour augmentation?

Yes. Prostaglandins have no place in labour augmentation.

Using an infusion (drip) tends to restrict the labouring woman's movement. Can the oxytocin be administered as a one-off injection?

Unfortunately not. This drug has to be administered continuously and in well controlled (if necessary) incremental rates. A drip holder with castors for easy mobility will almost always be available if the woman wants to be mobile and if this is deemed to be safe.

36. Pain relief in labour

Introduction

Labour is painful: there is no argument about that.

The perception, of course, differs widely among individual women but many will tell you that labour was the most intensely painful experience of their lives.

The need for pain relief differs among individuals. The range is from those who are absolutely resolute that they do not want anything chemical or otherwise throughout labour to those who actually demand to be "put out", an option which is of course unavailable in any labour ward repertoire.

There are four broad groups of pain relief in labour:

- general measures: which include mobility, breathing exercises and warm baths (as in water birth)
- light self-administered methods, which include the TENS machine and using entonox ("gas and air")
- systemic opiates, including diamorphine and pethidine (there are other related synthetic drugs used less often, which are just as effective)
- the so-called "regional analgesia" in the form of an "epidural".

Of all these, the epidural method is superior by a long way. It is the only method where complete pain relief can be promised and delivered. In a small minority of women, this is unfortunately not achieved. Moreover, in a small number of women, the epidural is not suitable or may even be contraindicated.

There are no absolute contraindications for any of the other methods. Water birth may be unsuitable for some (*see* Chapter 40, "Water birth").

Overall, pain control in labour should be tailored according to the needs and wishes of the individual. One aspect that we have always regarded with dismay is a restrictive birth-plan. It is not unusual to find a birth-plan prepared antenatally which states categorically that "I do not wish to be offered an epidural under any circumstances at any stage of labour".

Such statements are commonly a result of pregnancy classes, where some so-called experts impose their personal opinions on unsuspecting and trusting women. Any such individual who influences such a decision deserves condemnation in the strongest terms.

It is the duty of anybody in that position to present the facts and facts only to his or her clients and allow them to make up their minds. In the area of pain relief, the enduring wisdom is for the women to be open-minded and to consider all the options, depending on her needs at the time. This is as long as she knows what each of the options entails. Those are the facts she should be offered in the antenatal class and the facts presented here.

Pain in labour

Is pain an essential part of labour?

It would be presumptuous of anybody to try to answer this question in a few short sentences. Labour and delivery are unique and very personal experiences. The concept of "whose body is it, anyway?", so flagrantly abused in various settings, is probably quite valid in labour. This is a physiological process where the individual undergoing it ought to have the final word on how she wants to go through it. A purely medical perspective is that no pain is ever necessary for any process: physiological, pathological or therapeutic.

Over the centuries, the primary and immediate aim of a physician was and remains to relieve pain and make the individual comfortable. This is why doctors will almost always positively encourage labouring women to have effective pain control in labour. However, if the woman feels that relieving pain will somehow make the birth experience somehow less profound, this view will be respected. After all, as the cliché above goes: whose body is it, anyway?

Is labour always painful?

There is only a small percentage of women who experience very little or no pain at all in labour. The overwhelming majority of women find labour painful or very painful. It is very difficult to grade such a subjective thing as pain and making comparisons of the amount of pain among individuals is a futile exercise. Suffice to say, most women feel that labour pain is severe enough to require strong pain control. The individual woman concerned may decline this as a matter of choice.

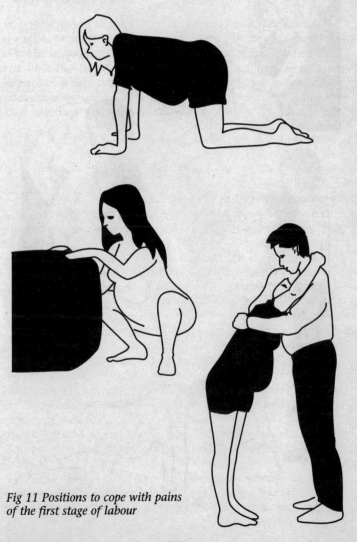

Fig 11 Positions to cope with pains of the first stage of labour

*Fig 11 Selection of positions to cope with
pains of the second stage of labour*

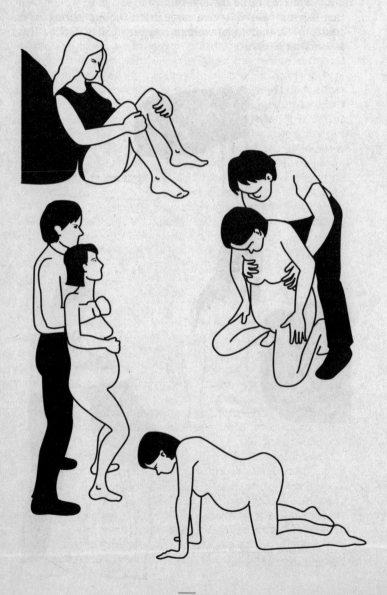

Non-medication pain relief

Are there any methods of pain control in labour which are not medication-based?

Yes. The most popular one to date is the TENS machine. TENS stands for Transcutaneous Electrical Nerve Stimulation. This is based on the theory that by repeatedly stimulating sensory receptors in the skin using light electrical impulses, the pain arising from the womb and cervix will be inhibited. TENS works well for some people but is probably only effective in the latent phase and in early labour. Very few women find it sufficiently effective in established labour, unless it is supplemented with something else. It is also used by some women in the immediate period after delivery to control after-pains. The main attractions are its non-invasive nature and being non-pharmacological.

Other non-pharmacological pain control methods are hypnotism, the use of which is not widespread; and psycho-prophylaxis, in the form of exhaustive antenatal education about pain in labour. This may positively influence the perception of pain.

Gas and air

How good is "gas and air"?

Entonox – or "gas and air", as it is popularly known, is a mixture of oxygen and a gas called nitrous oxide. It is the latter component that is aimed at the pain.

This is a rapidly acting agent but the action lasts only a short duration. Probably the main attraction of gas and air is the fact that it is inhalational (no needles involved!) and is self-administered. This means the mother can have it if and when she wants it.

Many women find it quite helpful but are rather frustrated by its short duration of action. This means, if a woman uses it exclusively, she has to keep breathing on it practically continually. Others find it disagreeable because of the sedative effect it produces. In fact, some woman fall asleep between contractions because they have been pulling energetically on the gas and air. The majority of women will probably be of the opinion that at the height of labour pains, especially with pushing in the second stage of labour, gas and air is hardly adequate.

Does "gas and air" have any adverse effect on the baby?
No.

Pethidine and diamorphine

What are the injectable painkillers used in labour?
Pethidine is the most common injectable analgesic (painkiller) used. Debate still rages on the effectiveness of this drug in controlling pain. There is no question that pethidine has a strong sedative effect and there is quite a large section of the obstetrics and midwifery fraternity who believe that pethidine actually works through sedation rather than true pain relief.

A lot of women in labour have reported finding pethidine totally inadequate. The most common side-effect of pethidine is nausea and vomiting. In many units, an anti-emetic drug to counter this is routinely administered with pethidine. Other units have a policy of administering an anti-emetic only if the labouring woman complains of nausea and/or vomiting.

Pethidine can be given repeatedly every three hours or so, depending on requirements.

Are there any other injectable pain control drugs?
Yes. Diamorphine is another popular choice. The drawback is that this very powerful narcotic cannot be given repeatedly, as the problem of dependency sets in rather rapidly. In most units, it will be administered as a one-off at the onset of painful contractions or at any time in labour when the mother is in marked distress because of the pain. Another positive aspect of diamorphine is the fact that it causes less nausea and/or vomiting when compared to pethidine.

Other injectables that have been used in labour but are less common include meptazinol (meptid) and pentazocine. They are both morphine-related (i.e. opiates). They have no particular advantage over pethidine.

Are there any particular concerns about the use of pethidine and other similar injectable drugs in labour?

The main concern is its effect on respiration. While the depression of respiration on the labouring woman is so mild that it is of little or no concern, the effect on the fetus is a different story. Since these drugs cross the placenta to affect the fetus, the newborn may have such marked respiratory depression that he or she may require special help. The respiratory depressive effect becomes an issue after birth and not before. However, the general sedative effect on the fetus may have such an effect on the heartbeat to the extent of forcing intervention of some kind. In fact, in most cases, that intervention is later found to have been unnecessary.

Is there any way of reversing the respiratory depressive effect of these drugs on the baby?

Yes. A drug called naloxone can be injected to reverse the unwanted effects of diamorphine and the other related drugs on the baby. This works quite quickly and is safe. However, while it is extremely effective in countering the effects of diamorphine, it is only partially effective in the case of pethidine, meptazinol or pentazocine. Rarely, with these drugs, additional respiratory support may be required for the first few hours to allow the baby's body to completely rid itself of the drug.

Are there circumstances where the use of these injectable painkillers may be undesirable?

On the same note as the unwanted effect on respiration, it may be less than ideal to use these drugs in a labour where a premature baby is going to be delivered. This is because the immature organs do not process the drug as efficiently and the effect will be marked and longer-lasting on these fragile beings.

Epidurals

What can one say about epidural analgesia?

This is a method of pain relief that involves the injection of a local anaesthetic in the lower spine. This acts on the nerve roots that control pain sensation in the lower abdomen, the pelvis and the lower limbs. The effect is freedom from labour pains. A fine flexible catheter is left in place to allow repeated top-ups of the local anaesthetic as and when the effect starts to wear off.

Alternatively, the anaesthetic may be infused continuously rather than intermittently through this fine catheter.

How effective is the epidural in controlling pain?

The epidural is by far the most effective method of pain control available for a labouring woman. In fact, the epidural is not in the same league as the other pain control methods as it the only method which can render the person completely pain-free. No other method currently available can achieve this.

Does the epidural work every time?

Most times. Unfortunately, for a small minority, the epidural may not work very well and they will continue to feel pain. The most likely failure of an epidural is a scenario where only an isolated area remains unaffected. This is commonly called a "window". Because the rest of the region is completely pain-free, the window area is felt quite acutely. It is often difficult to solve this problem, short of replacing the catheter. One has to emphasize the fact that epidural failure is an uncommon event.

Does the epidural have any additional advantages?

Yes. The pain control is so effective that if a caesarean section becomes necessary in the course of labour, the epidural will usually be adequate for the procedure. Only a top-up is usually required. This is, of course, if the labouring mother is not averse to the idea of staying awake for the operation.

Needless to say, a working epidural is more than sufficient for forceps or ventouse delivery.

Is anything special required for the epidural?

To insert the epidural catheter requires expertise and this is done by an anaesthetist. Trained midwives will give top-ups or monitor the infusion.

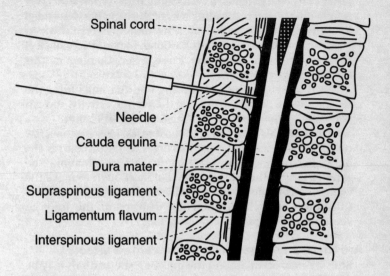

Fig 12 Cutaway of spine, showing where/how an epidural is inserted

Are there any unwanted effects from the epidural?

There are occasional unwanted effects, all of which can be solved easily. An immediate unwanted effect could be an "ascending epidural", where the effects extend upwards to affect the chest and the respiratory muscles. This will produce respiratory difficulties, which will require a change in position to a semi-sitting or propped up posture and, occasionally, respiratory support. It soon resolves. Fortunately, this is an exceptionally rare occurrence.

The epidural also tends to lower the blood pressure and that is why an intravenous infusion will always be started before the epidural, to offset this effect.

What about its effect on the duration of labour?

The epidural does not reduce the strength or frequency of contractions. Therefore, it does not influence the length of the first stage of labour one way or the other.

There is, however, irrefutable evidence that it tends to prolong the second stage of labour. Ironically, this is a direct result of its effectiveness in controlling pain. When the cervix is fully dilated and the leading part of the baby has descended low enough to allow for pushing and delivery, with an effective epidural, the labouring woman may not actually feel the urge to push. This may cause a lengthening of this (second) stage of labour.

This is overcome by the attending midwife supervising the second stage where, by palpating the uterine activity, she can encourage the woman to push whenever there is a contraction. This works well, in most cases. However, in a few cases, the absence of the painful urges to push removes the only effective motivating factor. In such a situation, the exhortations of the midwife may not be enough to make the woman push effectively to achieve delivery. This is the situation where an instrumental delivery in the form of ventouse or forceps becomes more likely.

Are there any other delayed unwanted effects?

Bruising may occur around the injection site and this may be sore for a day or two.

In a few instances, especially if catheter insertion involved several attempts before eventually succeeding, there is a small risk of a haematoma (blood-clot) forming and, even more rarely, an abscess. This will present in the form of worsening low backache (within one two three days). Appropriate treatment will be required.

It is widely believed that backache is common following an epidural. Is this true?

This is one of the most unfortunate myths. Backache does occur after an epidural, but is by no means common.

Apart from the potential causes described above, there are a few other possible causes. Probably the most common cause of prolonged low intensity low backache following an epidural is that caused by bad posture. When an epidural is very effective, the labouring woman may assume a posture that puts considerable strain on her back for several hours. Because she is pain-free, she will remain oblivious to that strain. Once the epidural wears off, she will start feeling the effect of that posture. It may take several weeks before she is completely free of pain. Unfortunately, this will inevitably be blamed on the epidural.

What about headache following an epidural?

Again, in a few instances, headache soon after delivery may be a direct consequence of an epidural. This normally results from what is known as a "dural tap". This simply means the needle had extended into another space (the sub-arachnoid), causing the fluid in this space to leak.

The headache is usually frontal but may also be felt at the back. It is normally felt on rising from a lying position or on standing up. She will also complain of nausea and/or vomiting, occasionally sensitivity to light (photo-phobia) and neck stiffness.

Maintaining a flat position is very effective in keeping her free of pain but is normally not a practical solution for a new mother. In such a case, treatment using a "blood patch" is very effective and quick. This involves injecting the patient's own blood (about 10–15 ml) into the site of the epidural puncture. This complication is very uncommon.

Is there a possibility of paralysis as a direct result of an epidural?

No.

In years gone by, severe neurological damage taking weeks, even months, to recover was occasionally reported. This involved injection of other chemicals (not the local anaesthetic used in epidural) and also involved injection of those chemicals in the sub-arachnoid space (not epidural). Childbirth that has been improperly managed has a far greater potential of producing neurological damage than an epidural ever can.

Are there any circumstances where an epidural is specially recommended?

An epidural is first and foremost a method of pain relief. There are, however, circumstances in labour when it has additional advantages by facilitating successful vaginal delivery and preventing potential complications.

It is strongly recommended in pre-eclampsia as it improves blood supply to the womb (which may be tenuous in such cases) and hence the baby. It also effectively combats one of the principal causes of worsening blood pressure, i.e. pain.

It is also strongly recommended in the case of a breech presentation or twin delivery. In the latter case, it is especially useful if the second twin is in an abnormal lie, where some kind of manipulation may be required.

It is also quite useful in preterm labour where the fetus is rather delicate, and in medical conditions such as heart disease, where maternal exertion may be a bad idea. It also prevents maternal exhaustion and distress in prolonged labour.

Are there any other benefits from the epidural?

An indirect benefit is that of removing the need to use any other drugs for pain which inevitably reach the baby and may have various effects on him or her. The drugs (local anaesthetics) used in an epidural have no effects on the baby whatsoever.

The lowering of blood pressure is a worrying thing. How is this handled?

This is never a serious problem. The infusion given just before inserting the epidural is usually an adequate measure against this. Even if the blood pressure fall was found to be severe enough to require further action (which is very rare), an injection of ephedrine quickly and effectively reverses this effect.

Are there any contraindications to epidural analgesia?

Yes. Some heart conditions are considered a contraindication to using epidural analgesia. These include aortic stenosis (where the valve that leads from the heart to the artery known as the aorta is narrowed) and pulmonary hypertension (where the blood pressure in the arteries supplying the lungs is abnormally high). In these cases, such patients are usually delivered by caesarean section and pain relief in labour is not an issue.

Other situations where "epidural" may not be recommended is current use of anticoagulant medication. This is because of a theoretical increase in the risk of bleeding. It is also contraindicated in the presence of an infection in the vicinity of the injection site, such as an abscess, or even in the case of a systemic infection such as septicaemia.

The greatest and most important contraindication is maternal wishes NOT to have one.

Oral pain relief

Are there any pain relief drugs taken orally that are used in labour?

No. They would not work anyway because absorption from the stomach during labour is patchy at best.

Effectiveness of pain relief

What is the final word on pain relief in labour?

There cannot be any final word when it comes to this very subjective aspect of labour. There are, however hard facts that any pregnant woman anticipating labour needs to know.

Methods that do not use any kind of drugs are available. They are usually only really effective in the latent and early stages of labour. The TENS machine is the most common and well known.

Gas and air works fast and the effect wears off rapidly. It has to be used continuously to be really effective. It makes you sleepy and its effectiveness is limited and probably outright inadequate in established labour.

Injection (systemic) painkillers such as diamorphine and pethidine are the most widely used painkillers in labour. Virtually all cause nausea and/or vomiting. They are also quite sedating. Opinion among women differs widely on their effectiveness; some find them adequate and many others think they are almost totally useless.

The epidural is by far the most effective method of pain relief in labour. In most cases it renders the woman completely pain-free. Drawbacks include being confined to bed and it may prolong the second stage of labour. It is extremely safe with occasional temporary side-effects. In a very few instances it doesn't work.

37. Abnormal labour and fetal distress

Introduction

Labour does not always proceed according to expectations. Moreover, in the majority of instances, the difficulties are neither predicted nor anticipated.

In normal labour, there is a short latent phase characterized by abdominal discomfort, low backache and irregular tightenings, which get progressively stronger and more painful. This experience varies widely. Once labour is established, the principal guiding parameters of progress are the dilatation of the cervix and the descent of the baby's leading part (in most cases, the head) into the pelvis.

By the time the cervix dilates to its maximum (10 cm), the first stage of labour is completed and the second stage commences. This stage, which should be much shorter than the first, includes maternal efforts for the first time, in the form of pushing and actual delivery. There is, of course, the third stage of labour, which is concluded by delivery of the placenta (afterbirth).

As anyone can envisage, there are many things that can go wrong to turn a routine labour process abnormal. The uterus may not contract effectively, making labour abnormally long; it may contract too vigorously, causing fetal distress; the cervix may fail to open beyond a certain point; or the leading part may not descend beyond a certain level in the pelvis effectively arresting labour. Many other things can go wrong, as we shall see shortly.

For many of these problems, remedial measures are available. For some, labour may have to be abandoned, resorting to caesarean section. Once labour is established, delivery is inevitable.

However, as a golden rule, nobody can guarantee anybody a vaginal delivery at the onset of labour. Every labour can potentially go wrong. Between 10 and 20 per cent of all pregnancies are delivered by caesarean section. Only half of these are planned (elective); the rest are emergencies, mostly because of problems in labour.

Abnormal labour

What is abnormal labour?

To understand what is meant by the term "abnormal labour", one has to know what normal labour is. This can be described as a process of labour which lasts for an optimum length of time, neither too long nor too short, passes without causing undue distress to the mother, and the baby is delivered in good condition. Any departure from this can be termed an abnormal labour.

Many people will take issue with rapid labour being classified as abnormal. What is wrong with it?

Extremely rapid labour is potentially dangerous. This is because it can lead to injury to the baby because of its rapid passage through the birth canal. The injuries – especially to the brain – can be quite serious.

Very rapid labour (also termed "precipitate labour") may also lead to heavy, even dangerous bleeding after delivery (postpartum haemorrhage). There is also the fact that the labour may start when the mother is not in hospital, or even at home. She may therefore have no help, a potentially dangerous scenario. Rapid labour may also cause injuries to the birth canal. Nasty tears to the perineum have been known to result from precipitate labour.

Prolonged labour

What are the causes of prolonged labour?

Arguably, the most common cause of prolonged labour is inefficient contractions. If the contractions are weak, irregular or uncoordinated, they may be unable to facilitate dilatation of the cervix and push the baby further down the birth canal.

This problem is most often overcome by using an oxytocin infusion. Oxytocin is actually the natural chemical that is produced in the brain and stimulates contractions.

Are there any other causes of prolonged labour?

If the fetus is of above average size and if it is large relative to the size of the mother's pelvis, there is potential disproportion. If the disproportion is only slight, the strength of the contractions may overcome it. Sometimes, however, the disproportion is considerable and labour fails to progress beyond a certain point.

It is usually not easy to conclude that vaginal delivery is not achievable during labour and the realization that there was disproportion is usually retrospective after a prolonged labour culminating in a caesarean section.

Apart from size, are there any other fetal causes of prolonged labour?

Yes. An abnormal position of the baby's head can make for slow progress of labour.

Normally, the head will be facing downwards with the neck of the baby bent forward and the chin resting on the chest. If the head descends into the pelvis with the neck extended and facing upwards ("stargazing"); there could be trouble in the form of a protracted labour. This state of affairs increases the possibility of instrumental delivery (forceps or ventouse) or caesarean section.

Can the cervix be to blame in prolonged labour?

Yes. Occasionally, in spite of strong, regular contractions, the cervix does not continue to dilate beyond a certain point. The cause of this is, in most cases, obscure.

Occasionally, the cervical resistance may be due to scarring resulting from previous surgery or injury.

When labour has been induced, it is important to ensure adequate cervical preparation before stimulating contractions. If contractions are stimulated before the cervix is ready (i.e. while it is still long, firm and closed), there is a risk that it may not dilate, a situation that could culminate in an otherwise unnecessary caesarean section. This is why application of prostaglandin preparations (gel, tablets or pessaries) is sometimes necessary before stimulating contractions.

Fetal distress

What is fetal distress?

Even in the medical fraternity, there is no firm agreement as to what this term means, despite its common use.

In essence, it refers to a state of the fetus brought about by insufficient oxygen reaching the fetus. If oxygen deficiency is severe and prolonged, permanent damage to the baby could result. This is why any hint of possible fetal distress is taken seriously.

What are the causes of fetal distress?

There are several potential causes.

Fetal distress is commoner during active labour but could occur before labour onset even though this is uncommon.

"Placental abruption", which is a condition where the placenta (afterbirth) detaches from its base partially or wholly, is one of the more common causes of pre-labour fetal distress.

Vigorous fetal activity sometimes leads to a cord accident, which may be in the form of a knot or entanglement of the cord around a limb. This could lead to partial occlusion of the vessels in the cord, leading to distress.

Other causes of distress before labour onset remain obscure, even after the baby is delivered.

What about causes during labour?

Any activity that reduces the blood supply to the fetus will cause fetal distress.

If the cord is compressed – either as a result of being around a fetal limb, neck, trunk or simply by being compressed by the fetal head against the pelvic side-wall – features of fetal distress will follow. Correction to this can occur spontaneously as a result of fetal movement or the cord sliding away from the pressure point, hence relieving the compression. Sometimes this does not occur and a rescue procedure needs to be carried out.

Is hyper-stimulation of the uterus a cause of fetal distress?

Yes. This can occur spontaneously or following the infusion of oxytocin. If the uterus contracts strongly, with the contractions being prolonged and coming close together, this will reduce the amount of blood (and therefore oxygen) that is getting to the placenta and ultimately to the baby.

If this state of affairs is sustained over several minutes, fetal distress will ensue.

Can hyper-stimulation be overcome?

Yes. This is overcome quite easily simply by stopping the oxytocin infusion, if this was the cause.

If it occurs spontaneously, an intravenous injection of a tocolytic drug can be given and this will very quickly eliminate the over-stimulation. These drugs are also available in an inhalational (aerosol) form but this method is associated with a slight delay in action.

Tocolytic drugs simply relax the muscles of the womb to negate the effect of sustained strong contractions.

Can the placenta detach in labour before delivery?

This can happen but is a very unusual occurrence.

It will cause fetal distress, the gravity of which will depend on the extent of placental separation. It could lead to a caesarean section unless labour is the second stage, when instrumental vaginal delivery may be the preferred option.

Can the uterus rupture?

This is a very serious complication that is, fortunately, rare.

It is serious for the mother because the blood loss that ensues can be life-threatening. For the fetus, this occurrence causes very severe acute fetal distress, where the only hope of saving the baby is delivery within minutes of the rupture occurring. Delivery in this situation is almost always abdominal (caesarean).

The uterus could rupture as a result of over-stimulation of an already weakened womb. Mothers who have had many babies are at particular risk of this complication. Over-stimulation may be spontaneous, probably combined with another factor such as a big baby. It could also result from administration of an oxytocin infusion.

Rupture of the uterus may occur in the presence of normal contractions in cases where there is an abnormally weak scar on the uterus following previous surgery.

When a uterus ruptures, the baby is usually lost. Even the few that survive are at high risk of ending up with brain damage, because of prolonged oxygen starvation lasting several minutes.

Lying on one's back is regarded as unwise in labour. Why is that?

The heavy uterus will be lying on top of the major blood vessels in the mother's abdomen. This may be severe enough to reduce the amount of blood flowing through these vessels.

This will result in inadequate oxygen delivery to the uterus itself and hence to the baby. It could lead to fetal distress. Propped-up, sitting up and left side positions are considered more ideal, as far as the baby's welfare is concerned.

How is fetal distress recognized?

If fetal distress occurs before the onset of labour, the mother may get a warning in the form of suddenly reduced or complete disappearance of fetal movements. In cord accidents, the fetus may react by suddenly increasing movements. The mother may therefore experience uncharacteristic vigorous fetal activity. In many cases, pre-labour fetal distress may go unsuspected and unrecognized, sometimes with catastrophic results.

What about fetal distress in labour?

This is where the essence of fetal surveillance during labour is demonstrated. Many cases of fetal distress will have no warning whatsoever and it is only the fetal monitoring which will give a clue that something may not be right.

Electronic fetal monitoring in the form of cardiotocography (CTG) is now the standard form of fetal surveillance in labour in most countries.

How does CTG monitoring help in detecting fetal distress?

CTGs monitor the unborn baby's heartbeat and how this is behaving. The contractions are also monitored and their frequency, timing and duration are recorded. Standard CTGs do not measure the strength of contractions.

By looking at the pattern of the heartbeat both in isolation and in relation to the uterine contractions, it is possible for a midwife or doctor to identify signs of fetal distress.

Does this mean CTG monitoring needs to be continued throughout the entire duration of labour?

Not at all. Different units operate different policies on this matter. However, the scientific evidence available indicates that properly timed intermittent monitoring is just as good as continuous monitoring in its ability to detect fetal distress. This applies to low-risk pregnancies, which are the majority.

For high-risk pregnancies – such as in cases of intrauterine fetal growth restriction or previous unexplained stillbirth – all agree that continuous monitoring is the appropriate policy. This is because the behaviour of such babies is less predictable and this measure will be reassuring to the parents, who will be inevitably anxious.

Is CTG diagnostic?

No. All it does is point towards the probability of fetal distress.

A normal CTG is always reassuring whilst a suspicious or frankly abnormal CTG is not always significant. In fact, the majority of CTGs classified as unsatisfactory or suspicious will turn out to be false scares, with babies being born perfectly healthy with no hint of distress.

Does this high rate of false scares on the part of CTG not lead to increased, unnecessary intervention?

Indeed it does. Nobody doubts that the CTG has single-handedly increased the rate of caesarean section quite substantially. However, one needs to remember that this technology has also saved the lives of millions of babies. The increased rate of intervention is probably a small price to pay for the greater good.

Is there any way of verifying the findings of a suspicious CTG?

Yes. The standard next step is to obtain a small sample of blood from the baby to have it analyzed for oxygen saturation. This is much more definitive. The blood is obtained by scratching the leading part of the baby (usually the scalp). A drop of blood is collected in a fine capillary tube and put in a machine which gives results in less than one minute. In the majority of cases, the results are reassuring but in some, the results will confirm the fetal distress suspected earlier, therefore calling for expedited or immediate delivery.

Will every abnormal result following a fetal blood sample lead to caesarean section or instrumental delivery?

Not really. The action taken will depend on the degree of abnormality. If the reflected distress is only mild, action such as changing the position of the mother, stopping or reducing the rate of oxytocin infusion and giving oxygen to the mother may be all that is required. With that, improvement on the CTG may soon be apparent and, if need be, a repeat sample is taken after some time to reassure everybody concerned.

If there is significant distress, then delivery by the quickest means possible will be carried out. This may be a caesarean section but it may also be by forceps or ventouse vaginal delivery, if this is feasible.

What is the significance of the baby opening his or her bowels during labour?

When the fetus opens its bowels, passing the green stuff called meconeum, there is usually some concern as to whether it might be significant.

Passing meconeum before labour is uncommon but becomes more common, the further the pregnancy advances beyond forty weeks. In fact, for those pregnancies reaching forty-two weeks, roughly half of the babies will be found to have already passed meconeum when the "waters" (membranes) are broken.

This old meconeum tends to have a yellow tinge and any midwife will distinguish old from fresh meconeum. It is the latter that is usually (but not always) significant.

So, what is done when the fetus passes meconeum?

This may indicate some degree of fetal distress. It is therefore regarded as a wise measure to do continuous CTG monitoring for a baby that has passed meconeum, particularly so if the meconeum is thick and fresh.

If the CTG is normal, the doctor may opt to do nothing other than continued monitoring and observation. If the CTG is equivocal, fetal blood sampling for analysis may be carried out.

Suppose fetal blood sampling is technically not possible for one reason or another or the parents object to it – what then?

If suspicious findings such as an abnormal CTG and passage of thick fresh meconeum cannot be verified, then a caesarean section becomes inevitable. This is not a situation in which one can afford to take risks – better be safe than sorry.

Would you say premature fetuses are at increased risk of distress in labour?

Not particularly, no. Small-for-dates babies whose growth during pregnancy has been sub-optimal are a different case. These babies are prone to fetal distress because of their inherent "weak" state and the common problem of reduced amniotic fluid, and therefore the increased risk of cord compression.

What is the risk of permanent brain damage as a result of fetal distress?

The oxygen deprivation needs to be severe and prolonged for this eventuality to occur. This is therefore a rare consequence of fetal distress in labour. Even for babies that are born floppy with a delayed cry and who end up in special care baby units for several days, the vast majority of them make a full recovery.

It is those unfortunate babies where the insult to the brain goes unsuspected and therefore unrecognized for prolonged periods in pregnancy where cerebral palsy eventually results. The same applies to acute episodes of serious conditions such as uterine rupture or severe placental abruption.

38. Forceps and ventouse (vacuum) delivery

Introduction

Can't deliver! Won't deliver!

When it comes to the crunch, quite a few women utterly believe this.

The second stage of labour when the mother-to-be has to summon all her energy reserves and is being exhorted by the midwife and her partner to "Push!" "Keep it coming!" "Again, again!" "Hold your breath" etc. can be an overwhelming experience.

Occasionally it all becomes too much, so she descends into full-blown maternal distress. This will normally happen after a prolonged first stage, especially if pain control was sub-optimal. She is exhausted, she is in a lot of pain and she is called upon to perform a monumental and very intensive task. It can be a tall order. Help is then offered in the form of instrumental delivery. This could be by one of a variety of designs of forceps or the ventouse, where a suction cup is used, as we shall explain shortly.

Maternal distress is, however, not the only indication for using instruments to facilitate delivery. It could be fetal distress in the second stage, an unfavourable position of the head for delivery, and a few other indications.

There are circumstances where instruments cannot be used, where the remaining option is caesarean delivery.

The instruments – in the right hands – are extremely safe and complications are rare and usually transient. Debate flares up from time to time among the obstetrics fraternity about which is a better instrument, the ventouse or forceps. In the UK, historically, the forceps were the most commonly used instrument. Since the mid-1980s the ventouse has made significant inroads into most labour suites and statistics towards the end of the '90s show that it is by far the most used instrument: a quiet creeping coup.

The general reasons for the take-over are more to do with the fact that it is regarded as kinder to the mother and probably easier to use even by relatively junior obstetricians. On the issue of safety, both the ventouse and forceps are extremely safe and the argument in comparison is largely an exercise in splitting hairs. Specific questions on these instruments are answered here.

Forceps

How long have forceps been in use in obstetric practice?

Nobody knows for sure because various designs of forceps have been found in archives from different civilizations in different parts of the world. It is certainly an instrument that has been around for many centuries. The various models in use today are variations of a design first introduced in the middle of the nineteenth century.

How frequently is the forceps used for delivery in hospitals?

Statistics from various countries and even various hospitals in the same country differ widely. In English-speaking countries, forceps deliveries account for 10–20 per cent of all hospital deliveries. This means every woman who walks through the delivery suite doors in labour has at least a one in ten chance of having her baby delivered using forceps. From the early 1990s, forceps as a method of instrumental delivery has been steadily losing out to the ventouse (vacuum) extractor. In non-English speaking countries this started a few decades ago. In some, forceps are rarely used.

Why is it necessary to use the forceps for delivery in some instances?

There are several indications for resorting to the forceps. These could be maternal or fetal and, rarely, both.

Maternal indications for use of forceps include:

- Maternal distress or fatigue. Sometimes the pains of labour in the second stage are such that the mother cannot cope at all. It may then be decided that to expedite delivery, help with forceps is called for. On the other hand the second stage may be prolonged and, with repeated pushing, the mother may be totally exhausted and unable to carry on. Forceps can then be used to conclude the delivery.

- Maternal heart or respiratory diseases. There are some heart and/or respiratory conditions that can be badly – even dangerously – exacerbated by exertion. Pushing in the second stage of labour can be quite physically demanding. To prevent this, women with such conditions are electively planned for forceps delivery. In some cases, caesarean section may be opted for.

- Failed ventouse. In some instances, an instrumental delivery may be under way and ventouse may be chosen. In the course of delivery, this may be unsuccessful and the attending obstetrician may assess the situation and elect to conclude the delivery using forceps. However, this is unusual.

Is asthma an indication for forceps deliver?

Unless an asthmatic has an attack during labour, this condition by itself is not an automatic indication for forceps or ventouse delivery.

What are the fetal indications for forceps delivery?

The most common is presumed or confirmed fetal distress. Sometimes there may be clinical features strongly suggestive of a distressed fetus. If the attending obstetrician feels that a recourse to confirmatory tests is going to delay delivery unduly, forceps delivery may be resorted to. Sometimes it turns out to be a false scare, a classical example of erring on the side of safety.

Another fetal indication for forceps delivery is an abnormal position of the head, making spontaneous delivery difficult. In this case, the forceps are used to rotate the head into a favourable position before applying traction to achieve delivery.

It may be used in breech delivery to facilitate delivery of the head.

Some experts advocate use of forceps in delivering premature babies, with the express aim of protecting the head, which is relatively fragile.

Do forceps have any role to play during caesarean section?

Yes. In a few instances, forceps are used to facilitate delivery of the head out of the uterine and abdominal cavity during a caesarean section.

Are there any contraindications to using forceps for delivery?

Yes, there are several:

- if the fetal head is still high in the pelvis, forceps should not be used, as the manoeuvre is unlikely to succeed and may be dangerous. If immediate delivery is required in this situation, then a caesarean section is the only feasible option
- if the leading part of the baby is anything other than the head (see above for breech)
- if, on applying the blades of the forceps, a perfect "lock" is not achieved
- if it is not possible to discern the landmarks of the baby's head on examination
- if the attending obstetrician is not trained in the use of the instrument
- if the labouring mother does not wish to have them used.

What are the requirements for forceps delivery?

The requirements for a forceps delivery are as follows:

- the mother has to lie on her back with her legs in stirrups. This is called the lithotomy position.
- the urinary bladder is emptied, unless the fetal head is very low, when this may be unnecessary
- adequate pain control: if an epidural has been used, this is more than adequate. If not, the region around the birth canal is numbed by injection of a local anaesthetic in strategic areas
- an episiotomy has to be applied. This is always the case regardless of the number of deliveries in the past
- the cervix has to be fully dilated and membranes ruptured.

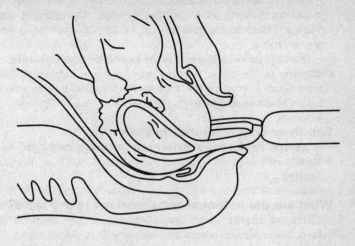

Fig 14 Forceps around a baby's skull

How many types of forceps are there?

If you challenged an obstetrician to name at least half the "types" of forceps used in the obstetric world, the chances are he or she will fail. There are so many. However, there are only two main groups of forceps. One is the type used for traction only (this is the most common) and the other group is the type used for rotation and traction. The latter are very infrequently used, mainly because situations requiring their use are uncommon and secondly because they are not very popular with obstetricians and probably only a proportion of obstetricians are adequately trained in their use.

What are the potential complications of using forceps for delivery?

Most of these are soft tissue injuries to the mother.

There may be bruising or even lacerations to the perineum and vagina.

Occasionally, injury to the vaginal wall escapes detection and presents a few hours later as a painful and progressive haematoma (blood-clot) under the vaginal skin.

Injuries may be sustained to the bladder and/or urethra. This may show in the form of urine retention and, rarely, a fistula (an abnormal communication between two different body parts, such as a channel between the bladder and vagina – the most common type of fistula – or the vagina and rectum).

If an episiotomy applied turns out to be small, relative to the size of the baby, traction may cause an extension tear, sometimes involving the anal sphincter. This is a relatively major tear requiring careful repair.

Can there be any injuries to the cervix?

If all the prerequisites have been strictly adhered to, this should not happen. A completely dilated cervix cannot be injured.

What are the potential complications to the fetus?

There are almost always forceps marks on the sides of the face. These are temporary and fade within a day or so.

Occasionally bruising, even light laceration may occur.

Rarely, swelling consisting of a scalp haematoma (blood-clot) may develop, following a difficult forceps delivery.

Isolated cases of intra-cranial haemorrhage (bleeding inside the skull cavity, i.e. into or around the brain) have been reported over the years. This appears to be an exceedingly rare occurrence.

Temporary facial nerve palsy on one or both sides has also been reported but is also rare.

Ventouse

What is the history of the ventouse and how long has it been in use?

The ventouse – or vacuum extractor, as it is otherwise known – has been used intermittently for delivery for almost three centuries. However, its place in mainstream obstetric practice was secured in the early 1950s and it now sits alongside the older instrument, the "forceps", with equal status.

How does the ventouse differ from the forceps?

The two instruments achieve the same goal through two different ways. With the forceps, a firm grip secures the head of the fetus and the operator applies steady traction to bring it down. Maternal efforts and/or uterine contractions may facilitate the process but are not always necessary.

With the ventouse, a metal or silastic (soft) cup is applied to the scalp. Vacuum is created in the cup, exerting a grip on the scalp skin. If it is a metal cup, the scalp skin is sucked into the cup, while with the soft rubber (silastic) type, the cup moulds itself on the fetal head to fit like a cap. Controlled traction is then applied but this has to be synchronized with uterine contractions and maternal effort. This is an important safety feature of the ventouse.

Are there any important differences between a metal cup and a silastic (soft) cup?

Not really. They are both equally efficient and just as safe as each other. The metal cup has been around for much longer and the silastic cup only since the early 1970s. However, many obstetricians probably prefer the soft silastic cup, because it is more user-friendly and – in theory, at least – has less potential to cause harm to the mother or baby.

Fig 15 Position of ventouse on head

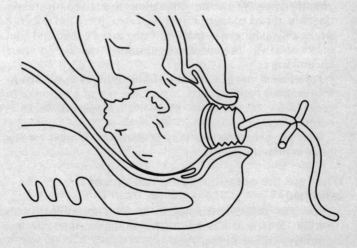

The trend appears to be to use ventouse in preference to the forceps. Is there any particular reason for this?

Studies show that the ventouse is generally gentler to the mother, causing fewer injuries. Also importantly, it can be used on an incompletely dilated cervix if an immediate delivery is called for.

Ventouse, especially the silastic type has another very important feature. It has an inbuilt safety feature in that the amount of vacuum that is set allows for a certain maximum amount of traction force. This is usually safe for the baby. If this is exceeded, the cup simply comes off and the efforts of the over-enthusiastic doctor will have done no harm. Moreover, attempts to reattach the cup after this are usually unsuccessful.

Another attractive feature of this instrument is that an episiotomy is not always necessary. This is always a pleasant surprise to an exhausted mother.

Are there circumstances where the forceps may be preferable to the ventouse?

Yes, definitely.

If delivery needs to be achieved very urgently, then forceps is the best instrument. This is because preparation for it is relatively short (there are no parts to assemble); it does not absolutely require uterine contractions to succeed (the uterus does not always cooperate when you want it to) and does not necessarily require maternal effort (she may be tired and "out of it" totally!). Forceps are significantly quicker in these circumstances.

Forceps will also be the best instrument in preterm delivery, if instruments are required. In fact, the use of a ventouse in pregnancies of less than thirty-five completed weeks is contraindicated.

Forceps is the only instrument that can be used for the head in breech delivery.

What are the potential complications of the ventouse?

These are generally similar to those encountered with forceps. It is generally felt that maternal injuries are less common with ventouse.

As for fetal complications, scalp haematoma is probably more common with ventouse than with forceps.

A complication that is unique to the ventouse but which is exceptionally rare is loss of hair in infancy for the baby.

The most common feature, which parents notice immediately, is the swelling on the baby's head where the ventouse cup has been applied. Metal cups produce a bigger swelling. It takes up to seventy-two hours for this swelling to disappear. It does not appear to trouble the newborn unduly, because the feeding and sleeping pattern is never disturbed.

Should the labouring woman have a choice of the instrument to be used on her?

There should be no problem with this, as long as she is well informed and both types of instruments are available and ideal for the circumstances. Of course, the operator must have the expertise in employing either.

Would one say these instruments are safe?

Definitely. If and when used appropriately by a well-trained operator, these instruments are very safe and extremely useful. Every case where one of these is used for delivery is a potential caesarean section and the labouring woman on whom these have been used should consider herself "rescued" from a caesarean delivery.

39. Caesarean section

Introduction

Caesarean section as a method of delivery has come a long way, even when viewed from as recently as the 1950s.

It can now be declared in absolute terms that caesarean section is a very safe procedure that should be carried out without hesitation in the presence of a valid indication. But this is where debate rages. Has caesarean section achieved a level of safety where it can be offered on demand? This question is not the mainstay of this chapter. In here, we have attempted to present broad and specific details about this very common surgical procedure.

It is extremely important to remember that, whatever degree of technical refinement achieved in performing it, caesarean section is and will remain a major surgical procedure. Any arguments for a more liberal approach towards caesarean section should never lose sight of this fact. On the other hand, those mothers who feel that they are well informed and would like to deliver by caesarean section regardless deserve the right of a sympathetic ear, though not necessarily an affirmative nod. Between 10 and 20 per cent of all pregnancies are delivered by caesarean section. In the UK, the average is 14 per cent, while in some parts of the USA and South America, the rate is consistently above 25 per cent and rising.

While childbirth in developed countries is now a very safe undertaking, as far as the mother is concerned, caesarean section is a riskier delivery method in terms of both death and illness.

Although the figures are very small (a death rate of less than 0.1 per cent), vaginal delivery remains a far safer way of having a baby today. In twenty or thirty years' time, quite plausibly, this statement may belong to history.

History and safety of caesarean sections

What is the history of caesarean section?

Nobody knows for sure. It is certainly known that caesarean delivery (which means abdominal delivery) has been practised in various civilizations for over 2500 years. History shows a specific law in the Roman empire in the year 715 BC known as *"Lex caesarea"*, which demanded the abdominal delivery of a baby if the mother died during pregnancy or labour. The term *caedere* means "to cut" in Latin.

How safe is caesarean section?

It is very safe. When compared to a century ago, the safety of caesarean section has improved light-years. It has improved enormously, even when compared to the mid-1930s.

Compared to vaginal delivery, caesarean section – even in developed countries – has significantly higher complication rates. For this reason alone, caesarean section is and should be resorted to only when necessary. At least, this is the argument still holding sway as we enter the twenty-first century.

Why is caesarean section safer today, compared to the past?

There are several reasons why there has been tremendous progress in this area.

Operation techniques have evolved over time to reach a stage where optimal approaches have been adopted.

The safety of anaesthesia has improved quite dramatically in the last few decades. Both regional (spinal or epidural) and general anaesthetic are now much safer compared to only fifteen or twenty years ago.

The control of infection – another major scourge of surgical procedures – is much better now. This is a result of an effective creation of a sterile environment necessary for operations as well as the development of antibiotics. Many people forget that antibiotics have only been around since the late 1920s.

Blood services are much more reliable now. Since excessive blood loss is one of the more serious potential complications of this operation, reliable blood replacement is an important facet. Nowadays, blood and blood products are readily available and safe.

The operation

How is a caesarean section done?
It is easy for doctors and midwives, who live with this common operation in their daily working lives, to assume that everybody knows what happens. In fact, many woman confront it with no idea as to what it involves. Basically, a caesarean delivery will involve cutting open the abdomen and then the uterus to deliver the baby. It is therefore an abdominal delivery as opposed to the usual vaginal delivery.

How is the abdomen opened?
By far the most common incision is the "transverse" one, made just above the bikini line. It is also known by various other names, but the wound and ultimately the scar will look the same, more or less.

Less commonly used is the "midline vertical" (up and down) incision. This extends from just below the navel to just above the pubis. It accounts for probably less than 5 per cent of all caesarean skin incisions. Needless to say, the more common transverse incision gives significantly better cosmetic results.

Does the term "lower segment caesarean section" refer to the common skin incision?
No. This is likely to be found on the consent form. If left unclarified, the woman may assume it refers to the skin incision. In fact, it refers to the incision on the uterus. Its mention is not an act of mere pedantry on the part of the doctors, as it has a very important implication: we shall see this shortly.

How is the womb (uterus) opened?
The most common incision is the lower segment transverse incision. This is because it is an easier approach, bleeds less, is easier to repair and gives the strongest scar.

Historically, the incision used was a vertical upper segment one. It is in the historical context that this old method has come to be known as "classical caesarean section". This is used only in exceptional circumstances, such as extreme prematurity (where it may be easier and safer for the baby).

Another kind of approach is a lower vertical incision, also used in special circumstances only.

More than 90 per cent of all caesarean sections are performed through a lower segment transverse uterine incision.

Why caesareans are performed

What are the indications for caesarean section?

There are many different indications, both maternal and fetal. Listed below are some of the more common maternal indications.

- Maternal pelvis: if the birth canal is deemed too narrow to allow safe passage of the baby, a caesarean section will be the only option. This state of affairs may be recognized following previous experience (labour that was very difficult or that never progressed beyond a certain point), in which case the caesarean section will be planned electively. It may otherwise be discovered in the course of labour and caesarean section is resorted to.

- Previous caesarean section: this is not always an indication for repeat caesarean section, except in a situation where the reasons for the previous caesarean section are still there, such as a narrow pelvis.

- Medical conditions: presence of serious medical conditions – such as heart failure or serious respiratory conditions – is sometimes deemed an indication for caesarean delivery in order to circumvent the stresses and strains of labour. More often, instrumental (vaginal) delivery in the form of forceps or ventouse is opted for.

- Abnormal placental position: a low-lying placenta (a condition known as "placenta praevia") is an indication for caesarean delivery.

- Placental abruption: if the placenta detaches partially or wholly during pregnancy or labour, emergency caesarean section may be performed, especially if there is hope of saving the baby.

- Previous plastic or corrective surgery to the vagina: if childbirth risks undoing the previous surgery, then the only way of getting around this problem is to perform a caesarean section.
- Failure to progress in labour: if labour appears to be getting nowhere in spite of everything, abdominal delivery may be the only option.

What are the fetal indications?

Fetal distress is the most common fetal indication for caesarean section. This may be perceived or confirmed. The tendency is to err on the side of safety.

- Breech presentation: when breech is the leading part of the baby, there is a high likelihood of caesarean section. A significant minority of breech-presenting babies are delivered vaginally. (*See* Chapter 33, "Breech presentation", for further details.)
- Multiple pregnancy: a significant proportion of twins are delivered by caesarean section. This is usually because the first twin is presenting with a part other than the head. It could also be performed because one or both twins' well-being is causing concern. Virtually all high-order multiple pregnancies (triplets, and so forth) are delivered by caesarean section.
- Abnormal lie: it is not only breech which is the positional indication for caesarean section. Sometimes the baby is found in a "transverse" or oblique lie, where the fetus is lying across so the head is on one side and the bottom on the other. This is incompatible with vaginal delivery and a caesarean section will need to be done if the mother is in labour. If she is not, an expectant management is adopted, with hope that the baby will assume a favourable position.
- Cord prolapse: if the "waters" break in early or mid-labour and the umbilical cord prolapses, a caesarean delivery is the only option.

Is maternal preference a valid indication for caesarean delivery?

Maternal request or demand in the absence of any medical indication is a good example of abuse of services. An obstetrician who agrees to such a demand is not doing any woman a favour.

Anaesthesia

How many modes of anaesthesia for caesarean section are there and how do they differ?

There are two main types of anaesthesia: general, where the patient is rendered both pain-free and unconscious (asleep) and regional, where the patient is pain-free, her lower body is paralyzed but she is fully awake.

A general anaesthetic is used when rapid induction of anaesthesia is required (it is usually reliably quicker), in case of difficulties with regional anaesthesia or where there is contraindication for this – and, of course, if and when the mother concerned does not wish to be awake during the operation.

Regional anaesthesia, which is either spinal or epidural, is probably used more often for caesarean section, though this differs from hospital to hospital and country to country. There is evidence that the majority of mothers prefer this method of anaesthesia.

What is the difference between spinal and epidural anaesthesia?

This is purely the space where the local anaesthetic is injected in the spine. Both are quite effective but an epidural (commonly used for labour) takes effect much more slowly. An epidural is therefore not ideal where a rapid induction of anaesthesia is required.

Does epidural or spinal anaesthesia have any particular advantage over a general anaesthetic?

Most people will say yes. Firstly, it allows the mother to be awake and therefore witness the birth of her baby. She can hold the baby within minutes of delivery while the surgeons are continuing with their work.

Secondly, her partner is allowed to be by her side, if she is awake. This allows for the family atmosphere to be maintained at this very crucial and emotive time in their lives. It all augurs well for bonding.

Additionally, complications are fewer with regional anaesthesia, compared to general anaesthesia.

Why is spinal or epidural termed "regional" anaesthesia?

Because the effects are confined to only a particular section of the body and the upper half is left untouched.

What are the potential complications of regional anaesthesia?

The most common is a drop in blood pressure, and this is easily dealt with.

Occasionally, patients have post-spinal headache, which may last a few days and can be quite debilitating as it is felt with change of posture (usually from a flat position to a sitting or standing position). This can also be effectively dealt with.

Rarely, an abscess or blood-clot (haematoma) may form at the injection site. The symptoms are progressively worsening backache within a day or so of the procedure. It occurs with the epidural rather than spinal.

Occasionally, after starting the operation, it is discovered too late that the spinal or epidural is not fully effective and the patient is in some pain. There is then no choice but to resort to giving a general anaesthetic. This can be quite upsetting for someone who had wanted to stay awake. Fortunately, this is uncommon.

What are the potential complications of general anaesthesia?

"Aspiration" is the feared complication of a general anaesthetic. The unconscious patient undergoing the operation may vomit and breathe the vomited stuff into the airway. This can result in her being quite ill for days afterwards. This is why any mother who is to undergo a caesarean section will be given an injection of a drug to reduce the production of acid in the stomach and an antacid drink to neutralize the acid that is already there.

The other common complication is lowering blood pressure. As with the regional anaesthesia, general anaesthesia can lower the blood pressure.

What are the potential complications of the caesarean section itself?

It is important to keep things in perspective.

The safety of caesarean section has improved dramatically over the years. However, it remains a major operation, with the potential for serious complications. This means, when necessary, the doctor will not hesitate to do it but, by the same token, when it is not really indicated, the doctor will resist the temptation to do it.

Apart from complications which are attributable to the anaesthesia as described above, other things which may happen include:

- Haemorrhage: this can be so severe that it requires multiple transfusions. In extreme cases – which occur from time to time – the bleeding may be such that a hysterectomy has to be done as a life-saving measure.

- Injury to adjacent structures: during a difficult operation, structures such as loops of bowel and the urinary tract (bladder and ureters) may be injured. Normally, if recognized, injuries can be repaired relatively easily. If, however, they go unrecognized, they can lead to serious complications requiring a repeat operation and a long recovery period.

- Infection: infection of the lining of the womb (endometritis) may follow a caesarean section. This has the potential for serious consequences, as eventual healing may produce a weak scar which may not withstand a subsequent pregnancy or labour. Again, this is uncommon. Infection is sometimes confined to the abdominal wound but this also means a prolonged and uncomfortable recovery period. The resulting scar may also be unsightly. Many units have a policy of giving preventative antibiotics before or during a caesarean section to reduce the possibility of infection afterwards.

- Thromboembolism (and/or pulmonary embolism): this is a condition where a clot or clots form within the veins and may be dislodged, travel and end up in vessels within the lungs, with sometimes very serious consequences. Since pregnancy is in itself a condition that promotes blood clotting, a major operation during pregnancy increases the risk of thromboembolism.

- Respiratory problems: lung collapse with pain and breathing difficulties may follow any major surgery, including caesarean section. Pneumonia may also occur.

- Bowel problems: intestinal ileus – where a loop of bowel is filled with gas, causing very uncomfortable abdominal distension – sometimes occurs and may last up to two days or so. Constipation is another minor potential complication.

If a woman opts to stay awake during the operation, what should she expect in terms of the experience of the operation?

The squeamish should not worry! The area of the operation is always screened off and it is only when the baby is delivered out of the abdomen that she may see a hint of blood as the baby is held up for her to see. Some women only want to see the baby after he or she has been cleaned and put in clothing. Staff will never object to such a request.

During the delivery of the baby, most times, pressure is applied on the upper part of her abdomen to ease delivery. This is only felt as pressure and not pain. It lasts about fifteen to thirty seconds. Remember, the baby is delivered within five minutes of starting the operation and the rest of the time (twenty to thirty minutes) is spent putting everything back together again.

Post-operation

Barring complications, what is the post-operation period like?

The vast majority of women having a caesarean section will have no complications of any kind. They can expect to be sitting up within hours, they will be on their feet within 24 hours and will be up and about by three days.

What is the length of stay in hospital, following a caesarean section?

This may range anything between three and seven days. The average is five.

If the skin has been repaired using stitches or staples which need removing, this is usually done between days five and seven, depending on the type of incision that was made. It is not unusual to allow the mother home before the stitches are removed and to have the midwife visit her at home to take them out on the scheduled day. This is if there are no problems, the mother has adequate help at home and this is her wish.

What about going back to work after a caesarean section?

This depends on the type of work that the woman does. If it is a desk-bound job which is not physically demanding, she may be able to go back to full-time work within six weeks of delivery. If the job involves physical exertion, then twelve weeks is probably the minimum interval she requires. Every woman should pace herself and listen to her own body in whatever activities she wants to try.

Caeseareans in subsequent pregnancies

How does caesarean section influence the method of delivery in a subsequent pregnancy?

If the indication for a caesarean section was for a one-off reason – such as fetal distress, abnormal fetal lie or presentation, or maternal distress – then the standard advice is to try for a vaginal delivery, next time around. This is on the proviso that there is no new complicating factor.

Most women succeed in having a successful vaginal delivery, second time round. For a significant minority, however, the attempt is unsuccessful and they end up having a repeat caesarean section.

If the indication for caesarean section first time around was an unchanging factor, such as a narrow pelvis, then any future delivery will be by a caesarean section.

What if a woman has had two caesarean sections?

The method of delivery following two caesarean sections is always a caesarean section. Of late, there have been divergent opinions that, in carefully selected cases, a trial of vaginal delivery can be attempted. In fact, this has been successful in a substantial number of cases. This is, however, unlikely to take a foothold in standard obstetric practice, because most women with such a history do not appear keen on the idea.

What is the acceptable interval following a caesarean section before trying for another baby?

There is no evidence that any time is too soon to conceive, following a caesarean section.

However, if she happens to conceive within three months of having a caesarean section, the chances are that she will end up with another caesarean delivery. This is because many obstetricians are anxious about the strength of the scar after such an abnormally short interval. This is doubly so if there had been post-operative complications, such as infection of the womb. Cases of such rapid conception following caesarean section are uncommon.

How many caesarean sections can a woman safely have?

There is no definite number. There is a myth among many people that anything beyond three caesarean sections is life-threatening! This is certainly not true. What is true is that each subsequent caesarean section makes the next one potentially more difficult. There may be so much scar tissue and distortion of the normal anatomy that chances of injury to other structures – especially the bladder, ureters (tubes that carry the urine from the kidneys to the bladder) and bowel – are increased substantially.

There is also the issue of increasing risk of the placenta abnormally adhering to the old scar. This may be so serious as to lead to severe uncontrollable haemorrhage requiring a hysterectomy. Every individual's circumstances are different and the obstetrician will give advice regarding future fertility on the basis of those unique individual circumstances. What is common to all is that the potential for serious complications increases with each subsequent caesarean; it is the extent that differs from person to person.

40. Water birth

Introduction

Practically every obstetric unit in the UK provides this service today. The majority of women who become pregnant will have heard of it and those who seek alternative labour and delivery methods take interest in this, one of the truly different methods.

Water birth is meant to offer an alternative to the drug-based pain relief methods. It is also supposed to offer a possibility of a less stressful labour, in allowing more freedom of movement and changing position, because of the buoyancy of the body in water. Moreover, the water birth units in hospitals are set up in such a way as to create as near to a home atmosphere as possible. It is actually possible to hire the pool and have the labour and delivery taking place in your actual home, provided the safety conditions (as we shall see) are met.

All in all, water birth is a very attractive option for some pregnant women. However, it is crucial that any enthusiasm for the pool is tempered with a healthy dose of realism. The water will not give the same degree of pain relief as an epidural, for one. It is quite possible that a mother who has opted for the pool may find labour pains so stressful that she needs to leave the pool to get more effective pain relief. If this happens (and it does happen), she should not feel that nature has let her down. We are all different. In addition, even when she is happy with the experience, other labour complications may develop which may lead the midwife to advise abandoning the pool.

As in all areas of pregnancy, any strategy should be approached with an open mind. Tunnel vision about pregnancy, labour and delivery leads to disappointment, more often than not.

The history of water birth

Is water a serious alternative to the traditional methods, or is it just a passing fad?

Water birth is not as new as one may be tempted to think.

The first documented birth in water was recorded in France at the beginning of the nineteenth century. This was purely accidental and there is no evidence that it was adopted then as a viable alternative to traditional methods of labour and/or delivery. More than 150 years later, obstetricians in the then Soviet Union started researching this method and it quickly became part of mainstream obstetric practice. It soon spread to virtually every part of the developed world and, today, many obstetric units in the United States, UK and the rest of Europe offer this service.

What if the mother wants a water birth as part of a home birth strategy?

This is a viable proposition.

If there is a big enough bathtub in the house – that is, one that can comfortably accommodate two people – and where there is a reliable hot water supply, then there is no reason why this possibility cannot be explored. Of course, the midwife who will monitor the labour and conduct the delivery should be satisfied that all the other prerequisites for a safe home delivery are in place.

Presently, there are several companies which offer pool rental services. The "birthing" pools are purpose-built and a spacious room in the house can be converted into a temporary delivery room. The advantage of these pools is that they are usually quite spacious and there is an inbuilt thermostatic control of water temperature, which allows for a constant ideal temperature level.

The flip side is that they tend to cost a considerable sum of money to hire.

The benefits of water birth

What are the benefits of labour in water?

The main claimed benefit is the soothing and relaxing effect of the warm water, which in turn reduces the sensation of pain.

Secondly, since the atmosphere is decidedly non-medical, this may engender a positive experience of the whole labour and delivery process.

It is claimed that, by being in warm water for such a prolonged period, the perineal and vaginal tissue become so supple that trauma (both in the form of a need for episiotomy and accidental tears) is reduced. There is no conclusive evidence to support this.

What are the benefits to the baby?

In concrete terms, none.

It is true that no painkilling drugs are given to mothers who are labouring in water. This means that these babies are born free of any potential side-effects of these drugs (mostly sedation). However, this cannot be claimed to be an exclusive benefit of water birth, since there are many women who labour the traditional way and opt not to have any of these drugs.

The assertion that delivery under water allows for a smoother entry into the world appears plausible but it is difficult to assess, let alone quantify the purported advantage.

When water birth does not work

Are there any contraindications to labouring in water?

There are several. The most important are as follows:

- presence of a major medical condition such as kidney failure, heart disease, diabetes or hypertension
- premature labour
- placenta praevia or any other significant vaginal bleeding prior to labour
- abnormal fetal position – such as transverse or oblique lie – which may make successful vaginal delivery improbable.
- lack of or inadequate facilities or absence of an experienced professional (midwife) to monitor the labour or conduct the delivery.

What are the most common reasons for women labouring in water leaving the pool?

The most common reasons are:

- prolonged labour
- maternal distress (mostly because of pain)
- fetal distress
- maternal request.

Why would maternal request feature so prominent among the reasons for abandoning water birth?

In most cases, it is because the experience does not live up to her expectations. She may find the pain unbearable and the relaxing effect inadequate to overcome this.

As for maternal distress, it is upon the attending midwife to assess and recommend leaving the pool if it becomes obvious that the mother is not coping. This will allow for a more effective method of pain control to be adopted.

Preparing for a water birth

If one is considering a water birth, what are the preparations?

A midwife will have an exhaustive discussion of this method of labour and delivery with the parents-to-be. All questions should be asked and answered.

Importantly, the pregnant mother should be encouraged to spend prolonged periods in warm water, to form her own opinion of the experience. She should remember that, on the day, it will be different, as there will be pain. Also, the process could last six hours, even more.

Nearer term, the usual obstetric assessment will be made to ensure there are none of the factors which will contraindicate labour in water (see above).

At the onset of labour, before entering the pool, a shower is taken and the midwife ensures the rectum is empty. This is done by administering a gentle enema if necessary.

Cardiotocographic (CTG) monitoring will be done for at least thirty minutes prior to entering the pool, to ensure that the baby is fine.

What kind of water is used?

Ordinary tap water is used. Some practitioners advocate salinizing the water, for example by adding sea-water. This is claimed to make the tissues of the birth canal even more supple. This claim is not backed up by evidence.

What is an ideal temperature?

Water should be kept as close to the normal body temperature as possible. For the thermostatically controlled pools, this temperature is set to fluctuate in a narrow range of about 35–38°C.

The ambient temperature should also be warm but not stuffy.

What is the problem of water being hotter (or colder, for that matter)?

Very hot water may bring about quick exhaustion to the labouring woman. It is important to remember that, for the majority of women, labour lasts several hours. Early exhaustion may lead to her having to leave pool.

There is evidence also that very hot water may diminish the strength of the contractions. In early labour, it can stop the contractions altogether.

When water is merely lukewarm, it will be uncomfortable and the relaxing effect will be lost.

When is the ideal time to get into the pool?

The optimal time is when the labour is established. This is confirmed by the presence of regular strong contractions as well as a cervical dilatation of at least 4 cm.

Too early an entry may lead to an apparent prolonged labour, which may lead to a forced abandonment of the pool, either for an alternative mode of pain relief or for augmenting labour with an oxytocin (Syntocinon®) infusion.

A very late entry into the pool will mean that she will not get the intended full benefit of labour in water.

Sometimes the latent phase of labour can be very painful. What is wrong with entering the pool then?

There is nothing wrong. However, the mother has to be aware of two important facts.

Firstly, that the latent phase of labour can last many hours, sometimes a good eighteen hours or more before true labour is established. The uncertainty of the duration of this phase should be made clear.

Secondly, if the latent phase of labour is found to be unbearably painful, it may imply that when actual labour commences, the soothing effect of warm water is unlikely to be sufficient to control the pain.

It is said that one of the main advantages of labour in water is that it reduces the rate of obstetric intervention. Is this proven?

Unfortunately not. Properly conducted studies indicate that there are no differences in the rate of intervention in the form of instrumental (forceps or ventouse) delivery or caesarean section.

Since infusions are prohibited if labouring in water, is there no risk of dehydration?

Not really, since drinking (but not eating) is allowed during labour.

What additional pain relief can one get if labouring in the pool?

Many women find that the relaxing and soothing effect of water is sufficient. However, if additional pain relief is required, many units will allow entonox ("gas and air").

No injectable opiates such as pethidine or diamorphine can be administered. If this is deemed necessary, then she has to leave the pool and water birth is abandoned. An epidural in water is contraindicated, too.

What if pethidine or diamorphine have been administered in the latent phase of labour?

Then an interval of about four hours (or more) has to be ensured before she enters the pool. This is mainly because of the sedating effect of these drugs, a state which is incompatible with a prolonged stay in water, considering the additional relaxing effect of the water itself.

Delivery

What is the advice regarding breech or twins labour and delivery in water?

This is controversial. Many units regard both these situations to be high risk and therefore unsuitable for water birth. Others take a more liberal view regarding breech labour, where this may be conducted in water. Very few will allow breech delivery in water and, for this, the woman has to leave the pool. This is mainly for practical reasons, as proper assistance in breech delivery in the pool can be quite problematic, and therefore unsafe for the baby.

There are even fewer practitioners happy to allow twins labour in water. Fortunately, mothers requesting this are fewer still.

What is the advice regarding delivery under water?

This remains a difficult question. Many units will allow delivery under water, if the mother wishes. However, because of the uncertainty regarding the safety of this undertaking, some units will allow labour in water but delivery has to be conducted outside the pool.

Even in those units which allow underwater delivery, some midwives are unwilling to conduct delivery under water and therefore the mother may be unable to have her wish, for this reason. The issue of safety for this kind of delivery is likely to remain unresolved, since a proper scientific study in this area is probably impractical.

If delivery is conducted under water, how long should the baby be left submerged?

If the temperature has been kept constant and as close to the body temperature as possible, the baby is unlikely to start breathing under water. The risk of inhalation of water is therefore minimal. This assertion is borne out by the widespread experience around the world.

However, if the water had been allowed to cool significantly below the body temperature, the baby is likely to gasp in reflex on coming into contact with the relatively cold environment. This is one of the main reasons why strict water temperature control is essential.

Experience shows that a baby born in water with appropriate temperature is relaxed and makes no effort to breathe, since the placenta is still supplying him or her with adequate oxygen.

Prolonged submersion may, however, be inadvisable, since the placenta may start to separate, risking hypoxia (oxygen insufficiency) for the baby.

Should suction of the baby's mouth and nose be commenced immediately after delivery?

If the baby is born under water, suction should never be started while the baby is still submerged. If one wants to do this, the head of the baby may be brought above water and suction performed.

What is the advice regarding delivery of the placenta?

Most practitioners advocate that the third stage (i.e. delivery of the placenta) should be conducted outside the pool.

This has three theoretical benefits. Firstly, it may reduce the risk of heavy postpartum haemorrhage. Secondly, it allows for a more accurate estimation of blood loss post-delivery; and thirdly, it prevents a potentially serious – even fatal – complication of water embolism (where water finds its way into the bloodstream). It has to be emphasized that no case of water embolism has been reported in relation to water birth. However, all the ingredients for such a complication are there and hence placental delivery outside the pool is regarded to be a worthwhile precaution.

Would you say the popularity of water birth is an important gauge of women's opinion about natural birth?

There is nothing natural about labour or delivery in water – at least, not for human beings! Anybody promoting water birth on this theme is promoting falsehood. However, there is no denying that the availability of this service is an important development which has enriched the experience of labour and offered choice to thousands of women. It is an important alternative.

41. Problems occurring after delivery (puerperium)

Introduction

The incredible euphoria of a new baby is followed soon after by a myriad problems which bring one back to earth, sometimes with a bang.

Most problems are minor, short-lived and easy to cope with. When my wife and I had our first son, I went to work complaining of our sleepless nights, to which a colleague airily remarked in reassurance, "Oh, not to worry; that will end in about eighteen years or so."

A wailing baby in the small hours is unfortunately not the only thing that can wreak havoc in the postnatal period. There could be problematic vaginal bleeding and infection, which could be in the genital tract, urinary tract, chest or the lactating breasts.

There are also mood problems commonly known as postnatal depression. Postnatal psychosis is another possible problem of a different kind. This has been known to lead mothers to commit infanticide. Though uncommon, these are clearly very serious complications, which call for careful evaluation and very aggressive management. All these are discussed below.

Apart from infections and psychological problems, other potential disorders are neurological, blood-clotting disorders and injuries to the pelvic girdle sustained during delivery. Likewise, these are covered fully below.

The puerperium

What is the puerperium?

This is the period following delivery. It lasts six weeks but this figure is really only for convenience and is not marked by any particular milestone. The puerperal period is a continuum with changes taking place, both physically and emotionally, following the period of pregnancy and eventual delivery.

What happens in the puerperium?

For the majority of women, this period passes relatively smoothly, with realization of their hopes and adjustments to motherhood as they had expected. For a very significant minority, things do not go according to expectations. Problems can range from the relatively minor to quite serious and complex ones, as we shall see below.

Pain after delivery

What causes perineal or vaginal pain after delivery?

For those women who achieve a successful vaginal delivery, be it spontaneous or with some instrumental assistance, an episiotomy may be applied to ease delivery. This is repaired immediately but, for the first day or two, the area may be quite sore.

Alternatively, in the course of delivery there could be a tear (which is also repaired immediately after delivery) and/or bruising in the vaginal and vulval areas. These could produce soreness, which tend to make sitting and walking rather uncomfortable. The healing is quite rapid and usually the pain is gone within three or four days.

Are there any other sources of pain?

Haematoma (blood-clot) formation is another significant source of perineal or vaginal pain occurring shortly after delivery. The pain is usually progressive, starting only a few hours after delivery. If it remains undiagnosed for a lengthy period of time, it may lead to urine retention. Examination will readily reveal the swelling, usually in the vaginal canal.

If the injury leading to the haematoma formation is high in the genital tract, the haematoma may form in the pelvic cavity and an ultrasound is the readily available means of establishing the diagnosis.

Haematoma

What causes haematoma formation?

Usually it is the trauma of delivery that causes rupture of blood vessels underneath the vaginal skin. Accordingly, there is no surface evidence of the damage and that's why it may remain undetected for hours, even days.

Alternatively, a haematoma may result from an inappropriately repaired episiotomy or tear. Laceration to the cervix may also lead to a pelvic haematoma.

What is the treatment for a haematoma?

The clot has to be accessed and drained. The bleeding vessels are then secured with absorbable stitches. Most affected women are quite amazed at the instant and almost total relief obtained after such a seemingly simple procedure.

What happens if the haematoma is in the pelvis?

If this is not progressive – which is usually the case – the preferred approach is conservative management. Pain associated with a pelvic haematoma is usually adequately managed using ordinary pain-control medication. The haematoma will clear up with time. The only risk, albeit small, is that it could get infected, where a change of plan becomes necessary (see below).

What if the pelvic haematoma is progressive?

If the haematoma appears to be getting bigger, with evidence from serial – usually daily – ultrasound scans and/or falling blood count (haemoglobin), then there is no choice but to perform an operation to stop this. A laparotomy (where the abdomen is opened) will be performed and the clot evacuated. The bleeding points are sought and secured. It is a major operation which will prolong the new mother's hospital stay for probably four to seven days.

Haemorrhage

How common is delayed postpartum haemorrhage?

Significantly heavy bleeding occurring more than twenty-four hours after delivery affects around 1 per cent of all new mothers. The technical term is secondary PPH (postpartum haemorrhage). It may occur any time in the first six weeks following delivery, but is most common between the first and second week. Secondary PPH after the first four weeks is quite uncommon.

What causes secondary postpartum haemorrhage?

The cause is not always identifiable.

The two known causes are:
- retained products of conception – where some bits of placenta or membranes are not expelled
- infection of the lining of the womb.

How common is the problem of retained products after delivery?

It is less common than one may be tempted to imagine. In fact, a lot of cases purported to be retained products following ultrasound scan turn out not to be this. Following this apparent diagnosis, evacuation of the uterine contents is done and, as it turns out in many cases, only clots are retrieved. Because of this, many obstetricians regard ultrasound in a person with symptoms of secondary PPH to be an ill-advised venture, since it is likely to lead to a uterine evacuation procedure – mostly under a general anaesthetic – which in many cases turns out to be unnecessary.

How will one recognize secondary postpartum haemorrhage (PPH) caused by infection?

There are usually clinical features that may point towards this possibility. These may include pelvic pain, fever and general malaise. Then again, they may be completely absent.

Tests are usually done, including a blood count and vaginal swabs to look for the culprit bacteria. These may be inconclusive. In fact, the value of taking vaginal swabs in a woman who is bleeding from the uterus is doubtful. Many experts argue that if one really wants to identify the infection, swabs have to be taken from high up in the uterus.

This is usually an impractical option, unless the woman is being taken to theatre for evacuation of the uterus.

So, how does one go about managing secondary postpartum haemorrhage where there is no readily identifiable cause?

A clinical judgement has to be made according to each individual's case. The management may include some or all of these: bed rest; oxytocic drugs to promote uterine contraction, antibiotics, uterine exploration for retained products and blood transfusion. Transfusion needs to be mentioned but in fact it is rarely required in secondary PPH.

Would one be justified in saying that, in secondary PPH, evacuating the uterus is not a means of first resort?

Absolutely. The clinician has a duty to ensure no unnecessary surgical procedures are carried out. Evacuation may actually aggravate the bleeding by dislodging the fragile clot plugs in the multiple potential bleeding points in the uterus. It is not always an easy decision.

Is there any possibility that secondary PPH can lead to loss of the uterus (hysterectomy)?

Yes, but this is a very remote possibility. When all conservative means of controlling the bleeding fail, the attending obstetrician may be left with no choice but to carry out a hysterectomy as a life-saving procedure. Emphasis has to be put on the fact that, in secondary PPH, this is very rare indeed.

Infection

Are there any predisposing factors to developing womb infection, post delivery?

Again, in most cases, there is no obvious predisposing factor. Occasionally such factors as prolonged labour, chronic undernutrition, anaemia or a weakened body immunity may be identifiable.

Occasionally the "flesh-eating bug" has been reported to cause postpartum infection. How common is this frightening occurrence?

This is very rare. However, when it occurs, especially if there is delay in diagnosis, it can be deadly.

When it occurs, it usually follows caesarean section. There may be destruction of extensive amount of tissue and treatment will involve surgical removal of this tissue as well as an aggressive antibiotic course in high doses. Fortunately, the offending bacteria respond well to antibiotics. The official term for the condition is "necrotizing fasciitis".

Would you say a caesarean section increases the risk of puerperal infection?

There is no doubt about this. Infection following caesarean section, especially emergency ones, is definitely more common than following vaginal delivery. This is the case regardless of whether we are talking about womb infection, pelvic infection or urinary tract infection. This is one reason among others why unnecessary caesarean sections should be actively avoided.

The risk of infection following caesarean section can be reduced by administering preventative antibiotics just before or during the operation. These are given intravenously. There is no place for oral antibiotics.

How common is pelvic abscess formation?

It is rare. Again, it is relatively more common after caesarean section when compared to vaginal delivery.

The abscess needs draining as the main form of treatment. This may be complemented with antibiotics for several days.

Can a puerperal pelvic abscess have long-term consequences?

Yes. This may be in the form of problems with future fertility and/or chronic pelvic pain. This is not because of failure to eradicate the infection but the aftermath of the infection, in the form of scarring and adhesions which may affect the free passage of the tubes. Such consequences are not common.

Is there any other form of pelvic infection occurring in the puerperium?

Yes. Though uncommon, it deserves special separate mention because of its distinctive form of management. This is septic thrombo-phlebitis. Pelvic veins may become infected, leading to clot formation within their cavities. It almost always follows caesarean section rather than vaginal delivery. Once diagnosed, medication to thin the blood will have to be commenced alongside antibiotics. Blood-thinning medication will be in the form of heparin injections (to begin with). This may be changed later to oral medication (warfarin), if required. Both these drugs are safe for breast-feeding.

In very rare instances, it may be necessary to insert a filter in the major abdominal vein to prevent more serious consequences while continuing with treatment.

What about "water" infections?

Urinary tract infection is not uncommon following delivery. This is understandable, considering the circumstances surrounding labour and delivery itself. There may be prolonged periods of stoppage of urinary flow in the bladder. Catheterization is also more common, usually to prevent over-distension of the bladder and to ease the descent of the baby into the pelvis. All these increase the risk of subsequent urinary tract infection. The infection hardly ever extends beyond the bladder.

The symptoms are usually frequency of voiding, urgency and a burning sensation when passing water. Occasionally there may be more generalized symptoms such as malaise and fever. This increases the possibility that the infection has extended higher, to the kidneys.

With symptoms like these, a urine sample is taken for urgent analysis and broad-spectrum antibiotics commenced. Relief is felt within a day or so, even though antibiotics will have to be taken for at least seven days, sometimes more, to ensure eradication of the infection.

Blood clots

What is thrombo-embolism?

Thrombosis or clot-formation within the veins is one of the potential complications of pregnancy. When a clot is dislodged and transported within the bloodstream to distant organs (usually the lungs), this is called thrombo-embolism. It can be a serious – even fatal – condition. In the Western world, it is one of the leading causes of maternal death.

How common is thrombo-embolism in pregnancy?

Deep vein thrombosis – commonly called by its short form, DVT – occurs in about 0.1 per cent of all pregnancies. It therefore means that, in an average general district hospital, with an annual delivery rate of about 3000 babies, they will expect to have three or four cases of DVT per year.

The risk of DVT increases with advancing pregnancy and is greatest in the early puerperium. It then gradually lessens. The veins usually affected are those in the lower limbs (calf or thigh) and, to a lesser extent, the pelvic veins.

The risk of pelvic vein thrombosis is significantly increased by caesarean section.

Is there anything that can be done to reduce the risk of thrombosis in the puerperium?

Yes. Getting on your feet quickly helps to reduce the risk of puerperal thrombosis. It is therefore imperative upon midwives looking after new mothers to encourage them to get on their feet as early as is practicable.

How is DVT treated?

A course of heparin injections will be commenced and this will continue for several days. The traditional heparin may be used or alternatively newer forms of what are known as "low molecular-weight heparin" may be used. Two brands of these most used in the UK are Fragmin® and Clexane®. They all do the same thing, but the administration regimes and monitoring are different. The patient will then be gradually switched to oral warfarin. Treatment will continue for several weeks, with regular clinical assessment and occasional blood tests to monitor the progress.

While treatment will almost certainly be commenced in hospital, after the condition has stabilized, treatment will continue on an outpatient basis. The patient is taught to self-inject heparin or her partner may do this.

An additional measure will be the almost continuous wearing of special pressure stockings (tights). These can be quite uncomfortable, but they are necessary if the clot was in the lower limbs.

Breasts

What sorts of breast problems occur after delivery?

The most common problem is marked breast engorgement, without infection. It may affect up to one in five new mothers. There is extreme discomfort and it may cause moderate fever. If there is no evidence of infection, all that is required is simple analgesics (such as paracetamol), adequate breast support, ice packs and – if the mother is not breast-feeding – fluid restriction.

What about infectious mastitis?

This is less common. It is estimated that about 2.5 per cent or one in forty new mothers will have infectious mastitis. A small minority of these will go on to develop a breast abscess.

Are there any predisposing factors to infectious mastitis?

Breast engorgement, nipple trauma and poor breast-feeding technique are some of the commonly cited factors increasing the risk of mastitis.

The cause or risk factor is not always apparent.

How can one recognize infectious mastitis?

Infectious mastitis commonly (but not always) affects one breast or the other. Simple breast engorgement mastitis without infection tends to affect both breasts, though to varying degrees. Apart from the discomfort, even pain, there may be other less specific symptoms, including malaise and fever. Examination of the breasts will almost always reveal inflammation of the affected breast.

What is the treatment for infectious mastitis?

Once recognized, broad-spectrum antibiotics should be commenced promptly. This should be complemented with painkillers such as paracetamol or stronger ones, according to need, as well as adequate breast support.

Women who are breast-feeding do not need to stop. If continuing to breast-feed is impractical, then breast expression to prevent engorgement should be done. This could be done manually or by using a pump.

The antibiotic course will be continued for a week or more.

Suppose the mastitis progresses into an abscess?

In this case, incision and drainage of the abscess is required. Adequate drainage means the procedure normally requires a general anaesthetic.

Drainage will be combined with an antibiotic course. Breast-feeding is usually difficult to maintain on the affected breast before the abscess is drained. However, after this, there is no reason to prevent recommencing.

What options are there for lactation-suppression if one does not want to breast-feed?

There are two alternatives if one wants to suppress lactation. One is to use non-pharmacological means (i.e. no drugs). The other is to use drugs.

General measures where no drugs are involved include breast support, simple analgesics and meticulous fluid restriction. Milk expression should be avoided, as this encourages production of more milk and will prolong the period of suppression.

Drugs used for lactation suppression are taken daily for a period of two weeks. Lactation may start again after completing the course, which will necessitate recommencing the medication.

There is really no evidence that using drugs is more effective than using general measures.

Joints and mobility

What are the pelvic joint complications of pregnancy and/or delivery?

Joints in the pelvis – mostly at the front, known as the symphysis pubis – may become lax or the bones may actually separate. This uncommon event tends to occur in late pregnancy or after delivery. There is pain, which is aggravated by movement, especially climbing stairs or rolling from side to side.

This can be quite severe and incapacitating. A wide support belt (brace) is available to try to stabilize the joints and prevent joint movement, which is the cause of the pain. In addition, measures such as rest and avoiding lifting are helpful. The condition almost always clears up entirely.

This may take a few days but may also continue for several weeks after delivery.

Are there any other joint complications?

Occasionally, during delivery, a fracture of the coccyx – which is the lowermost and smallest bone on the spine – may occur. This will cause pain on sitting down.

Treatment includes local infiltration with a local anaesthetic (temporary relief), heat therapy and rest.

A simple but ingenious device is a ring cushion for sitting in. This effectively takes the pressure off the affected area.

What is a "foot-drop"?

Sometimes for a variety of reasons, there could be neurological damage which may show in the form of foot-drop.

This, as the name suggests, is the inability to flex the foot upwards at the ankle joint. Consequently, the affected person walks with a limp and with the toes dragging or barely clearing the floor. There may be pain in the rest of the limb or numbness of the ankle and foot.

The cause is severe or prolonged pressure on the nerve, either at the level of the spine or lower down in the leg.

The problem clears up completely with time. In the meantime, splinting to relieve the foot-drop may be used. Passive physiotherapy, to keep the joint supple, is strongly recommended. In the few cases where the foot-drop is caused by protrusion of a disc in the spine, surgery may be required.

Depression and psychosis

What is "postnatal blues" and what cause it?

This is the mildest and arguably most common problem in the puerperium. It has also been called "third day blues" because it tends to happen around the third to fifth day following delivery. It is characterized by weepiness, feeling down, irritability and anxiety. There is no evidence of any underlying disease and most experts agree that it is brought about by the major changes to the system wrought by the arrival of a fragile, demanding and totally dependent being. The responsibility may initially prove too much, unleashing all these emotions.

So what does a mother suffering from postnatal blues require?

Support. The situation should be patiently and sympathetically explained to her. A partner has a crucial role to play, as well as the rest of the family. The midwife will be there to give expert advice, if this is required. The situation clears up in a matter of days. Only occasionally is a short course of sedatives required. A small percentage of affected mothers go on to have postnatal depression.

What causes postnatal depression?

There are no specific causes. It is known for certain that women with a previous history of depression in a non-pregnant state or following a previous delivery are more at risk. Recent or ongoing marital conflict has also been associated with postnatal depression.

What are the symptoms of postnatal depression?

There are similar to those experienced with postnatal blues, except they are far more pronounced. Moreover, the mother may complain of palpitations, lack of appetite and inability to sleep.

The most prominent symptom, however, is the feeling of profound lack of love for the newborn. Because of this, the mother may feel extremely guilty. She may also feel unable to love the other children, if she has any, and cannot feel any warmth towards other members of her family.

It is through such a sense of utter hopelessness that feelings of suicide are not uncommon. Even though actual attempts at this are rare, this symptom should never be ignored.

How is postnatal depression managed?

This requires intensive support for the affected mother. A psychiatrist is usually involved and takes the leading role in medical management.

Hospital admission may be necessary and, because the partner is crucial in the supporting role, if logistically possible, arrangements are made to enable him to stay with her. Attempts are made not to separate the baby from the mother.

Medication will usually be commenced and this could continue for several weeks, even months.

What role do hormonal preparations such as progesterone have in preventing postnatal depression?

For many years, progestogens were considered to be the logical form of treatment for this condition. This was based on the assumption that it is the sudden withdrawal of progesterone after delivery which causes depression. Experience and numerous studies have shown that there is no evidence that this has any effect. While it is still being used in some centres, the mother has a right to know that the expected benefit is not supported by any scientific evidence. Many obstetricians and their psychiatry colleagues alike simply don't offer this.

What can be said about puerperal psychosis?

As the name suggests, this is something entirely different from postnatal depression.

There is a change in the mental state and the new mother has wildly swinging moods, being euphoric one moment and at the depth of depression the next.

It is important to realize that the baby is at risk and even though he or she should ideally be kept with the mother, this should be coupled with adequate continuous vigilance to ensure he or she is not harmed by the mother. There are tragic experiences of such mothers strangling their babies.

Another potential problem not to be taken lightly is that of contraception. Because of mood swings, these patients are particularly prone to unprotected sex. This could easily lead to unplanned – and, in most cases, unwanted – pregnancy. This could complicate the picture enormously. It is therefore essential to ensure this aspect is addressed in the overall management strategy. The partner has a crucial role to play in this.

Where will a mother diagnosed as having postnatal psychosis be treated?

It is unusual to manage this condition at home. Hospital admission is almost always required and this could be in the psychiatric ward. Medication will be continued for as long as necessary. Almost all such patients make a full recovery.

Can postnatal psychosis recur in a subsequent pregnancy?

Yes. There is slight increase in risk of a recurrence. There are no known effective measures to reduce this risk.

42. Postnatal sex and contraception

Introduction

How soon after delivery a woman resumes an active sex life differs quite widely among individuals. This is because of varying circumstances which may be cultural, her physical state (is there a healing episiotomy or tear?), her psychological state (relaxed, very stressed or with postnatal depression), her home situation (is there a partner? is he supportive?) and many others.

Even though the advice in the older teaching was that intercourse should not occur until at least six weeks have elapsed after delivery, the majority of women ignored it. Six weeks is the accepted puerperal period but this advice was always ill-founded because it does not have any scientific basis.

Since many couples virtually cease to have sex in the final weeks of pregnancy, to impose an arbitrary moratorium after the birth is seen by many to be unacceptable and with good reason.

However, any couples resuming sexual intercourse in the postnatal period have issues to consider, one of which is the possibility of pregnancy. This is particularly crucial for bottle-feeding mothers (the majority in the Western world). This and the other issues related to sex and contraception in this period are clarified below.

Resuming sexual intercourse

When is it OK to resume sexual intercourse after delivery?

This depends on the newly delivered mother's particular concern. The general answer is, therefore, whenever she is physically and psychologically ready.

Is there any risk in resuming sex soon after delivery?

There are two main concerns. Firstly, the area around the birth canal is likely to be tender after delivery, making it difficult to have a satisfying sexual act. There is also the post-delivery vaginal discharge (lochia), which may be rather off-putting. This takes a few weeks to stop completely. From the medical point of view, there is the theoretical risk of precipitating an infection of the raw womb lining. This is because the bacteria that reside in the vagina may hitch a ride on the spermatozoa, ending up in the womb and even the pelvis. If one has to have intercourse in this early period, the use of condoms is therefore recommended.

It is said that sexual desire is quite low in the period after delivery and takes time to come back, especially if one is breast-feeding. Why is this?

This is not universally true. However, a mixture of psychological adjustment to the new role as a mother and the sheer physical exhaustion that this role engenders may place sex low on the list of priorities. It is thought that the role of hormonal changes in this state of affairs is minor. However, it is true that levels of the sex hormone oestrogen are low, especially for those who are fully breast-feeding. This may cause relative dryness of the vagina, which may make sex uncomfortable or outright painful. This is easily overcome using an oestrogen vaginal cream.

What is the average interval before newly delivered mothers resume sexual intercourse?

This differs widely among different cultures. Experience in the Western world shows that most women have resumed sex by the end of six weeks.

How soon can a woman conceive after delivery?

This depends on a number of factors. The most important among the natural factors is whether she is breast-feeding or not. A fully breast-feeding woman has a 90 per cent chance of not ovulating and not having a period, at least in the first four to six months. In developing countries, this has proved to be a fairly reliable form of contraception on its own. However, emphasis has to be put on the fact that it is not 100 per cent reliable and if a breast-feeding woman does not want to conceive, she has to use a supplementary form of contraception.

Is frequency of feeding of any relevance in increasing the effectiveness of breast-feeding in preventing ovulation?

Yes. Intervals between feeds should not exceed four hours, especially during the day and certainly not longer than six hours during the night. This is why breast-feeding is less reliable as the baby grows and starts demanding feeds less frequently and probably sleeps through the night.

Is recommencement of periods of any significance, regarding fertility?

Once the periods start again after delivery, the woman should assume that she is ovulating and therefore capable of conceiving. This is regardless of whether she is breast-feeding or not.

Methods of contraception

What methods of contraception are recommended for a breast-feeding woman?

There are several alternatives and we shall discuss them shortly. In summary, there are:

- both male and female barrier methods
- oral progestogen preparations
- injectable progestogen preparations
- intrauterine devices
- spermicidal preparations

and, finally

- natural family planning.

Which are the barrier methods?

The most widely used is the male condom. For a fully breast-feeding woman, properly used condoms should be sufficient in the first six months.

The female barrier methods include the diaphragm, the cervical cap and vaginal sheath (female condom). These, properly used, are equally effective for those who are fully breast-feeding. They are usually readily available from family planning clinics. However, it is important to remember that a diaphragm cannot be fitted until at least four weeks after delivery. The same applies to the cervical cap. With both of these, a spermicidal cream should be used as well.

What about the progestogen-only pill?

This is the most popular form of postnatal contraception among women who are breast-feeding. It is popularly known as the "mini-pill".

It has the advantage of not affecting milk production in any way. However, it calls for an element of discipline because, to work effectively, the pill has to be taken at regular times each day.

There may be irregular menstruation with its use. Overall, it is very effective when used appropriately.

What can be said about the injection form of contraception?

Depo-provera is the grand old duke of injectable progestogens. It is administered every twelve weeks and is an extremely effective contraceptive. However, like its oral cousin, the mini-pill, it can cause irregular vaginal bleeding, especially in the first three months. Thereafter, the tendency is to have no period at all. It does not interfere with milk production and is regarded to be safe for breast-feeding.

It is important to ensure that the injections are given on a strictly regular basis, for maximum effectiveness.

Are there any other ways of administering this hormone for contraception?

Yes. Apart from the oral and injectable progestogens, hormone implants (norplant) and a vaginal ring impregnated with the hormone are available. These are less popular but are known to be effective.

Where does the intrauterine device stand?

This device, widely but probably unfairly known as the "coil", is an excellent contraceptive.

Unbeknown to most people is the fact that there are three different types of intrauterine devices. The oldest is the non-medicated device, which is hardly used nowadays. The next is the medicated type (there is a variety of these). This is the most common type in use. The third, which has been available only in the last few years, is the progestogen-hormone carrying device.

All types of intrauterine devices have excellent effectiveness, with the progestogen device (Mirena) being more effective than the combined pill – hitherto, the most effective mode of contraception. In fact, this device is claimed to have a lower failure rate even when compared to female sterilization. Now, that is impressive!

Is the intrauterine device ideal to use in the postnatal period?

Yes. However, two words of caution.

There is a slight increase in the tendency of the device to fall out, if inserted in the period soon after delivery. If this happens and the loss goes unrecognized, there is a risk of pregnancy because the woman will be under the illusion that she is protected.

Secondly, for the plain (non-medicated) and the medicated devices (not the progestogen device), there is evidence that there is a small increase in the risk of pelvic infection. So, while it is perfectly all right for a woman in a monogamous relationship, it is not ideal for one who is likely to have multiple sexual partners, as the risk of pelvic infection is then quite real.

Are all intrauterine devices otherwise the same?

No. The progestogen-carrying device is certainly the most effective one.

It is actually so effective that, as stated earlier, it rivals sterilization, with the important exception that its effect is readily reversible. The medicated device is also quite effective, rivalling the combined pill in the medium- and long-term.

The progestogen-carrying device (one brand name being the Mirena) has one more important advantage. It almost invariably reduces the amount of menstrual blood loss. Some users stop having periods altogether. All the effects are, however, readily reversible on its removal.

And another thing. The progestogen device is actually believed to reduce the risk of pelvic infection. It has protective properties against this and therefore a woman who has this fitted is at an advantage in this regard.

Where do the spermicidal preparations stand as contraceptive methods?

For use on their own, they are pretty inadequate.

They are useful in supplementing the barrier methods mentioned above. Apart from disabling the spermatozoa, the common spermicide preparation (Nonoxynol) also kills most viruses, including HIV. It should not, however, be regarded as a protection against such infections.

Is there a worry that spermicide creams may increase the risk of genital infection?

There is really no evidence that this is true.

If one is averse to using artificial contraceptive methods, how reliable is natural family planning in the postnatal period?

Natural family planning is based on identifying the fertile period and abstaining from sex in this period to avoid conception.

This means it depends on regular reliable cycles and being able to identify the consistency of cervical mucus indicating ovulation. Both of those are either not there or highly unreliable in this post-delivery period. If the mother is breast-feeding, even partially, she may have no periods at all. Overall, the postnatal period is not the ideal period for using natural family planning.

Of course, one method of natural family planning is fail-safe whenever used – total abstinence. However, this is evidently not everybody's cup of tea.

What is the place of the combined oral contraceptive pill?

For a mother who is breast-feeding, this is a no-no.

The oestrogen component of the pill will have the effect of drying out the milk. The hormones are also passed into the milk and may have unwanted effects on the baby. It is not used unless the woman gives up breast-feeding first.

What is the contraceptive of choice for a woman who is not breast-feeding?

This woman has the freedom of the entire spectrum. Her concern should therefore be about the convenience, effectiveness and ultimately her personal preference. The consideration of milk production or effects on the baby is not in the equation.

The combined pill, the intrauterine device and the progestogen injection (Depo-provera) are the most effective.

Does a woman who is not breast-feeding need to start using a contraceptive straight away after delivery?

Yes, more or less. If she is sexually active in the immediate postnatal period, the possibility of conceiving is ever-present. Ovulation may occur as early as four to six weeks after delivery.

What about sterilization?

While only until a few years back, sterilization immediately after delivery was very popular, it is very infrequently done nowadays. There are a number of disadvantages associated with immediate postnatal sterilization.

One is that the chances of regretting the decision are significantly higher if it is done at this time.

Secondly, it is less safe as a surgical procedure as there is a higher chance of thrombosis complications.

Moreover, and probably most significantly for the majority, is the fact that the failure rate of sterilization at this time is considerably higher than at other times.

Recommended is what is known as "interval sterilization", where the procedure is performed several weeks after delivery. In the meantime, other temporary methods of contraception may be used. Unfortunately, even the six to twelve weeks interval is occasionally too long and some women find themselves pregnant before being sterilized.

Is there any contraindication to sterilization?

A decision on sterilization is an intensely personal thing. It is also a profound decision, by virtue of its permanent nature. Ultimately, a woman has to make the final decision, as long as she knows the facts. In this regard, doctors have a duty to advise where they feel the decision may be unwise and likely to be regretted later. This is their only role. Of course, some women take offence in being told that what they are proposing to do to themselves is not good – or at least the timing of it is not good. This should never make doctors shy away from their responsibility of giving what would be their best advice. Hostile reception of a doctor's advice is part and parcel of the job. And the interval is partly meant to allow the woman time to think things through.

What about reversal of sterilization?

This should never be relied upon as a fall-back plan. Firstly, it may not be available (many hospitals in the UK refuse to offer this on the NHS, except in very exceptional circumstances); secondly, even when offered, it may fail, as it does in 30 to 40 per cent of cases; and finally, it brings with it the risk of ectopic pregnancy, which in itself can be catastrophic.

What are the potential complications of sterilization?

It can fail in up to two in every thousand cases, which is really a low failure rate.

It may be technically impossible to perform it by the keyhole approach, necessitating a bigger operation, which means a longer (three to four day) hospital stay.

Other internal structures, such as the bowel, may be injured during the procedure, and pelvic infection is a possible complication.

While theoretically this looks a worrying list, in practice this is an extremely safe procedure and virtually everybody goes home the same day and resumes normal activities in less than a week.

Is there any alternative to sterilization for permanent contraception?

Yes. For those in steady relationships, male sterilization in the form of a vasectomy is just as simple, with an even lower failure rate. It can be performed under a local anaesthetic.

43. Breast-feeding

Introduction

In the 1980s and '90s, there has been a steady revival of breast-feeding which was virtually killed out by aggressive marketing by the giant multinationals producing infant formula. Even with this revival, most babies in developed countries are still bottle-fed.

This is made more poignant by the fact that bottle-feeding is more common in the lower socio-economic groups, which may indicate inadequate public health education or wrong mass education strategies.

Breast-milk is superior to formula milk: of that there is no doubt. It has several clear advantages, as we shall discuss shortly.

There are only a few contraindications to breast-feeding and these touch only a small minority of mothers.

Occasionally breast-feeding is not possible, in spite of good intentions and determined efforts by the mother. We discuss all these in this chapter. Apart from the advantages that the baby gets by being breast-fed, the mother also benefits. Contraception is more effective; she may remain amenorrhoeic (without periods) for months; weight gained during pregnancy is lost more rapidly and more easily; and there is the important issue of bonding, which is evidently stronger with breast-feeding.

There are many variables that need to be taken into consideration when deciding whether to breast-feed or not. All these are discussed below.

Milk production

Why is milk not produced during pregnancy?

It is because of the very high level of the hormone oestrogen in circulation during pregnancy. This inhibits the action of the hormone prolactin, which is responsible for milk production.

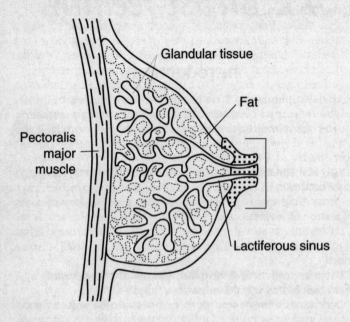

Fig 16   Cutaway of breast showing milk-producing glands

How soon after delivery is milk produced?

Soon after delivery, levels of oestrogen fall quite dramatically. This allows prolactin (the levels of which are already quite high) to stimulate production of milk. By forty-eight hours after delivery, milk starts to be produced and by the end of the fourth day, it is in full-flow.

Surely the baby cannot wait for forty-eight hours before starting to feed?

No; he or she does not have to. Shortly after delivery, the breasts produce a protein-rich fluid called colostrum. The baby can be put on the breast within minutes or hours of delivery and can feed on this. The act of suckling should actually be encouraged from as early as possible, because it positively facilitates milk production.

Are there any other important hormones in the production of milk?

Yes. Apart from prolactin, several other hormones play a lesser but still important role in milk production. They include insulin, cortisol, oxytocin and even thyroid hormones. Even oestrogen is important, in a negative way.

Oestrogen levels need to be low to facilitate the production and maintenance of lactation. This is why the use of the combined oral contraceptive pill (which contains oestrogen) and breast-feeding are incompatible.

So levels of the hormone prolactin have to remain high for milk production and breast-feeding to continue?

Surprisingly, no. After the first fourteen to sixteen weeks, the levels of this hormone fall to the non-pregnant level. However, as long as suckling is maintained, milk will continue to be produced.

Is there anything a mother should do to ensure adequate milk production?

Yes. Quite simply, she should ensure adequate fluid intake. The rest is sorted out by the interplay of the hormones in the body.

Feeding patterns

What is the "ideal" interval between feeds for a newborn?

In strict natural terms, feeding should be on demand. Hunger is a natural instinct and the baby will demand a feed whenever the need arises. This way, there is virtually no risk of overfeeding and, as long as the milk produced is adequate, no risk of underfeeding either. A new baby never demands a breast when he or she is not hungry and, even if it is offered in such circumstances, the tendency is for the baby to decline.

Is there any other acceptable feeding pattern apart from "on demand"?

Experience has shown that feeding every three to four hours roughly simulates the natural demand cycle and may be ideal for those mothers who want to fit feeding around their other activities. A mother should not expect the baby fed this way to be waiting contentedly for the regimented hour to strike. Rather, it is more of case of "where-have-you-been-all-this-time-Mummy-while-I-am-dying-of-hunger" wails. It does, however, work pretty well.

It is important for a new mother to know that roughly six hours out of every twenty-four will be spent on feeding the baby, whatever the method. This cumulative duration lessens gradually as the baby grows and is fed less frequently.

For a full-time working mother who wants to continue breast-feeding, are there any drawbacks?

A few. Firstly, it will most probably be necessary to mix artificial formula and breast-feeding. This is not considered ideal.

Secondly, the fact that there are prolonged periods without suckling will lead to reduced milk production. Suckling is crucial in maintaining milk production.

Thirdly, breast engorgement and considerable discomfort are inevitable with this kind of arrangement.

Is there any way around the problems mentioned above?

One can try. Expressed and stored milk to be used during the hours when mother is absent can reduce the need for formula feeding to a minimum. If the work environment allows, milk expressing can be done at work. This will help prevent engorgement and also maintain milk production.

How much milk is required by the baby per feed?

It has been calculated that, on average, a young baby requires 20 ml of milk per kilogram of body-weight. A baby weighing 5 kg (11 lb) will therefore need 100 ml per feed. Of course, there are considerable differences among babies.

What is the weight-change pattern of a newborn?

Virtually every mother knows that, after the birth the baby loses weight. The birth-weight is regained at around the end of the first week of life, though this may take slightly longer. Thereafter, at least for the ensuing three months, the baby gains an average of 30 grams per day. This means, in slightly over a month, the baby will put on a kilogram (2 lb) in weight. The weight doubles by three months of age and he or she will be three times the birth-weight by the time he or she is six to eight months old.

The benefits of breast-feeding

Why is breast-feeding encouraged so energetically?

Mother and baby bonding is quite clearly enhanced by this most natural of acts. But that is only one of the many benefits of breast-feeding.

What are the other benefits?

Human milk is natural and tailor-made for the human baby, so it has all the necessary ingredients in the right proportions.

Secondly, the act of suckling promotes contraction of the uterus and promotes its rapid reduction of size.

Thirdly, and most importantly, this milk is safe and virtually free. It is also convenient because it is readily available, clean and at the ideal temperature, thus avoiding the hassles of preparing a feed which characterize bottle-feeding.

Is it true that breast-milk has a protective element for the baby?

Yes. Both colostrum and breast-milk are rich in antibodies which provide the baby with passive immunity, thus protecting him or her against a variety of infections. There is evidence also that breast-fed babies are less prone to develop allergies.

Are there any direct benefits to the mother?

Yes. Apart from all the above, the mother may benefit directly in a number of ways.

Firstly, it allows for a more rapid return to a pre-pregnancy weight level.

Secondly, breast-feeding has a significant contraceptive effect, as it inhibits ovulation and therefore quite significantly reduces the chance of conceiving accidentally.

Thirdly, the risk of developing breast cancer later on in life is significantly reduced by breast-feeding.

Surely, from a nutritional point of view, bottle feeding cannot be inferior to breast-feeding?

Whichever way you look at it, it is. It is true that formula preparations have been altered to be as close to human milk as possible. Cow's milk has less vitamins A, B, C, D, & E, compared to human milk. Formula preparations are fortified with these vitamins to make up for the shortfall. However, the protective antibodies found in breast-milk are of vital importance. Also protective to the baby are a natural protein called lactoferrin and lysosomes (a form of protein which offers protection against a variety of bacterial and viral infections). All these cannot be found in cow's milk or formula preparations.

It appears from all this that bottle-feeding is dangerous?

Dangerous is an overstatement. However, it is important that a woman who can breast-feed is encouraged to do so by being made aware of the facts. However, if a woman is unable or unwilling to breast-feed then she should not be made to feel guilty. Formula preparations are an excellent substitute for breast-milk, even if not as good.

Physical concerns

There is usually some concern among women who have small breasts and who are going to be mothers for the first time about their ability to produce sufficient milk. What are the facts?

Breast size is a very poor guide to how much milk is going to be produced. Size is mainly determined by the proportion of breast tissue that is composed of fat (which has no function in milk production) rather than the milk-producing glandular tissue. The more fat there is in the breasts, the bigger the breasts.

Milk also continues to be produced during the actual action of suckling.

A woman with an ample chest should not take it for granted that she will flood the world with milk, nor should a not so well-endowed woman have sleepless nights worrying about starving her baby.

Another not uncommon concern is that breast-feeding may cause the breasts to change shape and be less firm as a consequence. Is this true?

In the Western world, the breast is established as a sexual organ. Keeping the breast as attractive to the opposite sex as possible is therefore an aspect that cannot be ignored. The idea that breast-feeding makes the breast sag is actually not based on fact. What is true is that pregnancy may bring about changes which may include increase in size, changes in shape and an appearance of reduced firmness. When these changes have occurred, breast-feeding will not make any difference. If the changes have not occurred with pregnancy, breast-feeding will not bring them about.

There is some truth in the contention that breast changes brought about by pregnancy are more pronounced in some races than others. Black women appear to have more pronounced changes while oriental women have the least; Caucasian women fall somewhere in between.

Cosmetic considerations should really not feature in deciding whether to breast-feed or not. It does not make any difference.

Are there any creams or lotions which can be used to ensure the breasts stay firm during pregnancy?

The changes to the breasts that occur during pregnancy are a direct effect of the hormones that are in high concentrations during pregnancy. The changes therefore come from within and applying anything to the skin outside will not make an iota of difference.

Feeding techniques

Regarding breast-feeding technique – how easy is it to master this?

It differs from person to person. In virtually every country in the world, midwives – or at least some of them – are trained to help first-time mothers master this art. To begin with, a midwife will ensure the baby is held properly to the breast

Incorrect latch

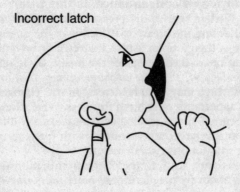

Correct latch

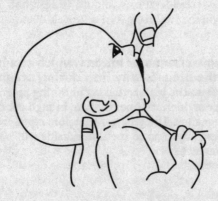

Fig 17 Breast-feeding – external of correct/incorrect latch

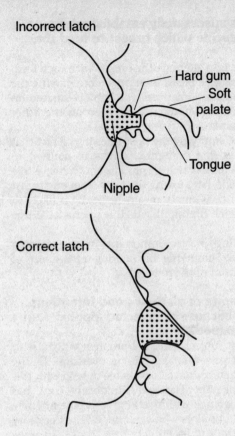

Incorrect latch

Hard gum

Soft palate

Tongue

Nipple

Correct latch

Fig 18 Cutaway showing incorrect latch (nipple on hard palate) and correct latch (nipple right down on soft palate)

and the appropriate amount of the breast is in the baby's mouth. This is commonly known as "fixing".

Sucking follows quite naturally after that. Once it is mastered, a woman often wonders what all the fuss was about. Mind you, the early process can be quite trying for some women, especially if there is also some delay in full milk flow and the baby is restless and irritable. Some women give up at this point. In virtually all maternity units, the proportion of mothers who are breast-feeding when discharged is smaller than that of those whose intention it was to breast-feed at delivery.

If breast-feeding is successfully established, how should a woman decide which breast to feed the baby on?

The standard advice is to alternate the breasts with each feed. It is important to ensure a breast is empty before moving the baby to the other breast. Sometimes, the baby is satiated on one breast, in which case he or she can feed on the other breast next time round.

The importance of emptying the breast lies in the fact that the milk that comes first (fore-milk) differs in content to hind-milk. The fore-milk is rich in protein and water, while the hind-milk is rich in fat. Moving the baby from one breast to the other before one is empty means he or she is likely to miss out on the fat-rich hind-milk which is so crucial at this stage of life.

Complete emptying is also important in maintaining lactation. Incomplete emptying has a long-term effect of reducing the amount of milk produced.

Some women, in spite of all their good intentions, fail to breast-feed because of inverted nipples. Can these women be helped?

This is an important subject. This is a problem which, with the right help and perseverance, can be overcome in the majority of cases. There are devices available to help with this problem. In the UK, the National Childbirth Trust has excelled in helping women with this kind of problem. There are breast-feeding counsellors who can offer all the necessary help, and all maternity units provide this service. In most countries, this kind of help is readily available. In developing countries, breast-feeding remains the norm and therefore the problem is rare.

In developed countries, there is some kind of paradox in that affluent middle-class women are more likely to breast-feed than women who are less well-off. Why is this?

This trend is true and is quite probably an indictment of public education in these countries. It almost certainly means the message is not getting through to the less well-off and that strategies in mass education need reappraisal to see what is being done wrong. However, the pattern is really one facet in a complex socio-economic picture and there cannot be an easy or quick fix.

Another disincentive to breast-feeding is the fact that breast-feeding in public is frowned upon, especially in the West.

This is a result of cultural trends. There have been attempts to overcome this difficulty. Most departmental stores and even some workplaces now provide mother and baby facilities, which include purpose-made areas for feeding babies. It may be a little harder on a public bus, where some people may feel inclined to disapprove, quietly or otherwise. It must be said that this antipathy is baseless and illogical but it is also a fact of life.

How long should a woman breast-feed for?

There can never be any hard and fast rules about this. Food supplements can be introduced into the baby's diet at about ten weeks but these should be in the form of fluids only, such as clear fluid and diluted fruit juice. Even though the gut can handle "soft" solids at this stage, these should not be introduced until around fourteen to sixteen weeks. Breast-milk is more than adequate for the first three months of life and therefore the need to wean a baby before then is simply not there.

Some women will wean the baby off the breast completely by six months, others at twelve months. Most will have stopped by eighteen to twenty-four months. Every individual should decide on the best arrangement in her case.

A baby is quite ready to be fed on full-cream cow's milk (not formula) by the age of twelve months. Skimmed milk should not be used.

44. Breast-feeding and taking medicine

Introduction

If a breast-feeding mother is prescribed any medicine, the fact that she is breast-feeding has to be taken into account. Many types of medicines do find their way (through the mother's bloodstream) into breast-milk. This means the baby will suckle the medicine.

There are three broad questions. Will the medicine affect the taste of the milk? Does the baby need this medicine? What effect does the medicine have on the baby?

In the section below we have attempted to cover as wide a range of common and not-so-common medicines as possible in answering these questions.

There are types of medicines that are clearly incompatible with breast-feeding. This is usually because of the potential of harming the baby. A few types change the taste of the milk, something that may lead to the baby declining the breast and consequently going hungry. Many other types of medicine are perfectly safe for the baby and have no effect on the taste of the milk.

For some, the effect is unknown and the advice is to stop breast-feeding, at least for the duration of the medication course.

Any breast-feeding mother should read the instruction leaflet accompanying the medicine, be it prescription or over-the-counter. If that information is missing (and if it is not covered here), then the doctor should be asked to provide this vital information.

The effects on babies

Should one be concerned about taking prescription or non-prescription medicine while breast-feeding?

Yes. Most drugs (medicine) do get into breast-milk. The quantities that get there range from insignificant to concentrated. Of course, some of these drugs are completely harmless to the baby. A breast-feeding woman should always check the safety of any drug, be it prescription or "over-the-counter", for compatibility with breast-feeding. We shall discuss the most common categories of drugs below.

Why would harmless drugs (to adults) suddenly be potentially harmful to babies?

Part of the reason is the fact that a baby's metabolism is still immature and therefore its ability to break down chemicals is not up to scratch. This means an otherwise innocent drug can accumulate to dangerous concentrations in the baby's system.

Antibiotics

What about antibiotics?

This is a vast group of drugs: some of which are quite harmless, some potentially harmful and others outright dangerous and therefore contraindicated.

- Penicillins: this group of antibiotics is harmless for use with breast-feeding. Penicillins appear in very low concentrations in breast-milk. Moreover, even high concentrations appear to be harmless to babies. The same applies to cephalosporins, erythromycin and trimethoprim.

  If antibiotics are prescribed to a breast-feeding mother, she should check whether they fall into any of these groups. If they do, there is no need to worry about taking them.

- Metronidazole: popularly known as flagyl. It is considered to be safe. Metronidazole, however, has a reputation of rendering breast-milk bitter. The baby may therefore not be too keen.

- Tetracyclines: even though tetracyclines appear in low concentration in breast-milk, they tend to be deposited in bone, and they may interfere with the growth of bones. In addition, deposition in tooth buds may lead to permanent discoloration of teeth. They are contraindicated.

- Gentamicin and other aminoglycosides: this group of antibiotics is only used in serious infections in hospital. They are given through the intravenous route. Only low concentrations appear in breast-milk. Moreover, absorption from the gut is poor. For all these reasons, they are considered safe with breast-feeding. However, they may cause diarrhoea in the baby, which is very rarely serious.

- Chloramphenicol: even though it appears in low concentration in breast-milk, it still has a potential of causing bone-marrow suppression in the baby. Moreover, in most cases there are safer alternatives. The general counsel is to avoid it if breast-feeding.

- Ciprofloxacin: this is one antibiotic that is considered to be definitely toxic. It should be avoided if breast-feeding. If it is necessary to use it, then breast-feeding needs to be suspended during its use and for at least forty-eight hours after the last dose, to allow the drug to be eliminated from the mother's system.

- Anti-TB medication: if the mother is on anti-tuberculosis medication, including Isoniazid, Rifampicin and Ethambutol, she should continue, as these are known to be safe for the baby. There is therefore no justification to prohibit breast-feeding in such a case.

- Sulphonamides: these could be prescribed on their own or as part of a combination (such as with septrin). These are regarded as safe unless the baby is premature or jaundiced, in which case they are best avoided.

Acyclovir is an antiviral preparation used for such conditions as "fever blisters" (cold sores) and genital herpes. Is it safe?

Even though some acyclovir will be found in breast-milk, it is safe for the baby, so treatment should continue, together with breast-feeding.

Antimalarials

If living or travelling to tropical countries where malaria is endemic, is Chloroquine safe to use?

Yes. So is Proguanil, another common antimalarial.

What about Mefloquine?

There is really no information as to its potential effects on the baby. However, on the basis of side-effects associated with it in adults, the advice is to avoid if breast-feeding.

Antacids and ulcer drugs

Antacids are used for peptic ulcers or even heartburn. Are they safe?

Most of them are safe but a breast-feeding woman should ensure she reads the manufacturers' recommendation, since new ones are continually coming out and this opinion is by no means universal.

What about drugs such as Zantac?

Zantac – the generic name of which is ranitidine – is the most widely used drug in the world for peptic ulcers. It is one of a group of drugs known as H2-receptor antagonists. Others include Cimetidine (tagamet). These are known to be safe and breast-feeding should continue.

What about Omeprazole (losec)?

This is also a popular drug used for peptic ulcers or simple heartburn. It is also known to be safe.

Anti-emetics

In case of nausea or vomiting, Metoclopromide (maxolon) is commonly prescribed. Is it safe?

Metoclopromide is one of the few drugs that are actually concentrated in breast-milk. It can make the baby sleepy but no other adverse effect has ever been reported. Since it is usually used for a very short time, the advice is to err on the side of caution by suspending breast-feeding during its use.

What about the other drugs used for nausea and vomiting such as Prochlorperazine (stemetil) or cyclizine?

Information as to their effects is not available and therefore they are rarely prescribed to breast-feeding mothers. When they are, breast-feeding will often be suspended.

Laxatives

Laxative use may be necessary sometimes while breast-feeding. What about them?

There are two broad categories of laxatives: those that are absorbed and those that are not (bulk laxatives).

Bulk laxatives are safe (they won't get to the baby in any way) but absorbable laxatives should always be avoided. The mother should check which category the prescribed laxative falls into.

Painkillers

Painkillers are often necessary. Which are safe and which aren't?

Paracetamol is the most common painkiller. It is found in very small quantities in breast-milk and there is no risk of it accumulating in the baby's circulation. It is safe.

Aspirin is a good analgesic but its use with breast-feeding is not advised. This is because modest amounts are found in milk and concentrations in the baby could reach a high level. There is a risk, admittedly exceedingly small, of Reye's syndrome, which causes brain and liver damage. This condition though rare, is extremely dangerous and could be fatal.

What about Diclofenac (voltarol)?

This is safe to use while breast-feeding. So are Ibuprofen (brufen) and mefenamic acid.

What about Indomethacin?

One of the more common painkillers and anti-inflammatories, Indomethacin is probably safe. However, because of its potency, if used, the baby should be observed carefully for any possible adverse effects.

Suppose strong painkillers such as morphine or pethidine need to be used?

This will almost certainly be for a very short time, probably twenty-four hours or less.

In normal doses and for such limited use, morphine is perfectly safe.

When pethidine is administered, the baby should be observed closely if being breast-fed, because he or she may become drowsy. This is accentuated by the fact that the drug is not eliminated from the baby's body as efficiently and effects tend to linger.

What about codeine?

Even though it is found in breast-milk, this is in an insignificantly low concentration. It is therefore considered safe to use if breast-feeding. However, some babies have been reported to become markedly sedated for prolonged periods, which could be worrying to the parents. The mother may wish to look for an alternative which doesn't produce this effect. Another painkiller called fentanyl is also safe.

Abused drugs

What about methadone?

This is almost exclusively used by those drug-dependents whose habit is being controlled with the eventual aim of trying to cure it. There has been one reported case of sudden infant death syndrome (cot death). Whether this was directly or indirectly associated with maternal use of methadone is not clear. Generally, if used in prescribed doses, methadone is theoretically safe to use while breast-feeding.

What if a person is abusing opiates such as heroin (diamorphine)?

In that case, breast-feeding should be avoided. Respiratory depression is a risk. The baby ought to be protected from the ravages of addiction and consequent severe withdrawal symptoms.

Anti-clotting drugs

What about drugs used in thrombosis?

Heparin is given in the form of injection. It does not appear in breast-milk at all and is therefore perfectly safe. The advice regarding newer forms of heparin-related drugs is more cautious and most manufacturers advise avoiding it if breast-feeding.

Warfarin is taken orally. It appears in breast-milk in insignificant quantities. It is safe.

Antidepressants

What about drugs used for depression?

The older antidepressants such as imipramine are probably safe as, in spite of long-term and widespread use, no adverse effect has been reported. However, small amounts appear in breast-milk and, because of their sedative effect, they can potentially cause infant drowsiness. Caution should therefore be exercised.

Prozac (fluoxetine) is now more popular and almost certainly more effective. There is insufficient information to give informed advice. Where it has been used, infant irritability and little else has been reported occasionally. If it is necessary to use it, then caution is advised.

What about diazepam, temazepam and the other related sedatives?

These drugs, when prescribed for anxiety, should be used only when absolutely necessary and the baby should be carefully observed. If they are to be used long-term, then it is probably best to stop breast-feeding. There is a real risk of accumulation and subsequent withdrawal symptoms. If temazepam is being abused, then breast-feeding is definitely contraindicated.

Anti-psychotics

What about those who suffer from puerperal psychosis and who are put on anti-psychotics such as haloperidol?

Anti-psychotics, including Haloperidol, Chlorpromazine and Flupenthixol, are found in small amounts in breast-milk. Caution regarding breast-feeding will be part of the management strategy of this difficult condition.

"Cytotoxics"

What if somebody is taking anti-cancer drugs?

If one is taking cytotoxic drugs for cancer treatment, breast-feeding should be avoided.

Organ transplant

Organ transplant is usually followed by long-term use of immuno-suppressant drugs. What is the advice in such a case?

Few women become pregnant following organ transplantation, especially of the kidneys. Breast-feeding should be avoided in women who are on drugs such as Cyclosporin or Azathioprine. In most cases, lengthy counselling will have taken place even prior to conception and such an individual is likely to be already well informed in these matters.

Hypertension

What if a newly delivered mother is taking antihypertensives?

Treatment for raised blood pressure is quite varied after delivery. Many drugs that are unsafe to use in pregnancy are perfectly acceptable with breast-feeding. Popular antihypertensive drugs that are known to be safe with breast-feeding include beta-blockers (such as Atenolol and Labetalol), Nifedipine, Hydralazine, Captopril and Methyl-dopa.

What about diuretics?

The popular diuretic Frusemide (lasix) is safe with breast-feeding.

Thiazide diuretics, on the other hand, have a potential for suppressing lactation, especially in high doses. These should be avoided whenever possible. They include bendrofluazide and clorothiazide.

Asthma drugs

What about drugs used for asthma?

Salbutamol and Terbutaline, the most common drugs used for asthma, are safe.

Theophylline and Aminophylline may cause mild infant irritability but are generally safe.

"Heart" drugs

What about digoxin?

Some people with heart trouble are prescribed long-term digoxin. This is safe.

Does the same apply to amiodarone?

No. Amiodarone contains iodine and is therefore unsafe to use if breast-feeding.

Epilepsy drugs

Epilepsy needs continuous treatment. What is the status of anti-epileptics regarding breast-feeding?

The most common anti-epileptics (or anticonvulsants, as they are better known) include Phenytoin, Carbamazepine and Sodium valproate. These are known to be safe. Phenytoin very occasionally causes sedation of the baby. If this happens, temporary suspension of breast-feeding is advised. If, on resuming breast-feeding thirty-six to forty-eight hours later, the problem recurs, then options should be re-evaluated.

Ethosuximide, another anticonvulsant, should not be used with breast-feeding. It causes hyper-excitability in the baby.

Newer anti-epileptics, including Vigabatrin and Lamotrigine, remain an unknown quantity as far as breast-feeding is concerned. The mother will need to make a choice between breast-feeding and using the drug. If she is keen to breast-feed and she is on one of these, then she will need to liaise with her doctor to explore the possibility of being switched to another drug of proven safety.

Itchiness

Skin itchiness is commonly treated with antihistamine preparations, which are sometimes available over the counter. Are these safe?

Orally taken antihistamines pass into breast-milk in small quantities. They may cause short-lived infant irritability but are generally safe to use.

Cough medicine

Cough preparations are available over the counter. Can they be used while breast-feeding?

Always check what a cough syrup contains. Those containing iodine – and there are several – should be avoided. Iodine is concentrated in breast-milk and there is a real risk of causing neonatal hypothyroidism, even goitre.

Migraine

Migraine is commonly treated with drugs made of or containing ergotamine. Is this safe with breast-feeding?

No. Ergotamine and breast-feeding should not be mixed. The drug, which passes into breast-milk, could cause infant vomiting and diarrhoea. More seriously, it could cause convulsions.

Contraceptives

Regarding contraception, where does "the pill" stand?

The combined pill containing both oestrogen and progesterone cannot be used for contraception if one is to breast-feed. This is not because of any direct adverse effect to the baby. Rather, it is because the oestrogen component of the pill will drastically reduce lactation, making breast-feeding impractical.

The progesterone-only pill, popularly known as the "mini-pill", is OK to use and is one of the recommended contraceptives for those who want to breast-feed.

Endometriosis

What about Danazol, used to treat endometriosis?

Danazol cannot be used during the period of breast-feeding. In any case, the need will not arise, since endometriosis goes into remission during pregnancy and this remission is sustained during the period of breast-feeding.

45. From the community

Introduction

Being hospital-based obstetricians, when we started compiling these questions – mostly from mothers we met in the course of our job – we realized that however comprehensive our list might be, something little but significant just might not be there. There are questions that we are quite plausibly not asked because of our setting, the hospital ward and clinic. Because of this, we approached national organizations that are dedicated to helping people with various pregnancy-related problems. Some of them responded positively by compiling lists of the most asked questions for us.

When you go through these questions, you realize how enriching this strand is. The questions have a decidedly "community" rather than clinical flavour. We have included them here because they give a different perspective to the subjects dealt with. We believe they will be eye-opening to many readers and may provide answers to questions that have been there in the backs of their minds.

The contact addresses of the organizations have been provided at the end of each section. There is, of course, a separate section subsequently of the various other organizations that deal with other pregnancy-associated problems. Wherever possible, a helpline number has been given as well.

Pre-eclampsia

Below are some of the frequently asked questions as compiled by "Action on Pre-eclampsia" (APEC). The association is a registered national charity, which provides support and information on all aspects of pre-eclampsia. Their contact address, e-mail and telephone numbers are given at the end of this section.

What is pre-eclampsia?

This is a pregnancy complication, which is mainly characterized by raised blood pressure (hypertension). Other features include a loss of protein in the urine and usually, but not necessarily, there is oedema or swelling, which may be generalized. A pre-eclampsia patient will therefore commonly have swollen feet, hands and even a puffy face. This condition can affect any pregnant woman but is more common in the first pregnancy or in a subsequent pregnancy in the case of a change of partner. Untreated, it can have severe consequences, including loss of the baby and even imperilling the mother's own life. One of its later complications is eclampsia (seizures), hence its name. The seizures are similar to "grand mal" epilepsy.

My mother or sister had pre-eclampsia. Does this mean I am likely to get it?

There is no evidence of a genetic tendency for this condition. As such, a family history cannot be regarded as a risk factor for pre-eclampsia.

How can I stop myself getting pre-eclampsia?

Pre-eclampsia cannot be predicted before conception. There are women who are at increased risk of developingpre-eclampsia. These include women who have a pre-existing hypertensive condition and those with such diseases as SLE. A good control of their respective conditions during pregnancy is a good thing, but even that does not influence their chances of their getting pre-eclampsia as the pregnancy advances. For the rest of the female population, there are no known ways of reducing or eliminating the chances of getting pre-eclampsia. It is important not to lose sight of the fact that pre-eclampsia is a relatively uncommon pregnancy complication, affecting roughly one in twenty pregnancies.

I have been told that my blood pressure is high. Can I bring it down by resting?

Unless the physical activities that you are engaged in are causing stress, rest will not lower blood pressure. If enforced inactivity is actually making you restless, it may end up causing a rise in the blood pressure. Bed-rest is recommended in moderate and severe pre-eclampsia primarily as a measure to optimize blood supply to the uterus and ultimately to the fetus. In pre-eclampsia, one of the most significant abnormalities is the reduction in the circulating maternal blood volume. Vigorous physical activities will inevitably shunt blood to the active muscle groups, which may reduce blood getting to the uterus to precarious levels. Bed-rest is meant to prevent this but it will not directly cause reduction in blood pressure.

Why do I need to go into hospital? I can rest much better at home.

The progression of pre-eclampsia is unpredictable. With some, the course is slow, over many weeks, even allowing for getting to term and spontaneous labour and delivery. For others it is quite different, with dramatic progression forcing an intervention and preterm delivery in a matter of days, sometimes by caesarean section.

In the early days after diagnosis, if the doctors are unsure as to the course your condition is going to take, they may play it safe and keep you in hospital for close monitoring. There may also be concerns about the fetal well-being and you may be detained in hospital for this reason. You will not be kept in hospital purely for bed-rest. When the condition is stable, the practice is to manage you at home, where you may be advised to rest and the community midwife will visit at scheduled intervals to do the necessary measurements and tests. The visits may range from daily to once or twice a week, depending on the degree of severity.

I had pre-eclampsia in my last pregnancy. Will I get it again?

For the majority, the answer here is that it is unlikely. On average, less than a quarter of those who have pre-eclampsia have a recurrence in subsequent pregnancies. Most cases of pre-eclampsia occur in the first pregnancy. However, when it occurs for the first time in a later pregnancy, the risk of recurrence subsequently is increased, probably to one in two. This may be because there is a latent hypertensive disease, where the pregnancy is only helping to unmask it. Such people should also be counselled of an increased possibility of chronic hypertension later on in life, to enable an effective surveillance and early diagnosis, if this turns out to be the case. As you can see, no standard answer can be given to this question. Each individual's chances of a recurrence should be quantified on the basis of her circumstances.

If I have pre-eclampsia, will I need to be induced or have a caesarean section?

When you have this condition, the chances of having labour induced or having a caesarean section are increased quite considerably. It is important to remember two things: one, that there is no cure for pre-eclampsia. The only effective and definitive treatment is delivery. Two, that all the measures taken during pregnancy are meant to lead to a stage when delivery can be achieved, ideally without putting the baby in jeopardy but with the mother's well-being remaining the primary priority. If the condition appears to be getting out of control, delivery will have to be effected. If induction of labour is deemed to be feasible and it won't cause undue delay, this may be opted for. If not, then caesarean section will be advised. On the other hand, things may remain under control and you may get to term and go into labour spontaneously, thus obviating the need for intervention.

Will my baby be all right?

Pre-eclampsia will not have any direct effect on the fetus as such. However, because of its effect on the circulation, the baby's growth may be restricted and it may be small. Moreover, there is an increased risk of premature delivery, usually as a result of intervention on the part of doctors. This is done to save the mother or the growth-restricted baby, sometimes both. Babies born small or prematurely (or both) suffer more illness. Pre-eclampsia does not cause abnormalities.

My doctor disagrees with my midwife about how often I need to be monitored. Who is right?

When such disagreements occur, the patient feels trapped in the middle and it can be alarming. Fortunately, this is uncommon. Any monitoring regime should be individualized. If, for instance, you have a blood pressure that has remained more or less stable over three or four weeks and there is little change in the test results, both of your blood and urine and the pregnancy is also progressing satisfactorily, you can be managed at home with the midwife going to check your blood pressure and urine once, at most twice a week. On the other hand, if your blood pressure is fluctuating, and therefore unpredictable and there is significant loss of protein in the urine and the fetal growth rate is also sub-optimal, the monitoring may be more intensive. An allowance may be made for you to stay at home, on the proviso that you rest and the midwife comes to see you daily. In addition, arrangements may be made for you to go to the hospital once or more every week for special monitoring of the baby. As you can see, there is a lot of room for individual tailoring of the monitoring regime. As such, sometimes the professionals differ in opinion on the suitability of a particular regime for a particular patient. If this happens, you should insist on knowing why a particular regime is recommended and not "the other".

Are there any long-term effects for me?

No. Once the pregnancy ends, in a few days at most, the syndrome of pre-eclampsia will also come to an end. Pre-eclampsia may affect various organs in the body but virtually all these effects are reversible. These organs' functions return to normal within days of delivery. In very rare cases, there could be neurological abnormalities that persist beyond this stage. If pre-eclampsia has led to brain haemorrhage (stroke), the damage may be lasting. This is very rare.

Is there any way of preventing pre-eclampsia from recurring?

There is no known effective way of doing this. You can only go on statistics, which indicate that your chances of having a recurrence are less than even for the majority of women.

Why wasn't I warned about pre-eclampsia before I got it?

It will almost certainly be because it could not be predicted in your case. There are many potential complications in pregnancy and pre-eclampsia is one of them. Since it affects only about 5 per cent of pregnant women, it means it is really of little or no interest to the remaining 95 per cent or nineteen out of every twenty. It is difficult to know who will be affected because the majority of women who get it will have no single identifiable risk factor. It is therefore unreasonable to "warn" every single pregnant woman about pre-eclampsia. This will amount to scare-mongering. Those with the known risk factors – such as pre-existing hypertension, certain kidney diseases and SLE – will almost certainly be counselled about pre-eclampsia. Information about pre-eclampsia is also available in the form of leaflets in virtually all antenatal clinics.

Why don't doctors know more about pre-eclampsia?

Doctors know a great deal about pre-eclampsia, but probably not the crucial facts as far as the patient is concerned. Over the years, there has been a great deal of research about this condition. Two main things remain elusive: what actually causes it and how to cure the condition during pregnancy.

Where can I get expert advice about my next pregnancy?

If you suffered from pre-eclampsia in your last pregnancy, your obstetrician in hospital will in most cases give you a postnatal appointment to discuss your future plans and what that may entail. This will normally be arranged for six to eight weeks after delivery. Part of the advice will be to ensure that you are bookedin early in your next pregnancy, so as to get the baseline measurements of your blood pressure and other things. That will also serve as an opportunity to go through the information that you have, to ensure that you are properly informed.

How can I persuade my doctor to offer me special care in my next pregnancy?

You don't need to. The reason why the postnatal session with your obstetrician is essential is to get all the necessary information about what the future holds. This will ensure that all those unfounded fears are banished. Appropriate care, which will chiefly consist of early booking and proper and appropriate regular surveillance, are all that is needed. This will ensure that if and when you do get a recurrence, the necessary action can be taken promptly. Remember, it is still an "if". As for the "when", it is also worthwhile knowing that pre-eclampsia, for the majority, is a disease of the second half of pregnancy.

I have had pre-eclampsia for the second time. Why wasn't I warned I could get it again?

When you have suffered from pre-eclampsia, part of the postnatal information that will be given is the roughly estimated risk of a recurrence. This is very crude and is nowhere near accurate. If, indeed this information was not given, then that is a significant omission. Sometimes, the information may take the form of, "Oh, it is unlikely that it will happen again," which is factually correct but which may have been taken to mean that it could never happen. It is important to ensure that the mother and the doctor are on the same wavelength when discussing such important matters.

Why does changing your partner make a difference?

It is a known fact that some women who have had problem-free pregnancies in the past suddenly develop pre-eclampsia when they conceive following a change of partner. Why this is the case is not clearly understood. However, the hypothesis goes to the suspected root cause of the problem, which is thought to be immunological. The interaction of maternal and paternal immunological factors in the placenta may lead to conditions that are conducive for pre-eclampsia to develop. While the former partner may not produce this reaction, the subsequent partner, purely by chance, may produce the ideal conditions for this to happen.

Yes, it is true that a change of partner may lead to pre-eclampsia for one who has not suffered it before, but it is not, strictly speaking, a risk factor. It is purely chance. Some women go through five or six partners, each union blessed with a child or two, with not so much as a whiff of hypertension.

Giving credence to the immunological interaction hypothesis is the fact that unions between very close blood relatives (consanguineous) very rarely lead to pre-eclampsia. . . not that we are suggesting anything!

Why did I get pre-eclampsia in my second or third pregnancy and not my first?

There is the issue of changed partner discussed above. If that does not apply to you, it may be that you are one of those with latent hypertension, where the pregnancy has just helped to unmask it through pre-eclampsia. This is plausible because the condition, even in its latent form, may not have developed yet in the first pregnancy, especially if there is a gap of a few years. Another aspect may be the type of pregnancy: are you carrying twins this time around? It is a known fact that multiple pregnancy increases the risk of pre-eclampsia. In other cases, an explanation remains elusive.

Should I warn my younger sister that she is at risk?

No. The evidence that this condition may run in families is very weak. Such advice would be misguided. Her chances of getting the complication are the average one in twenty, unless she has a specific risk factor. Being your sister is not one of them.

Will my daughter get it when she becomes pregnant?

Again, the answer should be in the negative. Your daughter will not be at increased risk of getting pre-eclampsia by virtue of being your daughter, with your history of pre-eclampsia during your pregnancy.

The contact address for **Action on Pre-eclampsia (APEC)** is:
31–33 College Road,
Harrow, MIDDX HA1 1EJ
Tel: 0208-427 4217 (Helpline)
Fax: 0208-424 0653
Email: apec@dial.pipex.com

Miscarriage

Below are some of the most asked questions as compiled by the Miscarriage Association. The association is a registered national charity, which provides support and information on all aspects of pregnancy loss. The contact address and telephone and fax numbers are given at the end of this section.

I miscarried at ten weeks but nobody seems able to tell me why it happened. Saying it is "just one of those things" doesn't help. I desperately need some answers but feel no one is bothering to find out what caused it.

The loss of your baby will never feel like "just one of those things". Sadly, despite the fact that around one in four pregnancies end in miscarriage, there is still much that we don't know about why miscarriages happen. Most women who miscarry go on to have a healthy pregnancy, so single miscarriages are rarely investigated and tests are usually carried out only on women who have had three or more consecutive miscarriages. Even then, many investigations fail to come up with an obvious and treatable cause.

Probably half of all early miscarriages – those in the first twelve weeks – are caused by a chromosome abnormality. This is usually a random event and is unlikely to happen again. Other possible causes are hormonal imbalance, problems in the immune system, infections and abnormalities or weakness of the uterus or cervix. Diet, smoking, alcohol and other environmental factors are also thought to have a part to play.

After trying for a baby for the last year, my pregnancy ended at just eight weeks in a miscarriage. It is now three months on and I still feel such a tremendous sense of loss. I know my partner feels I should be putting it behind me but I feel overwhelmed by the sadness of it all and unable to move on.

The sadness of miscarriage can be overwhelming, and especially so when it has been difficult to conceive and when the joy turns so quickly into sorrow. Many women find that they cope well in the first days or weeks, but seem to grieve more as time goes on and others, including partners, find it hard to understand.

Sometimes grief is sharpened by the return of menstruation: a reminder both of no longer being pregnant and of the miscarriage itself. Sometimes it is simply the approach of certain dates, such as the baby's calculated due date or an event you might have anticipated attending in maternity clothes. The progress of a friend's or relative's pregnancy can also be hard to cope with.

It may help if you can express your sadness openly – either to someone who understands, or in a poem or letter. Tangible memories can also help – perhaps planting a rose bush at home or in a garden of remembrance. Your sorrow will lessen as time goes on, even though you may always miss your baby.

How long after a miscarriage should you wait before trying for another baby? Everyone tells me something different.

The most crucial factor is how you and your partner feel, emotionally and physically. Assuming you are physically well, it is probably advisable to wait until you have had one period – usually four to six weeks after a miscarriage – before trying again. Having a date for your period makes it easier to estimate the development of a subsequent pregnancy. If you do become pregnant before this, however, there is no evidence that you are more likely to miscarry.

I have just had a miscarriage and I am so scared of getting pregnant again. Is there something I can do to make sure it doesn't happen again?

Pregnancy after a miscarriage can be a very anxious time, especially as there is no formula that will guarantee a healthy pregnancy. Do remember, though, that you are more likely to have a healthy pregnancy than another miscarriage, even if you have had several losses. Good care and support from your GP and perhaps an early scan can reduce anxiety and some research suggests that this in itself may be good for you and your baby.

In general it is a good idea to aim for a healthy diet and lifestyle both before conception and during pregnancy. Don't eat unpasteurized dairy products, such as Brie and Camembert, pâté or foods made with raw eggs. Ensure that meat is well cooked and fruit and salad vegetables thoroughly washed, and follow the Department of Health guidelines on taking folic acid. Try not to smoke and it is probably best to avoid alcohol, too, although an occasional glass of wine is not harmful.

I read in the paper that taking junior aspirin prevents miscarriage. Is this true?

Low-dose aspirin, often combined with another drug called heparin, is proving to be an effective treatment for women whose miscarriages are caused by a particular disorder of the immune system. It will not help in other situations, so don't take aspirin regularly unless it has been prescribed. If you have recurrent miscarriage, ask your doctor if you can be referred to a specialist centre for investigations and ask if they are testing for immune disorders. The Miscarriage Association has information on hospitals providing specialist facilities for recurrent miscarriages in the UK.

How long should I bleed after a miscarriage?

This differs from person to person and is influenced by a few factors. Generally, if this was an early miscarriage and was complete – that is, no products of conception were retained in the womb – the bleeding should last as long as a period, more or less. The average is five to seven days. As a rule in such circumstances, the bleeding continually subsides with each passing day. On the other hand, if the miscarriage was incomplete and a surgical evacuation was performed promptly, the bleeding period could be shortened to two or three days. Another scenario is where the miscarriage is incomplete but conservative management is opted for – that is, no evacuation is done. In such a case, the bleeding could be slightly longer, probably a week or more, but continues to be lighter with each passing day. Heavy bleeding days after a miscarriage usually indicates that some action is required, normally an evacuation.

Was the miscarriage my fault?

Miscarriage as a result of what the mother did is an exceedingly rare thing to happen. Many women ask whether it was because they had sex shortly before it happened. The answer here is invariably no. Some women will point to a physical activity they engaged in prior to the event such as hoovering, dancing etc. Again, the answer here is no. None of these can lead to a miscarriage. Still others question their lifestyle. Smoking has been associated with increased risk of miscarriage, but it is difficult to point to it as a direct cause. It is possible that, in the presence of another unfavourable factor, such as an immune disorder, smoking may tip the balance towards a miscarriage. There is no evidence that alcohol bingeing can lead to a miscarriage, even though it can have other very harmful effects on the fetus.

Will bed-rest help prevent a miscarriage?

In the olden days, bed-rest used to be suggested as a way of preventing miscarriage. There is really no evidence that it can do that. It will only be useful if you feel that you are physically stressed and you feel that a stint of bed-rest will alleviate this. For some people, bed-rest itself may cause psychological stress because it is so alien to their norm. Such people should avoid it as much as possible.

Is it true that, following a miscarriage, if I don't have a D&C, I will get an infection?

There is no truth in this at all. If, following a miscarriage, a clinical assessment indicates that conservative management is appropriate, then this is completely acceptable – even advantageous. There is no more risk of infection with this form of management when compared to a D&C (evacuation of the uterus). Sometimes a short course of antibiotics may be prescribed as a precaution if there is deemed to be a risk of infection. This is not common.

What is a blighted ovum?

This is a form of early pregnancy complication where there is no embryo growing. Instead, the gestational sac's contents are only water. Because the pregnancy tissue that produces the pregnancy hormone is growing normally, the woman may not be aware that there is anything amiss until eight to twelve weeks into the pregnancy. The most common warning sign is usually light vaginal bleeding, normally painless. An ultrasound scan will confirm the diagnosis. Why a baby fails to develop in such cases is poorly understood. It does not tend to recur.

The scan showed the baby was smaller than they think it should be. Why do I have to wait another two weeks before they do something?

For doctors to know for sure whether the apparent smaller-than-normal size is genuine, they need to track the rate of growth. For this, a minimum interval of two weeks between scans is absolutely necessary. If this was your first scan, it may be that your dates were incorrect or that you conceived much later than your dates suggest. A normal growth rate, as shown on a follow-up scan, will be a reassuring finding. This reassurance cannot be confidently given if the repeat scan is performed earlier than two weeks.

Do you advise having hormone injections? My doctor won't prescribe them but my friend had them and then had a baby.

Hormone injections because of a previous history of miscarriage are of no proven benefit. Research has shown that they do not improve the outcome. Historically these hormones were given on the assumption that these unexplained recurrent miscarriages were probably because of a deficiency of the crucial hormone that sustains the pregnancy in the early phase. This has been proven not to be the case. Any doctor who prescribes these is duty-bound to inform the woman about these scientific facts. A successful conclusion to a pregnancy where these hormones had been used may be ascribed to them, but this is a dubious claim indeed.

Can I insist on having investigations?

Investigations for recurrent miscarriage are notorious for drawing a blank. However, these will always be done after three or more consecutive miscarriages. They may be launched even after two when time is at a premium, i.e. in the older mother. It is different when it is an isolated miscarriage because the chances are that all will be well next time around. Demanding investigations into sporadic miscarriages, where there may be three or more, interspersed in normal full-term pregnancies, may also be misguided. This is because the specific investigations will almost certainly not be relevant to your situation. If the doctor is declining to perform investigations for you, there is usually an explanation for this and this ought to be given to your satisfaction.

I am having pain and vaginal bleeding. Am I miscarrying?

Pain in the lower part of the abdomen and vaginal bleeding are the main symptoms of an impending miscarriage or one that is already taking place. However, it is important to stress that isolated abdominal pain is rarely a sign of an impending miscarriage. Pain that is localized and continuous may be a sign of an ectopic pregnancy. Such a symptom needs to be investigated promptly. Painless vaginal bleeding is also regarded as a sign of threatened miscarriage. However, most of these will resolve and carry on as normal. Moreover, vaginal bleeding in pregnancy does not necessarily come from inside the uterus. It may be from the neck of the womb (cervix), especially if the bleeding was provoked by sexual intercourse. Such bleeding poses hardly any danger to the pregnancy. Again, this needs to be verified by a proper examination.

The **Miscarriage Association** can be reached at:
Miscarriage Association
C/o Clayton Hospital
Northgate
Wakefield
West Yorkshire
WF1 3JS
Tel: 01924-200 799 (Helpline)
Fax: 01924-298 834

Postnatal illness

This is a contribution from the Association for Postnatal Illness. This is a registered charity, which provides support to mothers suffering from the various types of postnatal illness. It is also aimed at increasing public awareness of the illness, and encourages research into the subject. Its services are free and an address and contact number are provided at the end of this section.

Baby "blues"

What are "baby blues" and how common is the problem?

This is the state of being emotional and upset, sometimes crying for no apparent reason, that many women experience three to four days after delivery. It affects up to 50 per cent of all mothers: that is, one in two. It is therefore a very common problem.

Some mothers with the "blues" will find that minor problems make them worry a great deal. Sometimes a mother feels just unwell with ill-defined pain. She tends to feel tired and lethargic most of the time. She may have difficulty sleeping.

What might be the causes of the "blues"?

This is thought to be a combination of factors, some biological and some psychological (emotional). A change in the hormonal levels is thought to be contributory. Some hormones are at very high levels during pregnancy and once delivery has taken place, this is no longer necessary and those levels fall quite sharply.

On the psychological front, it is true that many mothers are unprepared for the extreme weariness which often follows birth. There is the physical exertion of birth itself, which should ideally be followed by rest and quiet. Few mothers get either. The demands of the newborn ensure that both are at a premium. This may be made worse if the baby has even a slight health problem, such as mild jaundice or feeding difficulties. These cause a great deal of anxiety. These various factors combine to produce this very common postnatal problem.

Can anything be done to help a mother with the "blues"?

Support will be very important. An affected mother needs to be sympathetically reassured, especially if there is an added worry about the baby, who might have a minor problem that will clear up in a matter of days. Rest will be important and as much help as practicable should be given to allow her this. If such a mother wants to cry, she should be allowed to and the last thing one should say is that she should "pull herself together".

Affected mothers are often over-sensitive about what is said to them and therefore tact and empathy will be required on the part of medical staff, other care-givers and relatives.

How long should one expect the "blues" to last for?

They should not last more than a few days. In less than a week, these feelings start to fade and continue to do so before disappearing altogether, a few days later. Any persistence of such feelings should be treated more seriously because it could mean that the mother is suffering from a more serious form of postnatal illness, namely depression.

Postnatal depression

How common is postnatal depression?

It is estimated that a tenth of all newly delivered mothers are affected by depression to varying degrees. It tends to start after the mother has left hospital, normally within the first few weeks, but occasionally it manifests itself much later.

So, what are the symptoms of postnatal depression?

There is an overwhelming feeling of despondency, sadness and anxiety. The mother will cry frequently and for prolonged periods. She feels utterly unable to cope with the demands of the baby and the home. At the same time, she may feel fearful and anxious about her own health and that of the baby. Panic attacks are very common and the mother is often tense, unable to relax, and irritable. She feels unable to concentrate and will complain of poor memory. She may sit around all day staring vacantly into space. Simple tasks are perceived as confusing or insurmountable.

Is pain part of the picture?

Many mothers suffering from postnatal depression will complain of pain where there is no identifiable cause, apart from tension and anxiety. There is also difficulty in sleeping, which increases the general sense of fatigue.

Also common are loss of appetite and loss of interest in sex.

Does a sufferer experience all of these symptoms?

No, not necessarily. She may experience a few, most or sometimes all of the mentioned symptoms.

Are there any other effects?

Unrecognized or untreated, postnatal depression will inevitably lead to other problems. Personal relationships may suffer greatly. Since meeting people is a burden to the sufferer, she may avoid people to the extent of not answering the door or the phone. This might create offence in the unwary. Repulsing the partner's sexual overtures may be misinterpreted.

How is postnatal depression treated?

Features suggestive of postnatal depression should always be taken seriously and help should be sought sooner rather than later. A doctor's advice should be sought and, quite often, antidepressant medication will be prescribed. Support for such mothers is very crucial in their recovery and this can be given by an understanding member of the family, friend, a midwife, district nurse or health worker. Counselling, where available, can be very helpful. Overall, a genuine source of understanding, comfort and reassurance will be invaluable in the recovery process and the speed of it.

Are antidepressant drugs absolutely necessary?

While their use may not be absolutely necessary in every case, they are crucial in allowing for the necessary rest and they do actually make the patient feel better. They are not addictive and the mother should not worry that she might become dependent. When an assessment is made that they are required, it is probably best to take them.

Can treatment actually fail to work?

While the speed of recovery may differ, practically all mothers who suffer from postnatal depression recover completely. It is not known for postnatal depression to evolve into chronic depression.

Puerperal psychosis

What is puerperal psychosis?

This is the most severe type of postnatal illness. It is very uncommon and is characterized by an altered mental state with manic or depressive features or both (alternating). Admission to a psychiatric unit in hospital is almost always required.

What are the manic features of puerperal psychosis?

Manic features (or reaction) will include a manifestation of euphoria or excitement. The new mother is very jolly. There is rapid turnover of thoughts and before one is fully expressed, another one takes its place. Speech also follows suit and these patients characteristically talk very quickly, to an extent that it may be difficult to follow. The speech may soon become disjointed and impossible to follow.

She will be over-active and may not even find time to eat. Sleep is also dispensed with. Progressively, her activities may become destructive. There may be grandiose ideas, which may trigger a spending spree that can be ill-afforded.

She may become offended quite easily and this may prompt uncharacteristic obscene language, or sometimes aggressive behaviour.

What are the depressive features (reaction) of puerperal psychosis?

The mother feels down and dejected. She cannot bring herself to smile, laugh or relax, whatever the amount of encouragement to do so. She will spend most of the day in tears and has unpredictable feelings of panic.

She feels inadequate, incompetent and utterly unable to cope. This makes her feel guilty and ashamed. She feels unable to concentrate and will continually worry about poor memory. She may develop obsessional thoughts or rituals that may cause much distress.

Sleeping patterns may be altered, with inability to sleep being the more common feature, but others actually want to sleep round the clock.

Appetite may be decreased, but sometimes the opposite is the case. Probably most worrying is the mother's inability to feel affection for her baby and she may feel profound guilt as a result. She is unable to bond with her baby, as there are no maternal feelings at all. In severe cases, the mother may harbour suicidal thoughts and even the baby's life may be at risk.

What about the so-called schizophrenic reaction?

Sometimes patients with puerperal psychosis will exhibit delusions (false beliefs) and/or hallucinations (faulty perceptions). She may deny ever having had a baby or may claim that the baby is a monster. Others insist that they have been given the wrong baby. All sorts of delusions and hallucinations may be manifest.

How is this condition treated?

Treatment will depend on the severity and the various circumstances in each individual case. There are several facets that may be employed in the treatment but the mainstay will be supportive therapy and drugs.

Antidepressant medication may be prescribed and administered, first in hospital, then, with adequate improvement, as an outpatient. The family should support and encourage the patient to continue with medication and complete the recommended course. A network of support should be put in place and this may include a number of care-givers, including the midwife, health visitor, family doctor, obstetrician, psychiatrist and district nurse. Each will have their role to play.

Should a mother suffering from puerperal psychosis be separated from her baby?

Ideally not. Clearly, if adequate supervision to guarantee the absolute safety of the baby cannot be offered, then the baby may be cared for separately while ensuring frequent supervised union of mother and baby in the course of each day. Efforts should always be made to keep them together, as long as the safety of the baby can be absolutely guaranteed.

The **Association for Postnatal Illness** can be contacted at:
25 Jerdan Place
Fulham
London
SW6 1BE
Telephone: 0207-386 0868Monday–Friday 10am–5pm)
If writing, please include an SAE.

Breast-feeding

The Association of Breast-feeding Mothers is a registered charity which is dedicated to helping those mothers who are planning to or who are already breast-feeding. Help in answering questions and even counselling is available. Contact details are given at the end of this section.

Below are some of the most frequently asked questions (and their answers).

What are the implications for me and/or my unborn baby in continuing to feed my toddler while I am pregnant?

None. It is not uncommon for women to conceive whilst breast-feeding. It often takes time for them to realise they are pregnant, not least because the periods would not have resumed. This should help to reinforce the point that breast-feeding is not a reliable form of contraception in exclusivity.

However, if and when you find yourself in such circumstances, there are really no grounds for alarm as far as anybody's well-being is concerned. Your breast-fed baby, the unborn baby and you will not be adversely affected by this in any way. Of course, you will have to start thinking about weaning your baby off the breast, but this does not have to be done abruptly.

Can I smoke and drink or take any drugs while breast-feeding?

The wisest counsel is not to smoke if you are breast-feeding. Nicotine and a number of other harmful chemicals in cigarettes do get into breast-milk. There is also the fact that parents' cigarette smoking has been associated with increased risk of cot death. However, if it is not possible to quit smoking altogether, the next best option is to avoid smoking just before feeding. This is the time when the concentration of the harmful chemicals is highest. Also avoid smoking within the vicinity of the baby. This applies to non-breast-feeding mothers as well.

As far as alcohol is concerned, this too passes into breast-milk. It is therefore important to restrict the intake of this if you are breast-feeding. It is advised not to exceed fourteen units of alcohol per week. It is also important to remember that excessive alcohol intake can have a consequence of reducing milk production.

Some drugs, both prescription and non-prescription can have the potential of harming the baby. Whatever drug you are going to take, it is important to check with your doctor or pharmacist whether it is safe for breast-feeding.

When I have thrush, do both my baby and myself have to be treated?

Absolutely. If the baby has been noted to have oral thrush, which is not uncommon, your nipples can be infected from this. The reverse is also true. It is therefore important that treatment for thrush is given to both mother and baby.

Do I have to eat a special diet or avoid certain foods?

The beauty of breast-feeding is that it does not place any undue dietary burden on the mother. All you need is a sensible balanced diet. Moreover, those foods that are restricted during pregnancy – such as eggs, soft cheese and liver – can be eaten without any worry of harming the baby. It is true that a breast-feeding mother may feel hungrier than she usually does but this is hardly ever a problem. A breast-feeding mother tends to lose the extra weight gained during pregnancy more easily and usually more quickly.

Will I produce enough milk for my growing baby?

It is unusual – though not unknown – for a lactating mother to produce inadequate quantities of milk. The overwhelming majority of breast-feeding mothers experience no such problem. With a varied healthy diet and adequate fluid intake, there should be no such worry.

Why are my nipples sore?

The commonest known cause of sore nipples is poor fixing. If you have never breast-fed before, it is important that an expert is involved in guiding you at the outset. Many well-intentioned breast-feeding plans are thwarted early on because of lack of or poor guidance. As a result, the baby is perpetually hungry and fretful and the mother is tired and frustrated. The end result is quite often resignation and resorting to the bottle.

If you are unsure about your feeding technique, it is important to contact the health visitor, community midwife or even the GP and the appropriate help will be arranged for you. If you are still in hospital, there are usually dedicated breast-feeding counsellors and one will always be there to give help and guidance if and when required.

There are, of course, other less common causes of sore nipples, such as infection (usually thrush) and mastitis. Nipple stretching, which may happen if baby is repeatedly pulled off the breast while feeding, can also cause soreness. In the case of the latter all that is needed is to correct the feeding technique.

My baby seems to be feeding every couple of hours. Why is this?

It is important to remember that the best breast-feeding strategy is to feed your baby on demand. This will harmonize need and supply. Trying to regiment feeding times is counter-productive and will only result in a hungrier and more restless baby. The feeding patterns of different babies vary quite widely and it is misleading to compare your baby with someone else's or even your previous baby.

Generally, most babies will feed very frequently in the first few weeks. This should be considered as perfectly normal. With time, the frequency of feeding inevitably decreases. Every few weeks, there will also be increases in the frequency of feeding for a day or so. This is believed to be prompted by what are known as growth spurts. Many women are alarmed when these episodes occur out of the blue, thinking the milk supply is drying up. All you need to do when this happens is to adjust your own eating and water intake to respond to your baby's needs. Remember that this will last only a day or two at most.

My baby is always hungry. Will giving a bottle help?

Breast-milk provides all the food and fluid needs of your baby for at least four months. Giving a bottle will only have the effect of reducing your own milk supply and help thwart your efforts to feed your baby. The baby may seem to be demanding feeds very frequently but this will change with passing weeks and the baby will establish a pattern. There are simple ways of assessing whether your baby is getting enough and frequency of feeds is not one of them. If the baby appears contented after feeds, if there are plenty of wet nappies and stools are passed regularly and if the baby is gaining weight, then there is solid evidence that your baby is getting enough food and fluids and there is no need to worry.

Will giving a bottle stop my baby having colic?

If the baby is fretful, windy and appears to be in some discomfort as well as passing watery stools, there could be a whole range of causes. The bottle is not the answer. If the problem is persisting for the whole day, it may be wise to seek expert help so the cause can be investigated and established. Episodes of colic in an occasional evening are not uncommon but even these are not solved by giving the bottle. There are no specific remedial measures and all you may have to do is to ensure the baby is as comfortable as possible and it will soon pass.

I want to go out for the evening and I don't want to give formula milk. What should I do?

This has a simple solution, which is to express and store breast-milk. This can then be given to the baby when he or she demands a feed. A breast-feeding mother who is going back to work but wants to continue breast-feeding can use the same strategy. It is also useful if the mother wants to catch up on sleep and the partner or another adult member of the household is available to take over the feeding responsibility.

If you are considering expressing breast-milk, it is important that you get adequate guidance on how this is best done. A breast-feeding counsellor will happily do that. There are two main ways of expressing milk. One is hand expression, which is easy to master but time-consuming. The second is using a breast pump. There are three main types of pumps, which are hand-operated, battery-operated and electric pumps. Electric pumps are the most efficient but the initial financial outlay may be considerable.

Scrupulous cleanliness must be observed when expressing milk and it should be stored in sterile containers. To avoid wastage, feed-size bottles can be used so only the container to be used each time is thawed and if there is any left over, this must be discarded.

Expressed milk should be stored in the fridge, where it can stay for up to twenty-four hours. If there is a possibility that the milk will not be used within a day, then it should be put either in the freezer compartment of a refrigerator where the temperatures are below zero (0°C) where it will keep for up to a week, or in the deep-freezer. Here, with very low temperatures of around minus 16°C or lower, the milk will be safe for up to six months.

I am going back to work. Do I have to give up breast-feeding?

Not at all. For a mother going back to work, there are three main options. There is stopping breast-feeding, switching to formula milk in the intervals when you are at work and breast-feeding at all other times or using expressed milk during your absence and breast-feeding when you are at home. If you are keen to maximize the benefit of breast-milk for your baby, the last option will be the best. This strategy needs to be decided upon very early in the first two to three weeks of your baby's life. This gives you plenty of time to express and store sufficient quantities of milk.

Remember that you can confidently continue using breast-milk exclusively for up to four months before considering supplements. Just ensure that the milk is expressed and stored in the appropriate manner.

How do I thaw expressed breast-milk?

If the milk was in the freezer, it can be transferred to the fridge or at room temperature for slow defrosting. Quicker defrosting is achieved by placing the milk container in a large bowl of warm water. Once fully defrosted, the milk should be shaken to allow the cream to mix in again. A microwave should never be used to defrost breast-milk.

Once defrosted, the milk should be used within twenty-four hours, after which it should be thrown away if unused. It should never be refrozen.

Where can I get information about my rights at work (e.g. feeding breaks) while I am breast-feeding?

You should discuss your feeding plans with your work supervisor and the health visitor well before you are due to go back to work, to sort out the arrangements. This will not only ensure that you can do the feeding smoothly, but will also allow for minimizing disruption of your work as much as possible.

When will my baby sleep through the night?

Babies differ enormously in their sleeping habits and focusing on a specific figure could only lead to disappointment and frustration. There are three-week-old babies who only need a late evening feed – say at 11 o'clock at night – before sleeping for the remainder of the night. For the majority of babies, however, a full night's sleep is not achieved until eight to twelve weeks of age. For, some, unfortunately, this is still elusive when they celebrate their first birthday!

How long should I continue breast-feeding for?

It is important to plan well ahead on how long you would like to continue breast-feeding. This will depend on your individual circumstances. Factors such as your plans to go back to work, your circumstances at work (including the type of job and available facilities), your choice of contraception and your plans for future pregnancies will feature.

It is important to remember that for about four months, your milk will provide your baby with all the food and fluid needs. Supplementation should be planned from around this stage. To get maximal benefit from breast-feeding for both you and your child, you should be planning to breast-feed for well over six months if your circumstances allow. Many mothers breast-feed for a year and more and find it a positive and rewarding experience.

We hardly need to stress the fact that breast-feeding gives your baby the best possible start in life. It is also true that the benefits continue well after their breast-feeding 'career' is over. The same holds true for you. It is proven beyond doubt that a past history of breast-feeding significantly reduces the risk of both breast and ovarian cancer.

The **Association of Breast-feeding Mothers** can be contacted at:
P O Box 207,
Bridgewater, Somerset
TA6 7YT
Helpline: 0207-813 1481
Email: abm@clara.net
Website: http://home.clara.net/abm/

Active Birth

What is an Active Birth?

This is a concept whereby prospective parents actively participate in the birth of their baby, as opposed to being passive recipients of medical attention. It is a practice through which, in partnership with doctors and midwives, the parents take responsibility and control through informed choice of alternatives.

Principal features include encouraging upright positions, freedom of movement and natural breathing during labour. This is meant to maximize comfort, enhance ability to cope with contractions using natural resources and thereby complement the physiological process.

How do upright positions make a difference in labour?

Studies have shown that freedom of movement in labour helps significantly in coping with contraction pains. In the process, the need for drugs may be minimized or avoided altogether.

There is a theoretical advantage in the position as it promotes the natural alignment with the downward force of gravity. This may allow for good application of the baby's head on the cervix and possibly promote faster dilatation.

In this position, the uterine contraction forces work in tandem with gravity and therefore more efficiently. This may reduce the need for augmentation of labour through artificial stimulation of the uterus.

One of the commonest problems associated with a supine position (lying on your back) is compression of major blood vessels in the abdomen by the heavy pregnant uterus. This often leads to fetal distress. An upright position prevents this potential problem.

The positions encourage the easiest angle of descent and rotation of the baby through the pelvic canal thereby facilitating a more efficient labour.

Is it really beneficial to actually give birth in an upright position?

Lying on your back inevitably constricts the pelvic joints. This does not happen in upright positions. The freedom of the sacrum and coccyx to move back allows for the creation of more space in the pelvis, facilitating the easier passage of the baby through the pelvis.

The bearing down that is required during the second stage of labour (the delivery stage) is relatively easier to do in this position because of the help from gravity, akin to pushing a heavy object downhill as compared to along a flat surface.

Does an Active Birth benefit the baby?

By facilitating a more efficient labour, the baby's chances of suffering distress are reduced. Also, by reducing the need for pain-relieving drugs, the baby will not suffer the unwanted effects of these drugs, which include respiratory depression.

Overall, the reduced possibility of medical intervention will mean a faster recovery of the baby from the traumas of the baby after birth.

There are supposed to be several positions. Will I be able to remember them when labour is in full swing?

The Active Birth Centre encourages partaking in regular yoga classes, where positions are practised over several weeks, leading to term.

This will enable your body to create a physical memory, which will come back during labour. Your partner may also be at hand to remind you by suggesting positions to make you as comfortable as possible.

If you never got time to practise antenatally, don't be down-hearted. Birth is a natural and instinctive process and your body directs you to assume the most comfortable position, which is also the most beneficial during labour and delivery. The position will in most instances be one of the upright ones.

What if I find squatting or kneeling uncomfortable?

You can optimize the kneeling position by using a foam mat or thick soft cushions to kneel on. This is well complemented by using an inflatable "birth-ball" or bean bag to lean on. With squatting, you have to ensure there is lots of support to hold on to. There can be cushions under the heels as well. Other devices such as inflatable birth balls can be ordered from the Active Birth Centre.

There are other alternatives such as "all fours", upright kneeling or lunging while holding on to a chair or side of the bed. Other positions include sitting on a birth stool or standing and leaning forward on to support. This may be the side of a birth pool, bed or even the partner.

There is no doubt that being in water greatly facilitates changing of position. That is another alternative available.

Will I need any special equipment for an Active Birth?

The essence of Active Birth is that it promotes the merits of natural positions. Any additions will only be complementary. Such equipment as cushions, bean bags, floor mats, birth stools and the birthing pool will augment your comfort. Many hospitals will have these and if they are not there in your room, you can ask for them. However some hospitals do not have these and you may need to enquire about the possibility of bringing your own.

Some hospitals which do not have birthing pools will allow you to bring in a portable birthing pool, which you can rent from a number of dedicated places, including the Active Birth Centre. Check with your hospital in advance and make all the preparations with plenty of time to spare.

Remember, the calculated expected date of delivery is for guidance only and the baby may arrive two or even three weeks before.

Can I have an Active Birth regardless of where I labour (home or hospital)?

Your choice of place of birth should not interfere with planned Active Birth. Both home and hospital births are fully compatible with this. In fact, midwives who attend home births expect birth to be active. Many women or couples who opt for home birth do so in recognition of the freedom that this environment engenders. It is a familiar environment where the expectant mother is uninhibited, can move freely, make noise, use whichever piece of furniture for support, use the bath if and when she feels like etc. This gives a significant psychological boost to the eventual appreciation of the act of birth as a very enriching private experience.

If you are planning to labour in hospital, you may want to discuss with your midwife in advance the possibility of creating a home-like environment. This may include things like the preferred positions for labour and birth, what you may be able to bring in, your wishes regarding medical routines and intervention (you may wish these to be minimal) etc.

To this end, it may be useful to prepare a birth plan, which many obstetric units in hospitals encourage. This may enable you to achieve an Active Birth in hospital with as much assistance and as little disruption as possible.

Is a birth plan a good idea?

Yes. Hardly any midwife or doctor objects to a birth plan. It is meant to be a means of communication between yourself and the care-givers (midwives/doctors). This actually assists them to give you individualized and hence most satisfactory care. Take your time to gather your thoughts and prepare the plan. Discuss it with your midwife, who may be able to give you useful advice on your plan. Be open-minded and make allowances in your plan. Avoid things like "I don't want such and such under any circumstance": it creates an unnecessary sense of siege and there are better ways of presenting your dislikes.

A birth plan gives you peace of mind that you won't be asked to make difficult decisions while you are already in a state of distress, as all common possible scenarios are covered in advance. It also allows a care-giver who is unfamiliar (which is a possibility) to know your wishes and therefore assist you comfortably.

Will my midwife/doctor support me in having an Active Birth?

Most probably, yes. However the attitude towards Active Birth is variable. If your particular care-giver opposes your wish for an Active Birth, then they should give you a medical reason for their opposition. Of course, if you are not satisfied, you are perfectly within your rights to demand a second opinion. If the opposition is based onpersonal preference rather than medical reasons, you can demand a different care-giver.

This sort of opposition is not, however, common. You can actually requesta midwife who is experienced and supportive of Active Birth.

If you make all your plans in good time, you will have all the information you need and will avoid disappointment and frustration at labour onset. Apart from your midwife, it may be important to establish whether your local hospital provides for women who choose an Active Birth (most do). You may then ask for hospital statistics on such things as natural birth, epidural, water birth, Active Birth etc. Seek the help of your midwife in interpreting the data. Remember, statistics represent both availability and demand.

What can I do to prepare for an Active Birth?

The Active Birth Centre offers weekly yoga classes for physical preparation and breathing exercises. There is a national network of teachers which can be accessed on the internet or through the London centre. Try to attend these together with your partner, who should be your birth partner as well. The classes will also give information on the physiology of labour and birth and how Active Birth complements this. Information is also given on various potential interventions and what they entail.

A birth plan is important so take time to prepare one.

Make time to familiarize yourself with the intended place of birth, meet the midwives and generally satisfy yourself that you are comfortable and confident with the whole arrangement. If you are not, then you may have to seriously consider switching to another place. This is rarely necessary.

What are these Active Birth yoga classes?

These are weekly classes, which can actually be taken throughout the course of pregnancy. You can begin at any stage of your pregnancy. The classes are taught by qualified teachers, trained and experienced in antenatal and postnatal yoga. You are trained in – among other things – Active Birth positions and breathing awareness for labour and delivery.

The benefits are not only confined to the future. The gentle yoga benefits the pregnant body and mind. The common discomforts of pregnancy – such as backache, fatigue etc. – are alleviated. There is a general lifting of the mood through relaxation. The environment is also conducive to this as there is always a session of an informal chat and mingling at the end, which allows for exchange of ideas and experiences with other pregnant women.

There are stretching exercises combined with natural breathing, which help strengthen legs and the spine and make the muscles more supple. They also facilitate increased flexibility and promote toning of the pelvic floor.

Do Active Birth yoga classes continue in the postnatal period?

Yes. For the first few months after the birth of your baby, you will find them very beneficial. To facilitate this, crèche facilities are sometimes available, so you are encouraged to bring your baby with you. Gentle exercises and breathing are carried out to enable you to relax, loosen up and allow the inevitable tension to dissipate. The exercises are also designed to accelerate the body's healing process and aid the process of going back to the non-pregnant state. These classes also give you an opportunity to enjoy the company and camaraderie of fellow new mothers and swap tales of your experiences.

How easy is it to find a properly qualified Active Birth teacher?

The Active Birth Centre provides a list of qualified Active Birth teachers and Baby Massage throughout the United Kingdom and abroad. You can contact the Centre for the list which is also available on the Active Birth Centre Website (contact details at the end of this section).

What exactly is the difference between the Active Birth classes and the National Childbirth Trust (NCT) classes or the Parentcraft classes taught at my hospital?

These different classes are not and should not be seen as antagonistic.

There are a lot of similarities and the format is quite similar. Where they depart from each other is on the points of emphasis and depth and breadth of information given on Active Birth.

Parentcraft classes will concentrate on the routines as practised in that particular hospital unit. There is not much emphasis or encouragement in involving the partners in the classes. The partner's role in labour is covered only in theory. There may be little or no practical physical work. Parentcraft classes differ in content in different hospitals and some cover the aspects of childbirth more broadly than others.

Active Birth "couples classes" cover a very broad range of subjects to do with pregnancy and childbirth. Emphasis is put on giving unbiased comprehensive information, to enable the prospective mother and her partner to make an informed choice.

Areas such as pharmacological and natural alternatives for pain relief are exhaustively covered. It may not be possible to get the same depth of coverage on complementary therapies in other classes. Possible medical routines and interventions are covered as well as ways of being involved in decision-making.

The subject of breast-feeding is comprehensively covered to include the physiology of it, the common and uncommon potential problems and their solutions.

There are of course the yoga-based exercise classes, the practice of positions and the active involvement of partners in these as well as massage for labour, breathing and the required emotional support.

How can my partner be involved?

A partner can have a crucial role to play and there is ample scientific evidence that the partner's presence and participation can significantly improve the woman's perception of labour and childbirth as a positive and enriching experience. There is also evidence that it may reduce the need for pharmacological pain relief.

The partner can be there to offer physical and emotional support, ensure you are comfortable, help in moving and changing position, adjusting cushions etc. and can help and support you when you want to move about. He should also help in breathing together to keep steady rhythm and help you focus on this. You will have gone through those paces together again and again during antenatal Active Birth couples classes, and therefore he will know what to do.

Massage during labour is another invaluable role that a partner can play, as well as offering sips of water and carrying out other minor chores that arise. He will be there to liaise with the care-givers in advocating your wishes and allow you to participate in any decision-making that may arise. He will also be there with you offering support through any procedure or even any administration of drugs that may have to be undertaken.

At delivery, he may want to cut the umbilical cord.

If I need an epidural for pain relief, can I still have an Active Birth?

Epidural pain relief is not incompatible with Active Birth. This is why in the classes, comprehensive information is given on all manner of pain control in labour. If you are in a lot of pain, and distressed by it, an epidural may be the ideal mode of pain relief. This may allow you to rest, even get some sleep. With an epidural, only some adjustments may be required for active birth. You could try supported upright positions which you will have practised antenatally in the classes. An epidural does not have to completely ground you and if you make your wishes known to the anaesthetist administering it, you could still be fairly free to move about with support. A partner is particularly useful here. Epidural needs top-ups to keep the effectiveness optimal. You can time top-ups to allow wearing off during the second stage, so you can adopt your preferred position without the epidural being a hindrance.

Do I need to learn any breathing techniques for an Active Birth?

Not really. The yoga classes do focus on breathing to emphasize the role of natural breathing in each position. You are encouraged to use the natural spontaneous breathing cycle. You are also encouraged to avoid holding breath at the height of contractions. You are bound to memorize the practice and this will instinctively come back during actual labour. The assisting midwife will encourage you to breathe lightly (pant) at the time of "crowning" of the baby's head. This curtails the instinctive bearing down and therefore reduces the risk of tearing the perineal tissues.

If I am induced or my labour is augmented with a syntocinon drip, can I still use upright positions?

Yes. If you make your wishes known beforehand, the midwife will arrange for you to have the drip sited at an ideal position on your arm to facilitate freedom of movement. Even the baby's monitoring can be planned in such a way as to allow you that freedom. As a matter of fact, induced or augmented labour does not differ that much from spontaneous labour and it should not interfere that much with your birth plan. Your midwife will be there to support you throughout and ensure there is no unnecessary departure from your wishes.

Will I be disappointed if there is a complication and I cannot have Active Birth or if I need medical pain relief?

We always stress keeping an open mind. A blinkered approach to a physiological process such as labour is a mistake. Labour is unpredictable and even the apparently most low-risk pregnancy can end up requiring some kind of special intervention. With that approach to things, you should not be disappointed if things happen not to go according to your plans. You will know that you tried your best but some events may have occurred that were beyond your power to influence. Active Birth is a means and not a goal in itself. If it cannot deliver the baby's and mum's well-being, then the necessary alternative should be allowed to kick in.

Where does water birth come in?

Water birth can facilitate Active Birth quite enormously. As long as there are no contraindications, it is really worth considering. Discuss this thoroughly with your midwife or doctor. The buoyancy of water facilitates movement, and positions such as kneeling and squatting are easier to execute and maintain. The water is also relaxing and soothing as the temperature is maintained within a narrow limit around body temperature. The partner is also at hand for support and such things as massage. The atmosphere is generally less medical and more conducive to a relaxed labour process.

When should I get into the pool?

Conventional wisdom is that labour should be established before you get into the pool. This means, you should be having regular contractions and the cervix should be at least 4 cm dilated. This will ensure that you don't get in too early (quite possible in the latent phase of labour, which could last hours) and that you save the soothing effect of warm water for an active phase of labour, when the contractions are more painful and more difficult to cope with.

What can I do in the phase before it is ideal to get into the pool?

There are a few things that you can do to help you cope with the early phase of labour. Try to rest as much as possible, conserving your energy for later. You may find that being mobile helps but, if not, then use the upright positions as needed. Make circular, swaying or rocking movements of the pelvis with the contraction pains.

If at home, create a secure and comfortable environment where you won't be inhibited. Your midwife will help you to arrange this in hospital whenever possible.

Remember natural breathing. Don't hold your breath as a reaction to painful contractions. Rest as much as possible between contractions. Ideally, your birthing partner should be with you to offer emotional and physical support.

Allow yourself some fruit juice, glucose tablets, or a spoonful of honey every so often. This will help keep your energy levels up – something that will come in handy later on in labour.

You may consider massage by your birthing partner or the midwife using aromatherapy oils. You can also use homeopathic remedies. These are options you should explore fully well before you are due.

Can I actually have my baby in the birthing pool?

This is possible but there are a few factors that you will have to bear in mind. The midwife who is assisting you should be experienced in this and comfortable with the idea. There are some midwives who are happy to help look after you through labour in the pool but are not comfortable with conducting the actual delivery under water. That has to be established beforehand. Moreover, there are some hospital units which have a policy of not allowing underwater births. The practice in those hospitals is therefore to get out of the pool for the second stage. Again, this has to be established well in advance. Of course, if this does not match with your expecations, you can seek an alternative midwife or hospital.

Theoretically, birth under water is safe as long as all the conditions are met. The baby will not breathe under water (dive reflex) and therefore the risk of aspirating water into the lungs is not there. The temperature has to be strictly maintained and the baby allowed to surface immediately after birth. Prolonged immersion may allow the placenta to detach, which will cut off the oxygen supply to the baby, provoking a gasping reflex and therefore this is never allowed to happen. When appropriately conducted by an experienced midwife, this procedure should be safe. However, because these strict conditions may sometimes not be met, some units are cautious in allowing it.

There is also the fact that you may yourself prefer to leave the pool for the second stage, which is fine. Keep an open mind in all these things. If your instincts when the time comes are that you would rather have your feet firmly on the ground, by all means say so and the necessary assistance will be there.

The **Active Birth Centre** can be contacted at:
25 Bickerton Road,
London
N19 5JT
Tel: 0207-482 5554
Fax: 0207-561 9007
Email: mail@activebirthcentr.demon.co.uk
Website: http//www.activebirthcentre.com

Useful addresses

In the UK, like in other countries of the world, there are numerous organizations that are there to provide some form of help in a particular health-related area or subject. Some are statutory but many are voluntary organizations or groups aimed at self-help or support in their chosen area. Here, we have tried to provide contact details of some of those organizations. It is true that this is only a fraction of such bodies out there and a more detailed search from such places, as your local library or the Internet will yield a more comprehensive list. For a pregnant or newly delivered mother who may want to contact an organization missing from this list, the midwife will, in most instances, be able to give you the relevant contact details.

Action on Pre-Eclampsia (APEC)

31–33 College Road, Harrow, Middlesex HA1 1EJ
Helpline: (01923) 266 778
Tel: 0208-863 3271
Fax: 0208-424 0653

A very active organization, which offers advice and support for sufferers of pre-eclampsia or those worried about the condition. Apart from a Helpline, there are local contact groups and an information pack can be provided.

Action on Smoking and Health (ASH)

Devon House, 12–15 Dartmouth Street,London SW1H 9BL
Tel: 0207-233 1800
Fax: 0207-222 4343
Email: ashuk@ ash.org.uk
Website: http://www.ash.org.uk

An organization mainly aimed at providing information and publicizing health issues related to smoking for women. It publishes leaflets and regular bulletins. A visit to their Website will yield an abundance of information on this subject.

Active Birth Centre

25 Bickerton Road, London N19 5JT
Tel: 0207-482 5554
Fax: 0207-561 9007

A centre actively engaged in a number of activities related to Active Birth. These include running antenatal workshops imparting information on the subject, antenatal yoga exercise classes, postnatal and baby massage classes and a variety of other activities. Though based in London, there is a register of certified Active Birth teachers throughout the country and if contacted, they can put you in touch with one in your locality.

Aquabirths
15 Ayresome Terrace, Leeds LS8 1BJ
Tel: 0113-266 3658
Apart from manufacturing and hiring birth pools, advice on water birth is provided.

Association for Postnatal Illness
25 Jerdan Place, Fulham,
London SW6 1BE
Tel: 0207-386 0868
Fax: 0207-386 8885
This is a self-help group aimed at providing one-to-one support for affected mothers. It also promotes research into prevention and treatment of postnatal depression and other related diseases. Affected mothers and former patients are encouraged to join.

Association for Spina Bifida and Hydrocephalus (ASBAH)
ASBAH House, 42 Park Road,
Peterborough PE1 2UQ
Tel: 01733-555 988
Fax: 01733-555 985
Email: rosemaryb@asbah.demon.uk

For Northern Ireland:
ASBAH
73 New Row, Coleraine
County Londonderry BT52 1EJ
Tel: 01265-51522
Fax: 01265-320 929
Organization specifically aimed at promoting awareness of spina bifida, hydrocephalus and other related conditions and their complications. ASBAH advisors

are available throughout the country and they are able to advise on the whole range of problems related to these conditions.

Association of Breast-feeding Mothers
PO Box 207,, Bridgwater,
Somerset TA6 7YT
Tel: 0171-813 1481
Email: abm@clara.net
Website: http://
www.home.clara.net/abm
The association provides education on the subject and there is a network of local support groups. A directory of breast-feeding counsellors is available free.

Baby Life Support Systems (BLISS)
17–21 Emerald Street,
London WC1N 3QL
Helpline: 0500-151 617
Tel: 0207-831 9393
Fax: 0207-404 0676
Email: bliss@charity.nildram.co.uk
Among other things, BLISS offers information and support to parents whose babies need special care at birth for a whole variety of reasons.

Birth Crisis Network
Helpline: 01865-300 266
Women who have had a traumatic labour can contact the helpline where they will be put in contact with a local counsellor.

Birthworks

Unit 3F, Brent Mill Trading Estate,
South Brent, Devon TQ10 9YT
Tel: 01364-72 802
Fax: 01364-72 060

Birthworks offers assistance and advice about water birth and holistic childbirth. Portable birthing pools can also be hired from them.

Blue Lagoon Birth Pools

Beacon House, Woodley Park,
Skelmersdale, Lancashire WN8 6UR
Tel: 01695-556 642
Fax: 01695-51915

Organizes study days for prospective mothers as well as midwives and also runs a pool hire service. Information pack available free.

Brent Sickle Cell and Thalassaemia Centre

Central Middlesex Hospital
Acton Lane, London NW10 7NS
Tel: 0208-453 2262
Fax: 0208-453 2680

This is a walk-in information and counselling centre for sickle cell and thalassaemia. These conditions being more prevalent among people of ethnic minorities, information is available in a number of Asian languages (as well as from English). Screening services also available.

British Diabetic Association

Helpline: 0171-636 6112
10 Queen Anne Street,
London W1M 0BD
Tel: 0171-323 1531
Fax: 0171-637 3644
Email: bda@bbcnc.org.uk

For Northern Ireland:

British Diabetic Association

John Gibson House, 257 Lisburn Road,
Belfast BT9 7EN
Tel: 01232-666 646
Fax: 01232-666 333

For Scotland:

British Diabetes Association

34 West George Street,
Glasgow G2 2DA
Tel: 0141-332 2700
Fax: 0141-332 4880

The association, among other things, provides information and advice on diabetes including the specific subject of pregnancy and diabetes.

British Diastasis Symphysis Pubis Support Group

17 Muir Road, Ramsgate,
Kent CT11 8AX
Tel: 01843-587 356
Fax: 01843-587 356

Provides information on this painful condition to sufferers and professionals alike. A number of information sheets as well as a newsletter are available.

British Pregnancy Advisory Service (BPAS)

Austy Manor, Wootton Wawen, Solihull
West Midlands B95 6BX
Helpline: 0345-304 030
Tel: 01564-793 225
Fax: 01564-794 935

This charity provides a variety of pregnancy-related services including counselling and information on contraception, sterilization, fertility problems and many more.

Caesarean Support Network

55 Cooil Drive, Douglas,
Isle of Man IM2 2HF,
Tel: 01624-661 269

Provides information and advice on all matters relating to caesarean section. This could be from prospective mothers as well as those who had caesarean section in the past.

Centre for Pregnancy Nutrition

University of Sheffield
Dept. of Obstetrics & Gynaecology
Northern General Hospital
Herries Road, Sheffield S5 7AU
Helpline: 0114-242 4084
Tel: 0114-271 4888
Fax: 0114-261 7584
Email: Pregnancy.Nutrition
@Sheffield.ac.uk

The centre provides information regarding nutrition for the periods before and during pregnancy. The period after delivery especially for those who are breast-feeding is also covered.

Contact A Family (CAF)

170 Tottenham Court Road,
London W1P 0HA
Tel: 0207-383 3555
Fax: 0207-383 0259
Email: cafamily@org.uk

This is a nationwide network of parent support groups. The charity provides support to families who have children with special needs.

CRY-SIS

B.M.Cry-sis
London WC1N 3XX
Helpline: 0171-404 5011
Tel: 01634-710 913
Fax: 01634-710 913

Support group for families with excessively crying and/or sleepless babies. There is a network of volunteers and a caller to the helpline is put in contact with a volunteer in the locality.

Down's Syndrome Association

155 Mitcham Road, Tooting,
London SW17 9PG
Tel: 0208-682 4001
Fax: 0208-682 4012

For Northern Ireland:
Down's Syndrome Association

2nd Floor, 28 Bedford Street,
Belfast BT2 7FE
Tel: 01232-243 266
Fax: 01232-333 894

The association provides information and advice to parents and carers of Down's Syndrome children (and adults).

Exploring Parenthood – The National Parenting Development Centre

4 Ivory Place, 10a Treadgold Street
London W11 4BP
Helpline: 0207-221 6681
Tel: 0207-221 4471
Fax: 0207-221 5501
Email: parenthd@itl.net

The centre facilitates easy access for parents to appropriate professional advice, information and counselling on a variety of parenting problems.

Gingerbread

16/17 Clerkenwell Close
London EC1R 0AA
Helpline: 0207-336 8184
Tel: 0207-336 8183
Fax: 0207-336 8185
Email: ginger@lonepar.demon.co.uk

For Northern Ireland:
Gingerbread N. Ireland

169 University Street
Belfast BT7 1HR
Helpline: 01232-234 568
Tel: 01232-231 417
Fax: 01232-240 740

The organization, through a
network of self-help groups,
provides practical support for
lone parents.

Haemophilia Society

123 Westminster Bridge Road,
London SE1 7HR
Tel: 0207-928 2020
Fax: 0207-620 1416
Email: 100711.1677@compuserve.com

The society provides information
and practical help to people with
haemophilia and other clotting
disorders.

International Home Birth Movement

The Manor, Standlake, Witney,
Oxford OX8 7RH
Tel: 01865-300 266
Fax: 01865 300 438

This is a network of people
working for home birth. Help for
prospective mothers includes
woman-to-woman support.

La Leche League (Great Britain)

BM 3424, London WC1N 3XX
Helpline: 0207-242 1278

The charity provides information
and support to mothers who wish
to breast-feed and those already
doing so. Local mother-to-mother
support groups are available
throughout the country.

Maternity and Health Links

Old Co-op, 38-42 Chelsea Road,
Easton, Bristol BS5 6AF
Tel: 0117-955 8495
Fax: 0117-955 8495

The organization provides
support and practical help to
ethnic minority women who are
non-English speakers. This is
both in the antenatal and
postnatal periods.

Meet-a-Mum Association (MAMA)

Cornerstone House, 14 Willis Road
Croydon, Surrey CR0 2XX
Tel: 0208-665 0357
Fax: 0208-665 1972

MAMA offers support to those
mothers feeling lonely and overwhelmed or those suffering from
postnatal depression. Information
booklets and leaflets also
available.

Miscarriage Association

c/o Clayton Hospital
Wakefield, West Yorkshire WF1 3JS
Tel: 01924-200 799
Fax: 01924-298 834

Support and information on miscarriage and other related conditions such as ectopic pregnancy offered. Support groups throughout the UK.

Multiple Births Foundation Queen Charlotte's and Chelsea Hospital

Goldhawk Road, London W6 0XG
Tel: 0208-383 3519
Fax: 0208-383 3041
Email: mbf@rpms.ac.uk
Provides support to parents of multiples i.e. twins, triplets etc, including specialist advice.

National Childbirth Trust (NCT)

Alexandra House, Oldham Terrace,
Acton, London W3 6NH
Helpline: 0208-992 8637
Tel: 0208-992 2616 (Admin.)
Fax: 0208-992 5929
There is a support and information network throughout the UK. The NCT promotes informed choice in pregnancy care and childbirth. Also supports postnatal care including breastfeeding.

National Society for the Prevention of Cruelty to Children (NSPCC)

National Centre, 42 Curtain Road,
London EC2A 3NH
Helpline: 0800-800 500
Tel: 0207-825 2500
Fax: 0207-825 2525
The NSPCC actively works to prevent child abuse in its various forms.

Organisation for Sickle Cell Anaemia Research (OSCAR)

5 Lauderdale House, Goslin Way,
Brixton, London SW9 6JS
Tel: 0207-735 4166
OSCAR is a self-help organization, which runs a support group for Sickle Cell Disease. It promotes research into the condition and literature is available.

PARENTLINE (Helpline for Parents)

Endway House, The Endway
Hadleigh, Essex SS7 2AN
Helpline: 01702-559 900
Tel: 01702-554 782 (Admin)
Fax: 01702-554 911
This is a national network of helplines aimed at parents encountering all manner of parenting difficulties.

Perinatal Bereavement Unit

The Tavistock Clinic, 120 Belsize Lane
London NW3 5BA
Tel: 0207-435 7111
Fax: 0207-431 8978
Support, through specialist therapeutic intervention, to those affected in the longer-term by stillbirth, miscarriage and other pregnancy-related losses.

QUIT

Victory House, Tottenham Court Road
London W1P 0HA
Helpline: 0800-002 200
Tel: 0207-388 5775 (Admin)
Fax: 0207-388 5995
QUIT is dedicated to helping individuals give up smoking. Among other things, a booklet on

smoking and pregnancy is available.

Scottish Down's Syndrome Association (SDSA)

158/160 Balgreen Road
Edinburgh EH11 3AU
Tel: 0131-313 4225
Fax: 0131-313 4285

The association provides support to parents of affected children. It also works to promote public awareness of the condition.

Scottish Spina Bifida Association

190 Queensferry Road
Edinburgh EH4 2BW
Tel: 0131-332 0743
Fax: 0131-343 3651

Promotes public awareness of spina bifida and other related defects.

Soft UK – Support Organisation for Trisomy 13 (Patau's syndrome)

Tudor Lodge, Redwood
Ross-on-Wye, Herefordshire HR9 5UD
Tel: 01989-567 480

The organization provides support and information to prospective parents where a prenatal diagnosis of Patau's syndrome has been made. This also extends to those where the diagnosis is made after the birth of the affected child, live or stillborn.

Soft UK – Support Organisation for Trisomy 18 (Edward's syndrome)

48 Froggatts Ride, Walmley
Sutton Coldfield,
West Midlands B76 2TQ
Tel: 0121- 351 3122

The organization provides support and information to prospective parents where a prenatal diagnosis of Edward's syndrome has been made. This also extends to those where the diagnosis is made after the birth of the affected child, live or stillborn.

Support around Termination for Abnormality (SATFA)

73–75 Charlotte Street
London W1P 1LB
Helpline: 0207-631 0285
Tel: 0207-631 0280 (Admin.)
Fax: 0207-631 0280

This charity offers support and information to prospective parents facing antenatal diagnostic tests and to those who following diagnosis of abnormality face decisions about terminating the pregnancy. The support extends beyond the actual termination.

Terrence Higgins Trust

52-54 Grays Inn Road
London WC1X 8JU
Helpline: 0207-405 2381
Tel: 0207-831 0330 (Admin.)
Fax: 0207-816 4552
Email: info@tht.org.uk
Website: http://www.tht.org.uk

This trust actively works on providing help to individuals affected by HIV and AIDS.

Toxoplasmosis Trust
61 Collier Street
London N1 9BE
Helpline: 0207-713 0599
Tel: 0207-713 0663 (Admin.)
Fax: 0207-713 0611
The trust provides support to those affected by the disease and promotes public awareness of the condition. Information material available.

Twins and Multiple Births Association (TAMBA)
PO Box 30, Little Sutton
South Wirral L66 1BH
Helpline: 01732-868 000
Tel: 0151-348 0020 (Admin.)
Fax: 0151-200 5309
Website: http://
www.surreycc.gov.uk/tamba
TAMBA aims to give support to parents expecting or those who have twins, triplets and other higher multiples. Information material also available.

UK Turner Syndrome Society
c/o Child Growth Foundation
2 Mayfield Avenue, London W4 1PW
Tel: 0208-995 0257
Fax: 0208-995 9075
Email: cgflondon@aol.com
The society provides support to parents and individuals affected by Turner's syndrome through information and advice. It also promotes public awareness of the condition.

VBAC (Vaginal Birth after Caesarean Information and Support Group)
8 Wren Way, Farnborough,
Hampshire GU14 8SZ
Tel: 01252-543 250
Fax: 01252-543 250
Provides help and information to those women who are aiming for vaginal birth following previous caesarean delivery.

Women's Health
52 Featherstone Street,
London EC1Y 8RT
Tel: 0207-251 6580
Fax: 0207-608 0928
Women's Health strives to provide information on all manner of women's health problems to facilitate informed decision making on each individual's part.

Index